Advances in Vascular Stiffness: Part II

Advances in Vascular Stiffness: Part II

Editors

Paolo Salvi
Andrea Grillo

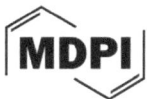

Basel • Beijing • Wuhan • Barcelona • Belgrade • Novi Sad • Cluj • Manchester

Editors

Paolo Salvi
Department of Cardiology
Istituto Auxologico Italiano, IRCCS
Milan
Italy

Andrea Grillo
Department of Medicine, Surgery and Health Sciences
University of Trieste
Trieste
Italy

Editorial Office
MDPI AG
Grosspeteranlage 5
4052 Basel, Switzerland

This is a reprint of articles from the Special Issue published online in the open access journal *Journal of Clinical Medicine* (ISSN 2077-0383) (available at: https://www.mdpi.com/journal/jcm/special_issues/OAFG3S3X4U).

For citation purposes, cite each article independently as indicated on the article page online and as indicated below:

Lastname, A.A.; Lastname, B.B. Article Title. *Journal Name* **Year**, *Volume Number*, Page Range.

ISBN 978-3-7258-2353-6 (Hbk)
ISBN 978-3-7258-2354-3 (PDF)
doi.org/10.3390/books978-3-7258-2354-3

© 2024 by the authors. Articles in this book are Open Access and distributed under the Creative Commons Attribution (CC BY) license. The book as a whole is distributed by MDPI under the terms and conditions of the Creative Commons Attribution-NonCommercial-NoDerivs (CC BY-NC-ND) license.

Contents

Mario Podrug, Pjero Koren, Edita Dražić Maras, Josip Podrug, Viktor Čulić, Maria Perissiou, et al.
Long-Term Adverse Effects of Mild COVID-19 Disease on Arterial Stiffness, and Systemic and Central Hemodynamics: A Pre-Post Study
Reprinted from: *J. Clin. Med.* **2023**, *12*, 2123, doi:10.3390/jcm12062123 1

Viviana Aursulesei Onofrei, Ecaterina Anisie, Carmen Lacramioara Zamfir, Alexandr Ceasovschih, Mihai Constantin, Florin Mitu, et al.
Role of Chemerin and Perivascular Adipose Tissue Characteristics on Cardiovascular Risk Assessment by Arterial Stiffness Markers in Patients with Morbid Obesity
Reprinted from: *J. Clin. Med.* **2023**, *12*, 2885, doi:10.3390/jcm12082885 15

Marjana Petrova, Alex Gavino, Yujie Li and Craig S. McLachlan
Comparison of Parameters for Assessment of Carotid Stiffness and Their Association with Carotid Atherosclerosis in Rural Australian Adults: A Pilot Study
Reprinted from: *J. Clin. Med.* **2023**, *12*, 2935, doi:10.3390/jcm12082935 30

Anna Giani, Rocco Micciolo, Elena Zoico, Gloria Mazzali, Mauro Zamboni and Francesco Fantin
Cardio-Ankle Vascular Index and Aging: Differences between CAVI and CAVI0
Reprinted from: *J. Clin. Med.* **2023**, *12*, 6726, doi:10.3390/jcm12216726 40

Simonetta Genovesi, Elena Tassistro, Giulia Lieti, Ilenia Patti, Marco Giussani, Laura Antolini, et al.
Wall Properties of Elastic and Muscular Arteries in Children and Adolescents at Increased Cardiovascular Risk
Reprinted from: *J. Clin. Med.* **2023**, *12*, 6919, doi:10.3390/jcm12216919 51

Ioana Mădălina Zota, Cristina Mihaela Ghiciuc, Doina Clementina Cojocaru, Corina Lucia Dima-Cozma, Maria Magdalena Leon, Radu Sebastian Gavril, et al.
Changes in Arterial Stiffness in Response to Blood Flow Restriction Resistance Training: A Narrative Review
Reprinted from: *J. Clin. Med.* **2023**, *12*, 7602, doi:10.3390/jcm12247602 65

Helga Gyöngyösi, Gergő József Szőllősi, Orsolya Csenteri, Zoltán Jancsó, Csaba Móczár, Péter Torzsa, et al.
Differences between SCORE, Framingham Risk Score, and Estimated Pulse Wave Velocity-Based Vascular Age Calculation Methods Based on Data from the Three Generations Health Program in Hungary
Reprinted from: *J. Clin. Med.* **2024**, *13*, 205, doi:10.3390/jcm13010205 81

Giacomo Pucci, Andrea Grillo, Kalliopi V. Dalakleidi, Emil Fraenkel, Eugenia Gkaliagkousi, Spyretta Golemati, et al.
Atrial Fibrillation and Early Vascular Aging: Clinical Implications, Methodology Issues and Open Questions—A Review from the VascAgeNet COST Action
Reprinted from: *J. Clin. Med.* **2024**, *13*, 1207, doi:10.3390/jcm13051207 92

Lisanne Tap, Kim Borsboom, Andrea Corsonello, Fabrizia Lattanzio and Francesco Mattace-Raso
Deterioration of Kidney Function Is Affected by Central Arterial Stiffness in Late Life
Reprinted from: *J. Clin. Med.* **2024**, *13*, 1334, doi:10.3390/jcm13051334 113

Michaela Kozakova, Carmela Morizzo, Giuseppe Penno, Dante Chiappino and Carlo Palombo
Diabetes-Related Changes in Carotid Wall Properties: Role of Triglycerides
Reprinted from: *J. Clin. Med.* **2024**, *13*, 5654, doi:10.3390/jcm13185654 . . . . **123**

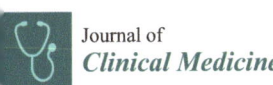

Article

Long-Term Adverse Effects of Mild COVID-19 Disease on Arterial Stiffness, and Systemic and Central Hemodynamics: A Pre-Post Study

Mario Podrug [1,2,*], Pjero Koren [1,3], Edita Dražić Maras [4], Josip Podrug [5], Viktor Čulić [3,6], Maria Perissiou [7], Rosa Maria Bruno [8,9], Ivana Mudnić [10], Mladen Boban [10] and Ana Jerončić [1,11,*]

1. Laboratory of Vascular Aging, University of Split School of Medicine, 21000 Split, Croatia
2. University Department of Health Studies, University of Split, 21000 Split, Croatia
3. University of Split School of Medicine, 21000 Split, Croatia
4. Infectious Diseases Department, University Hospital of Split, 21000 Split, Croatia
5. Otorhinolaryngology Department, University Hospital of Split, 21000 Split, Croatia
6. Department of Cardiology and Angiology, University Hospital Centre Split, 21000 Split, Croatia
7. Physical Activity, Health and Rehabilitation Research Group, School of Sport, Health and Exercise Science, Faculty of Science and Health, University of Portsmouth, Portsmouth PO1 2UP, UK
8. Université Paris Cité, INSERM, PARCC, 75015 Paris, France
9. Clinical Pharmacology Unit, AP-HP, Hôpital européen Georges Pompidou, 75015 Paris, France
10. Department of Basic and Clinical Pharmacology, University of Split School of Medicine, 21000 Split, Croatia
11. Department of Research in Biomedicine and Health, University of Split School of Medicine, 21000 Split, Croatia
* Correspondence: mpodrug@ozs.unist.hr (M.P.); ajeronci@mefst.hr (A.J.); Tel.: +385-21-491-805 (M.P.); +385-21-557-800 (A.J.)

Abstract: COVID-19-associated vascular disease complications are primarily associated with endothelial dysfunction; however, the consequences of disease on vascular structure and function, particularly in the long term (>7 weeks post-infection), remain unexplored. Individual pre- and post-infection changes in arterial stiffness as well as central and systemic hemodynamic parameters were measured in patients diagnosed with mild COVID-19. As part of in-laboratory observational studies, baseline measurements were taken up to two years before, whereas the post-infection measurements were made 2–3 months after the onset of COVID-19. We used the same measurement protocol throughout the study as well as linear and mixed-effects regression models to analyze the data. Patients (N = 32) were predominantly healthy and young (mean age ± SD: 36.6 ± 12.6). We found that various parameters of arterial stiffness and central hemodynamics—cfPWV, AIx@HR75, and cDBP as well as DBP and MAP—responded to a mild COVID-19 disease. The magnitude of these responses was dependent on the time since the onset of COVID-19 as well as age ($p_{regression\_models} \leq 0.013$). In fact, mixed-effects models predicted a clinically significant progression of vascular impairment within the period of 2–3 months following infection (change in cfPWV by +1.4 m/s, +15% in AIx@HR75, approximately +8 mmHg in DBP, cDBP, and MAP). The results point toward the existence of a widespread and long-lasting pathological process in the vasculature following mild COVID-19 disease, with heterogeneous individual responses, some of which may be triggered by an autoimmune response to COVID-19.

Keywords: arterial stiffness; central hemodynamics; COVID-19; vascular remodeling; long COVID-19 syndrome; autoimmune response

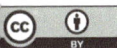

1. Introduction

In December 2019, the first official case of coronavirus disease (COVID-19) was detected in the Chinese city of Wuhan. Since its first breakout, the virus has swiftly spread over the world, and the World Health Organization (WHO) declared a pandemic in March

2020. At the time of writing, there had been 660,378,145 confirmed cases of COVID-19 with 6,691,495 fatalities globally (1). While COVID-19 was initially thought of as an acute respiratory illness, it is now recognized as a complex multisystemic disease with extensive and deleterious cardiovascular involvement [1,2]. In addition to direct consequences and complications due to acute COVID-19 infection, a recent study showed that 12 months after the onset of COVID-19 infection, up to 25% of patients who were otherwise healthy and free of underlying diseases exhibited the long COVID-19 syndrome [3].

Subclinical myocardial and vascular dysfunction have been linked to worse outcomes and an increased risk of death in patients with COVID-19 disease [4]. Even in patients with mild COVID-19 disease severity, the infection has been linked to impaired subclinical markers of cardiovascular and endothelial function [5]. It is presumed that COVID-19-associated vascular disease complications may be precipitated by direct endothelium damage [6] or immune-mediated vascular damage [7,8]. However, it is unknown to what extent structural alterations of the vascular wall occur in addition to endothelial damage. Even fewer data exist regarding the long-term effects of COVID-19 infection on vascular structure and function. Current fragmented evidence suggests that COVID-19 disease reduces systemic vascular function and increases arterial stiffness [9,10].

Arterial stiffness is a vascular aging phenomenon that refers to a loss of arterial compliance or changes in artery wall characteristics [11]. Arterial stiffness worsens with age and exposure to risk factors that hasten the stiffening process [12,13]. Various measures of arterial stiffness and central hemodynamics can reveal a decline in arterial elasticity brought on by structural wall changes in the arterial system. The most validated and direct measure of arterial stiffness is the carotid–femoral pulse wave velocity (cfPWV) (Townsend, Wilkinson et al., 2015). In addition, augmentation indices are indirect measures of arterial stiffness which are believed to capture the negative impact of systolic wave reflection on cardiac workload [14]. Finally, the central blood pressures refer to the pressure in the ascending aorta. These are the pressures that the target organs are subjected to, and they are lower than brachial cuff pressures due to arterial pressure amplification [15].

We hypothesized that even mild cases of COVID-19 disease could have long-term detrimental effects on arterial structure and function. To investigate this, we examined individual pre- and post-infection changes in arterial stiffness as well as systemic and central hemodynamic parameters in patients diagnosed with mild COVID-19. Baseline measurements were taken up to two years before a participant became infected, and post-infection measurements were taken two to three months after the onset of the disease.

2. Materials and Methods

2.1. Study Design

This is a pre–post study design in which measures of arterial stiffness and central hemodynamic were recorded in a group of participants before and after the COVID-19 infection.

All the recordings were made between October 2019 and April 2022 in the Laboratory for Vascular Aging at the University of Split School of Medicine.

To assess arterial stiffness and central hemodynamic parameters prior to COVID-19 infection, we utilized the stored recordings of enrolled participants from in-laboratory observational studies that applied the same measurement protocol as was used for the post-COVID-19 measurements. The post-COVID-19 measurement was performed between 8 and 12 weeks after the COVID-19 infection had ended, as evidenced by the absence of symptoms. This timeframe corresponded to 50 ± 2 to 90 ± 2 days after the onset of the first symptoms. The maximum amount of time between pre- and post-COVID measurements was set at 24 months.

2.2. Participants

The participants who had their arterial stiffness and central hemodynamic outcomes measured in our laboratory prior to infection with COVID-19 and who were afterwards infected with the virus were considered eligible for inclusion in the study. For all of those invited to the study, COVID-19 diagnosis was made by real-time Polymerase Chain Reaction test. During their first visit to the laboratory (pre-COVID measurements), all the participants underwent a medical history, and those with arrhythmias, cerebrovascular sickness, pregnancy, surgery amputation, oncology disease, psychiatric disease, infections throughout the trial duration, medical nonadherence, those that were unable to provide fully informed written consent or had any other serious medical condition that may affect data interpretation were excluded from the study.

While this was not originally our inclusion criteria, all of the participants reported mild severity of COVID-19.

In total, we invited 36 adults to participate in our study, with 32 (89%) agreeing to take part. All participants provided written informed consent to participate in the study, which conformed to the Declaration of Helsinki.

2.3. Study Procedures

Before undergoing testing, participants filled out a health history questionnaire, which inquired about personal and family medical history as well as medication use. They arrived for testing in a fasted state having abstained from food, caffeine, or smoking for at least 3 h and from exercise, alcohol and smoking for 24 h before testing. Those taking vasoactive medications (3 or 9%) maintained the same dosage throughout the duration of the study.

All study procedures were carried out in a quiet, temperature-neutral environment with the temperature range of 21–23 °C after participants had lain supine for 10 min.

To avoid possible confounding, each participant was recorded at the same time of day and with the same device during both visits.

2.4. Study Measurements

The arterial stiffness and central hemodynamics measurements were taken in accordance with the American Heart Association's recommendations for improving and standardizing vascular research on arterial stiffness (Townsend, Wilkinson et al., 2015).

Office blood pressure (BP) was measured during each visit using the validated oscillometric sphygmomanometer (Welch Allyn Connex ProBP 3400 digital blood pressure monitor with SureBP technology). The BP measurements were taken in a supine position after 5 min of resting and prior to PWV measurements. The participants did not change body posture between the two measurements.

Carotid–femoral pulse wave velocity (cfPWV); central blood pressures including: central systolic (cSBP) and diastolic (cDBP) blood pressures and pulse pressure (cPP); pulse pressure amplification; augmentation pressure (AP); augmentation indices: AIx calculated as AP/PP, AIx©75—AIx calculated as AP/PP and normalized to the heart rate of 75 beats per minute (bpm), and AIx index calculated as the ratio of late to early systolic pressure P2/P1; and heart rate (HR) were measured by either applanation tonometry using the Sphygmocor CvMS device (Atcor Medical, Sydney, Australia) or by the hybrid applanation tonometer—oscillometric device SphygmoCor Xcel (Atcor Medical, Sydney, Australia), as described previously [16,17]. While the validation studies comparing two devices indicated that they were comparable in terms of assessment of carotid–femoral pulse wave velocity (cfPWV) and augmentation index (AIx) [18,19], each participant was recorded using only one device to ensure that intra-individual changes are not affected by the type of device used.

A single operator (M. P.) carried out all of the measurements. For cfPWV measurements, recordings were performed on the right carotid and the right femoral artery. Central BPs and other parameters derived from the pulse wave analysis (PWA) were estimated after calibration of the pulse waveform recorded at the radial artery to mean and diastolic brachial pressures. We used the subtracted distance method to calculate the wave travel distance. The method was chosen over the direct method as per recommendation by the latest guideline [20].

2.5. Sample Size Considerations

Thirty-two participants are sufficient to detect moderate to strong effects on parameter changes using a simple linear regression model and strong effects when two-predictor linear regression model is used. Namely, using a two-predictor multiple linear regression model with $\alpha = 0.05$, $f^2 = 0.35$, and power of 80%, a sample size of 31 is required to detect a strong association between pre–post changes in vascular function/structure and potential predictors. For estimations based on a simple linear regression model, the sample size of 32 was sufficient to detect moderate to strong associations under assumptions of $\alpha = 0.05$, $f^2 = 0.27$, and power of 80%.

2.6. Data Analysis

To describe the distribution of a quantitative variable, we used mean and standard deviation (SD) or median and interquartile range (IQR), depending on the shape of the distribution. To decide if a distribution is asymmetrical, we used skewness and kurtosis tests for normality. The distribution of a qualitative variable was described with absolute and relative frequencies.

We utilized one-sample tests to determine whether a pre–post change in a parameter was statistically significant: either the parametric one-sample *t*-test or its non-parametric counterpart, the sign rank test, depending on the symmetry of the variable's distribution.

There were two sets of the regression models developed. We employed simple or multiple linear regression (MLR) models to identify predictors of the change from baseline (pre-COVID) for different arterial stiffness and hemodynamic parameters. These models were preferred as they use individual pre–post changes as the dependent variable. In addition, we built mixed-effects regression models to identify predictors affecting the values of a modeled parameter. Due to the fact that mixed-effects regression models employ repeated measurements of a parameter, these models had greater analytical power than simple or MLR models.

The model building was performed in two steps. In the first step, potential predictors—including age, sex, the amount of time that passed since the start of COVID infection, the amount of time that passed between the pre- and post-COVID-19 measurements, pre-COVID baseline values of a modeled parameter, and the type of device used to estimate its values—were used as single predictors in a simple linear regression or a mixed-effects model. For the final model, only those predictors that were significant at the 0.1 level or higher were considered ($p \leq 0.01$). Requirements for inclusion in the final model were significance at the 0.05 level or an increase in adjusted R^2 of at least 2% and a *p*-value of less than 0.2.

The above-mentioned potential predictors that were initially evaluated were selected to estimate the dependence of parameter values on the time that passed since the COVID infection and account for potential confounding variables. As an example, even though we did not anticipate any significant changes in vascular function over a 24-month period in the predominantly young participants (Table 1), we included the time between the first and second measurements as a potential predictor to control for its confounding effect.

We interpreted the strength of association between a predictor and a modeled parameter by applying the Cohen's effect size magnitudes for R^2 (small from 0.02 to <0.13, medium from 0.13 to <0.26, large from ≥ 0.26) to the adjusted R^2 of a single predictor model. [21]

As this is an exploratory study, no control for multiple testing was performed. The analysis was performed in STATA (version 17.0, Stata Corp. LP, College Station, TX, USA). We applied the significance level of $p = 0.05$.

Table 1. Demographic and clinical characteristics of participants, N = 32.

Characteristic	Statistics
Sex, N (%)	
Male	18 (56%)
Female	14 (44%)
Age (years), mean ± SD	36.6 ± 12.6
BMI, median (IQR)	28 (24.5 to 31.4)
Hypertension, N (%)	3 (9%)
Diabetes, N (%)	2 (6%)
Dyslipidemia, N(%)	0 (0%)
Familial history of CV disease, N (%)	7 (22%)
Smoking, N (%)	
No	17 (53%)
Yes	7 (22%)
Ex-smoker	8 (25%)
Smoking [cigarettes per day], median (range) *	5–10 cigarettes (1–10)

BMI—body mass index; * Calculated on N = 7 smokers.

3. Results

In this study, 32 participants were recruited; each participant visited the laboratory twice; and all of their data were collected. Table 1 shows their demographic and clinical characteristics at baseline prior to the COVID-19 infection. The participants were predominantly young (≤40 years) and healthy with only 9% (n = 3) of the cohort being hypertensive. None of the participants had dyslipidemia, and only two had diabetes (6%, one person was also hypertensive). The majority of the cohort was overweight or obese (69%) and did not smoke (78%).

The average time since the onset of COVID-19 infection in our sample was mean ± SD: 73 ± 10 days, with this time ranging from 51 to 92 days. The median time that elapsed between two measurements was 327.5 days (IQR, 129 to 458), with the range between 74 and 730 days. The majority of participants, 23 or 72%, were recorded with the SphygmoCor XCEL device.

In terms of the severity of COVID-19 infections, none of our participants have developed any of the cardiovascular, pulmonary, thromboembolic, or other COVID-19-associated complications, and there were no hospitalizations. Participants were evenly distributed according to the year they became infected (chi-square test, $p = 0.084$). There was no significant pre–post change in weight: median change 0 kg, 95% CI from −0.3 to 0.5.

When we looked to see if the mean individual pre–post changes were significantly different from 0, we found no significant pre–post change in any of the arterial stiffness or hemodynamic parameters tested ($p \geq 0.122$). We did, however, see an average increase of 0.19 m/s in carotid–femoral pulse wave velocity (cfPWV) from pre-infection values but at the significance level of 0.1 ($p = 0.052$). Table 2 shows the distribution of vascular parameters at baseline and after the infection.

Further analysis, however, revealed a widespread and complex pattern of confounders that affect the pre–post infection changes, and parameter values, in the majority of the assessed arterial stiffness and hemodynamic parameters (Tables 3 and 4). The size of these changes, as well as the direction in which they went, were dependent not only on the length of recovery time that had passed since the onset of the COVID-19 infection, confirming the existence of a response to the COVID-19 infection, but also, and more commonly, on cardiovascular health status at baseline (ascertained by age of an individual at baseline or the value of a parameter at baseline), as well as the amount of time that had passed between the two measurements. In accordance with the Cohen's interpretation of R^2, the majority of identified associations, regardless or the type of model, were moderate to strong [21].

Table 2. Distribution of arterial stiffness, and central and systemic hemodynamic parameters at baseline (pre-infection) and 2–3 months after the onset of COVID-19 disease (post-infection), N = 32.

Parameter	Pre-Infection	Post-Infection
Systemic Hemodynamics		
SBP (mmHg), mean ± SD	120 ± 9	119 ± 9
DBP (mmHg), mean ± SD	70 ± 8	71 ± 9
MAP (mmHg), mean ± SD	86 ± 8	85 ± 10
PP (mmHg), median (IQR)	47 (43, 54)	47 (43, 51)
HR (bpm), mean ± SD	65 ± 10	64 ± 7
Central Hemodynamics		
cSBP (mmHg), mean ± SD	107 ± 7	107 ± 9
cDBP (mmHg), mean ± SD	71 ± 8	72 ± 9
cPP (mmHg), mean ± SD	36 ± 6	35 ± 6
Carotid–Femoral Pulse Wave Velocity		
cfPWV (m/s), mean ± SD	6.3 ± 0.7	6.5 ± 1.0
Pulse Wave Analysis		
Aortic Augmentation (mmHg), mean ± SD	7 ± 5	7 ± 6
Aortic AIx, P2/P1 (%), mean ± SD	19% ± 13%	20% ± 16%
Aortic AIx, AP/PP (%), mean ± SD	123% ± 13%	126% ± 19%
Aortic AIx@HR75, P2/P1 (%), mean ± SD	15% ± 14%	15% ± 17%

AIx, augmentation index; AIx@HR75, augmentation index corrected for HR; cDBP, central diastolic blood pressure; cPP—central pulse pressure; cSBP, central systolic blood pressure; BP, blood pressure; cfPWV, carotid–femoral pulse wave velocity; DBP, diastolic blood pressure; HR, heart rate; IQR—interquartile range; MAP—mean arterial pressure; P1, first systolic peak; P2, second systolic peak; PP—pulse pressure; SBP, diastolic blood pressure; SD—standard deviation.

3.1. Arterial Stiffness—cfPWV

Regarding the cfPWV response to COVID-19 infection, defined as the pre–post change in this parameter, we found that post-infection values increased by 0.19 m/s (95% CI −0.04 to 0.41) but only at the significance level of 0.1 ($p = 0.052$). We also found no evidence that age, time since the onset of COVID 19, time between measurements, or cfPWV baseline values influence individual cfPWV responses. Individual pre–post changes were also significant at the 0.1 level according to the mixed-effects model (Table 4). However, age and time were moderately and positively associated with the cfPWV change since the onset of COVID infection at a group level. This model, which explains 32% of the intra-individual variability and 28% of variation at the group level, predicts an increase of 1.14 m/s in the average cfPWV value as a result of variation in the time since the onset of COVID-19 infection (51–92 days). The relationship between cfPWV and two predictors is shown in Figure 1. Although the age dependence is to be expected, we included it for comparison purposes. The change in cfPWV was not determined by the pre–post change in HR or the baseline HR value, nor was it affected by the change in BMI or the baseline BMI value ($p \geq 0.308$).

3.2. Arterial Stiffness—Augmentation Indices

As previously stated, no significant pre–post changes in augmentation indices were observed following the COVID-19 infection ($p \geq 0.244$). However, we discovered that the pre–post changes increased with age in AP and all of the AIx indices: Aix AP/PP, Aix P2/P1, and AIx@HR75 (Table 3). Except for the pre–post change in Aix P2/P1, which was moderately associated with age, this dependency was generally weak (Table 3).

Aside from age, which was found to be a common predictor of AIx pre–post changes, we discovered additional time-related predictors of these changes in Aix P2/P1 and AIx@HR75 indices.

Table 3. The predictors of the pre–post COVID-19 changes in systemic and central hemodynamic parameters and arterial stiffness parameters, as estimated by the linear regression models.

Pre–Post Change in:	Predictor	B (95% CI)	p-Value	Adjusted Simple Model R^2	Adjusted Final Model R^2
		Systemic and Central Hemodynamics			
SBP (mmHg)	Baseline value *	−0.46 (−0.68 to −0.24)	<0.001	21 §	21 §
DBP (mmHg)		no significant model			
PP (mmHg)	Baseline value	−0.35 (−0.68 to −0.02)	0.041	26 §§	30 §§
	Device, XCEL vs. CvMs	4.16 (−0.02 to 8.34)	0.051 †	12	
MAP (mmHg)		no significant model			
cSBP (mmHg)	Baseline value	−0.24 (−0.44 to −0.03)	0.026	3	3
cDBP (mmHg)		no significant model			
cPP (mmHg)	Baseline value	−0.36 (−0.71 to −0.18)	0.040	12	12
		Carotid–Femoral Pulse Wave Velocity			
cfPWV (m/s)		no significant model			
		Pulse Wave Analysis			
Aortic AP (mmHg)	Age	0.11 (0.02–0.21)	0.023	7	7
Aortic AIx, AP/PP (%)	Age	0.003 (0.0008–0.006)	0.013	10	10
Aortic AIx, P2/P1 (%)	Age	0.005 (0.002–0.008)	0.001	18 §	33 §§
	Time between measurements	0.0003 (−0.00003, 0.0005)	0.076 †	17 §	
Aortic AIx@HR75 (%)	Time from COVID	0.004 (0.001–0.006)	0.003	20 §	26 §§
	Age	0.002 (−0.0001, 0.004)	0.061 †	10	

AIx, augmentation index; AP, aortic augmentation pressure; B, unstandardized regression coefficient; cDBP, central diastolic blood pressure; cfPWV, carotid–femoral pulse wave velocity; cPP, central pulse pressure; cSBP, central systolic blood pressure; P1, first systolic peak; P2, second systolic peak; PP, pulse pressure; DBP, diastolic blood pressure; MAP, mean arterial pressure; SBP, diastolic blood pressure; * Refers to the pre-COVID value of a predictor; † The predictor is not significant, or is significant at 0.1 level, but its inclusion in the multiple linear model increased adjusted R^2 from 2 to 15%; § moderate and §§ strong association of pre–post changes with time from COVID or confounders, in accordance with the Cohen's effect size magnitudes for R^2 [21]; Variable is strongly correlated to the amount of time that passed between two measurements.

Table 4. Predictors of values of systemic and central hemodynamic parameters, as well as arterial stiffness parameters, estimated by the mixed methods regression models.

				The One-Predictor Model	The Final Model
Measure:	Predictor	B (95% CI)	p-Value	Snijders/Bosker's R^2 Level 1, Level 2	
		Systemic and Central Hemodynamics			
DBP (mmHg)	Time from COVID	0.20 (−0.01, 0.41)	0.063 †	8%, 9%	29% §§, 32% §§
	Age	0.32 (0.13, 0.51)	0.001	24% §, 27% §§	
cDBP (mmHg)	Time from COVID	0.19 (−0.02, 0.39)	0.082 †	7%, 8%	28% §§, 31% §§
	Age	0.33 (0.13, 0.52)	0.001	24% §, 27% §§	
MAP (mmHg)	Time from COVID	0.19 (−0.04, 0.42)	0.113 †	7%, 8%	31% §§, 34% §§
	Age	0.35 (0.17–0.53)	<0.001	27% §§, 30% §§	
		Carotid–Femoral Pulse Wave Velocity			
cfPWV (m/s)	Time from COVID	0.03 (0.003, 0.05)	0.030	13% §, 15% §	28% §§, 32% §§
	Age	0.03 (0.008, 0.05)	0.005	18% §, 21% §	
	Pre–post change in cfPWV	0.19 (−0.03, 0.40)	0.094 †	1%, 0%	

B, unstandardized regression coefficient; cDBP, central diastolic blood pressure; cfPWV, carotid–femoral pulse wave velocity; DBP, diastolic blood pressure; MAP, mean arterial pressure; † The predictor is not significant or is significant at 0.1 level, but its inclusion in the mixed model increased R^2; § moderate and §§ strong association of parameter values with time from COVID or confounders, in accordance with [21]; Level 1 defines how well the model describes changes at the level of the entire sample, whereas Level 2 depicts how well the model describes individual changes.

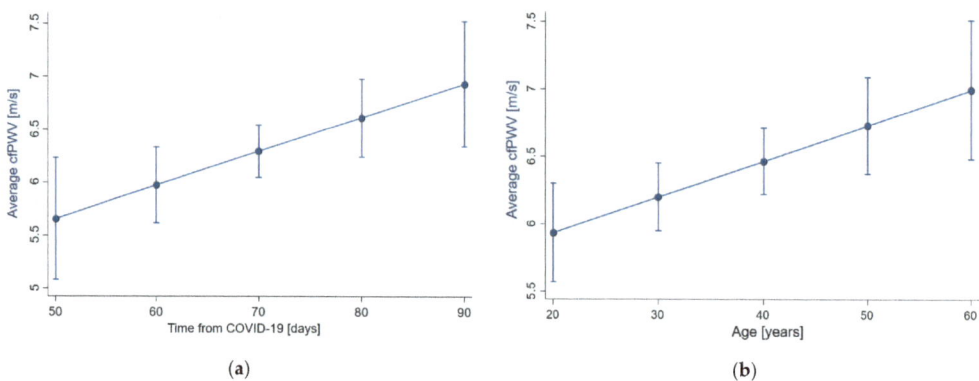

Figure 1. The relationship between the average cfPWV values in the sample and: (**a**) the time since COVID infection; (**b**) age, as estimated with the mixed-effects model ($R^2 = 27\%$ at the level of sample, $R^2 = 31\%$ for individual changes). Shown are predictive margins of cfPWV values with 95% CIs.

Time since the onset of COVID-19 infection was a moderate and positive predictor of pre–post changes in the AIx@HR75, accounting for 20% of their variance (Table 3, Figure 2). Within a range of 51 to 92 days after the onset of COVID infection, the AIx@HR75 pre–post change was predicted to move from −5% to +10%.

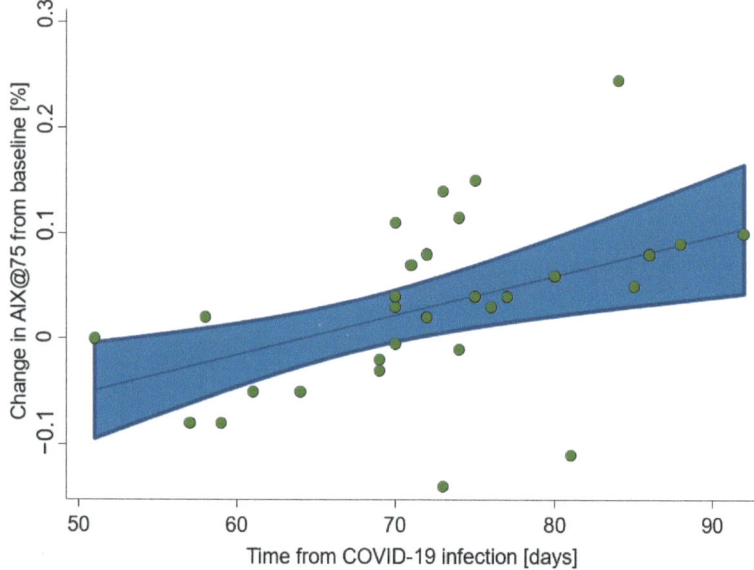

Figure 2. The change in AIx normalized to the heart rate of 75 bpm (AIx@HR75) from the baseline depends on the time that passed from acquiring COVID-19 infection. Shown are predictive margins with 95% CI estimated by the LR model ($R^2 = 26\%$) and the scatter plot of observation.

3.3. Peripheral and Central Hemodynamics

We found no significant changes from baseline in any peripheral or central hemodynamics parameters ($p \geq 0.122$).

Pre–post changes from baseline in SBP, cSBP, PP, and cPP were negatively dependent on their baseline values (weak—cSBP and cPP, moderate—SBP, strong—PP; Table 3). For example, given the range of baseline values for the PP parameter, the predicted post-COVID increase in PP ranges from +4 to −11 mmHg. It should also be noted that we also found a significant association of pre–post changes in PP with the time from onset of COVID-19, but at a 0.1 level of significance ($p = 0.098$). The variable was not included in the final model of pre–post PP changes because it did not meet our protocol's inclusion requirements.

Using the mixed-effects models, we were able to identify that age, and to a lesser extent the time since acquiring COVID-19, were positively associated with parameter values for DBP, cDBP, MAP, and cfPWV (Table 4). According to these models, the estimated change in average pressure values caused by variations in the amount of time that has passed since the beginning of the COVID-19 infection is as follows: DBP is envisaged to increase by 8.1 mmHg, cDBP by 7.6 mmHg, and MAP by 7.6 mmHg. As for individual pre–post changes, we were unable to identify significant mean changes nor the associations of these changes with any of the predictors listed above, nor were we able to find significant individual pre–post changes within mixed-effects models. Such a finding suggests that individual changes are likely heterogeneous and that that the effect that we identified at the group level is probably an average effect.

3.4. The Age Dependence of Pre-Post Changes in Investigated Parameters

We examined the pattern of pre–post changes in age dependence to see if there is a possibility that age modifies responses to COVID-19 infection. The scatter plots in Figure 3a–c depict a distinct pattern for those aged under and over 40. We demonstrated that the change in AIx P2/P1 from baseline for those over 40 years old is significantly greater than 0 (median 6%, 95% CI 0.7–24%, $p = 0.005$), whereas no significant change was observed for those under 40 years old ($p = 0.976$) (Figure 3a).

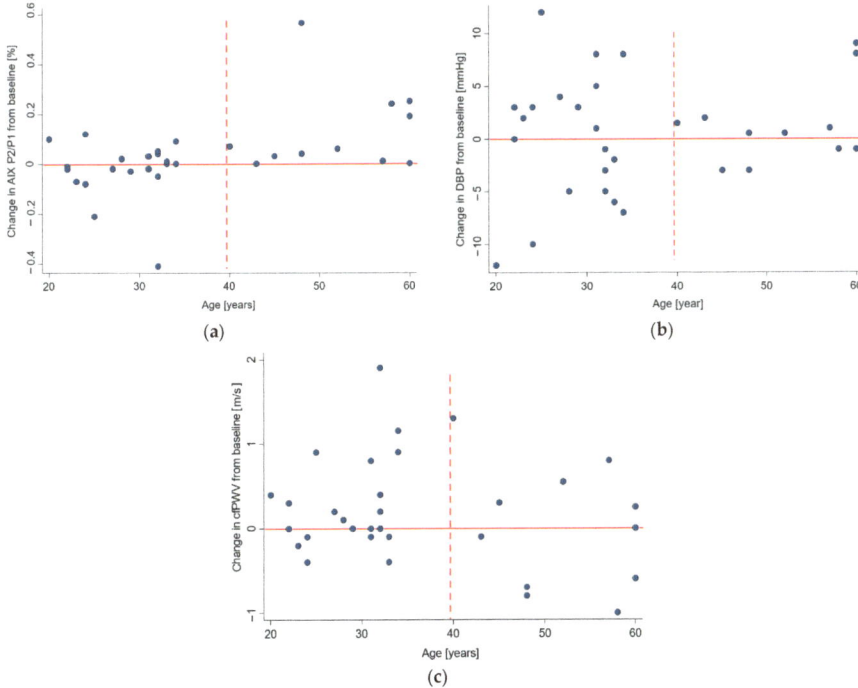

Figure 3. Scatter plots showing the relationship between age and pre–post change in: (**a**) augmentation index AIx P2/P1, (**b**) diastolic blood pressure, and (**c**) cfPWV. The horizontal reference line set at zero pre–post change, and the vertical dashed line set at 40 years that separates parts of a plot with apparently different dispersion patterns.

4. Discussion

This is the first study to compare pre- and post-COVID-19 infection levels across a wide range of arterial stiffness and hemodynamics parameters in the same group of participants. We discovered that the responses of the vascular system to a mild COVID-19 disease defined here as systematic, individual pre–post differences in investigated parameters, are not simple in the sense that COVID-19 on average either increases or decreases a parameter in infected patients by a comparable amount of measurement units. In fact, except for a non-significant trend for cfPWV, we were unable to detect any parameter with a mean pre–post COVID-19 change that differed from 0.

Instead, responses to COVID-19 infection are dynamic and depend on the time since the onset of COVID-19 infection. We identified such time-dependent responses in the arterial stiffness parameters—cfPWV and AIx@HR75, the central hemodynamic parameter—cDBP, and the systemic hemodynamics parameters—DBP and MAP; and we showed that their values increased with the length of time that passed from the onset of COVID-19 infection, independent of age or other confounders. In addition, the vascular impairment predicted by our models for observation period of two to three months post-infection is clinically significant as shown by an increase in cfPWV of +1.4 m/s, +15% in AIx@HR75, +8 mmHg in DBP, and +7.6 mmHg in cDBP and MAP.

The finding that the longer the period from COVID-19 infection the worse the vascular impairment was surprising, as we expected inflammation burden associated with COVID-19 to decrease with time. While we can only speculate on what causes this phenomenon, emerging evidence suggests that it stems from a failure to resolve autoantibodies observed during the acute phase of disease [22–24], or alternatively, that generating de novo pathogenic autoimmune responses post-recovery contributes to long COVID with evidence of residual inflammatory cytokines [25–27]. Hence, what we observed at the group level 2–3 months after infection, may be related to inflammation-induced arterial stiffening in some individuals [28], which is caused by inflammation from an autoimmune response or chronic inflammation that precedes one [29]. Furthermore, the heterogeneous responses observed in our study could be explained by the fact that inflammation in post-recovery was not triggered in all patients. Indeed, a recent study found that the circulating levels of anti-/extractable nuclear autoantibodies (ANA/ENAs) were higher at 3 months post-recovery in patients who had COVID-19 and were free from autoimmune diseases at the time of infection compared to healthy and non-COVID infection groups. High circulating ANA/ENA titers, which correlated with long COVID symptoms, were maintained up to 6 months after recovery but significantly reduced by 12 months. Even after 12 months several pathogenic ANA/ENAs were still detectable in up to 30% of COVID survivors. Furthermore, a retrospective study of 4 million participants found an increased risk of autoimmune diseases in patients with COVID-19 with an adjusted hazard ratio for different autoimmune diseases ranging from 1.78 to 3.21 [30].

All the time-dependent responses to COVID-19 disease were also affected by age in a way that each additional year at baseline added to vascular impairment post-infection. The effect of age was not the result of the time gap between pre- and post-COVID-19 measurements, as this confounding variable was controlled for in our analyses. In addition, we could not assign the effect of age only to the increased variability of investigated parameter with age [16], because in that case, pre–post differences would go in both directions—positive and negative, and we would not be able to find an increasingly positive relationship with age. Age, however, may modulate the response to a mild COVID-19 disease in arterial stiffness and central hemodynamics parameters in different age groups. Previous studies have suggested an age modulation of vascular responses to various triggers, including an infection [31,32], and the association of age with autoimmune inflammation [33]. While our results suggest the role of age as a modifiable factor in the response to mild COVID-19 disease, such a role should be further examined in studies with a larger sample size.

We detected the responses to COVID-19 disease in a variety of arterial stiffness measures and measures of its hemodynamic consequences, including: the direct (cfPWV) and indirect (augmentation index) measures of arterial stiffness as well as central (cDBP) hemodynamic parameter. Each of these three parameters represents a distinct aspect of the atherosclerotic process, which involves morphological and/or functional alterations to the vessel wall [34]. Therefore, the simultaneous detection of responses to COVID-19 disease in various vascular structure and function parameters supports the existence of a widespread and long-term pathological process in the vasculature following infection [35].

So far, only a handful of studies investigated the effect of COVID-19 infection on arterial stiffness and central hemodynamics. Most of them were case control studies with small sample sizes (10–22 per arm) comparing patients recovering from COVID-19 with controls [4,9,10]. Despite the possibly limited power of these studies, their results support our conclusions regarding the existence of vascular impairment after COVID-19.

The fact that cfPWV is increased in participants after the COVID-19 infection when compared to controls was found in several studies performed on: young healthy patients and their controls 3–4 weeks after the onset of COVID-19 (increase of 0.7 m/s) [9], acutely ill elderly patients (increase of 3.3 m/s) [4], as well as middle-aged patients that were compared to controls at 4 months (increase of 2.05 m/s) [36] and 12 months (increase of 1.15 m/s) after the COVID-19 onset [37].

Aix, like cfPWV, has been found to be higher in COVID-19-infected participants compared to controls. A 10% increase in the augmentation indices AIX AP/PP and AIx@HR75 has been reported in those infected with COVID19 when comparing 15 young adults 3–4 weeks after a positive COVID-19 test to healthy young controls. [10].

Finally, in terms of cSBP, at the 4- and 12-month follow-ups, COVID-19 patients have had a persistent increase of 10 mmHg in cSBP compared to controls [36,37]. In addition, Akpek et al. [38] reported an increase in systemic hemodynamics parameters during short-term follow-up in patients diagnosed with COVID-19.

Only one case control study did not find significant differences in arterial stiffness parameters—PWV and AIx75—at 4 weeks post-infection when young adults who were infected with COVID-19 were compared with their controls [39]. In addition, two small longitudinal studies reported results contradicting our findings. In the first study that followed 14 young participants from the first to sixth month post-infection, the authors reported a decrease in cfPWV (decrease by 0.82 m/s), SBP (by 11 mmHg), MAP (by 11 mmHg) with time; and no change in time was found for AIx@HR75 [40]. The second study followed 10 young adults for 6 months after the COVID-19 infection and found that SBP and DBP decreased throughout the study: with SBP decreasing by 15 mmHg and DBP decreasing by 10 mmHg [41]. Given that both of these longitudinal studies reported participant attrition on very small sample sizes, used inappropriate statistics (mean and standard deviation) to describe the distribution of limited data, and removed outliers from a small sample size [40], the reported results could be the result of methodological issues. On the other side, the lack of a uniform individual response to COVID-19 in the investigated parameters of vascular structure and function, which may be the consequence of age modulation (and possibly modulation by other factors), may have caused such results.

Our study had some limitations, the most significant of which was that the sample size only allowed us to detect moderate to strong associations. This means that even though we may have confidence in the significant associations observed in our study, we may have overlooked a relationship between the time since the onset of COVID-19 and several other parameters. For example, pre–post changes in PP were significantly associated with the time from COVID at the lower significance level of 0.1. As our sample size was limited by the number of recent pre-COVID recordings in our laboratory, we were not able to expand the sample size further.

Another potential drawback is the possibility that age and perhaps other factors relate to moderate responses to COVID-19 and that certain patient subgroups respond differently to COVID-19 than it was predicted in the overall model for that parameter. The fact that our models did not detect that individual pre–post changes in the tested parameters are significantly different from 0 but were able to detect in the mixed-effects models that parameter values depend on time from COVID-19, at the level of the entire sample, suggests that heterogeneous responses are possible. If this was the case, given that our results suggested an average response to COVID-19 disease, further analyses should be performed in studies with larger sample sizes.

Finally, because MAP in our study was estimated rather than directly measured, its estimation may be unreliable for some individuals [42], which could affect the accuracy of parameters derived from pulse wave analysis. However, since we were able to identify general patterns of change and interdependence, we do not expect this had a significant impact on the results.

The findings of this study demonstrated that there is a widespread and long-lasting pathological process in the vasculature following the mild COVID-19 infection which keeps deteriorating during 2–3 months post-infection. In light of the recent finding that up to 25% of otherwise healthy and disease-free patients exhibited the long COVID-19 syndrome 12 months after the onset of COVID-19 infection [3], and in light of the fact that vascular impairment increases the risk of future cardiovascular events, it is crucial that future studies explore these changes with larger sample sizes and with more synchronous population regarding the onset of COVID-19.

5. Conclusions

We found that various parameters of arterial stiffness and central hemodynamics respond simultaneously to the mild COVID-19 disease in predominantly healthy individuals. While we were unable to demonstrate this effect on all of the parameters tested, the worsening of values of those found to be responsive (cfPWV, AIx@HR75, cDBP, DBP, and MAP) points toward the existence of a widespread and long-lasting pathological process in the vasculature following the infection.

The detected responses to COVID-19 disease are not straightforward but rather deteriorate with the time since the onset of COVID-19 infection and age.

Within the period of 2–3 months following infection, our models demonstrated a clinically significant progression of vascular impairment.

Finally, we discovered that individual responses to COVID-19 are likely heterogeneous and possibly moderated by age.

Emerging evidence suggests that post-recovery autoimmune response to COVID-19 may be the cause of this phenomenon, although we can only speculate on its origin.

Author Contributions: Conceptualization, M.P. (Mario Podrug) and A.J.; methodology, A.J.; validation, M.P. (Mario Podrug), A.J., P.K., V.Č., M.P. (Maria Perissiou), R.M.B., I.M. and M.B.; formal analysis, M.P. (Mario Podrug) and A.J.; investigation, M.P. (Mario Podrug), P.K., J.P. and E.D.M. resources, A.J.; data curation, M.P. (Mario Podrug) and P.K.; writing—original draft preparation, M.P. (Mario Podrug) and A.J.; writing—review and editing, M.P. (Mario Podrug), P.K., E.D.M., J.P. M.P. (Maria Perissiou), R.M.B., V.Č., I.M., M.B. and A.J.; visualization, M.P. (Mario Podrug) and A.J.; supervision, A.J.; project administration, M.P. (Mario Podrug); funding acquisition, A.J. All authors have read and agreed to the published version of the manuscript.

Funding: The research was funded by the Croatian Science Foundation (No. IP-2018-01-4729). The Article Processing Charge was funded by the Split-Dalmatia County grant (No. 201900157031) and the City of Split Excellence Grant (No. OS520014).

Institutional Review Board Statement: The study was conducted in accordance with the Declaration of Helsinki and approved by the Ethics Committee of University of Split School of Medicine (No 2181-198-03-04-20-0096, 11/2020).

Informed Consent Statement: Informed consent was obtained from all subjects involved in the study

Data Availability Statement: The data presented in this study are available on request from the corresponding author A.J.

Acknowledgments: We thank included participants for their time and commitment to the study. We are grateful to the EU COST action VascAgeNet CA18216 for bringing the authors together.

Conflicts of Interest: The authors declare no conflict of interest. The funders had no role in the design of the study; in the collection, analyses, or interpretation of data; in the writing of the manuscript; or in the decision to publish the results.

References

1. Akhmerov, A.; Marban, E. COVID-19 and the Heart. *Circ. Res.* **2020**, *126*, 1443–1455. [CrossRef] [PubMed]
2. Barrantes, F.J. The unfolding palette of COVID-19 multisystemic syndrome and its neurological manifestations. *Brain Behav. Immun. Health* **2021**, *14*, 100251. [CrossRef]
3. Son, K.; Jamil, R.; Chowdhury, A.; Mukherjee, M.; Venegas, C.; Miyasaki, K.; Zhang, K.; Patel, Z.; Salter, B.; Yuen, A.C.Y.; et al. Circulating anti-nuclear autoantibodies in COVID-19 survivors predict long COVID symptoms. *Eur. Respir. J.* **2023**, *61*, 2200970. [CrossRef] [PubMed]
4. Schnaubelt, S.; Oppenauer, J.; Tihanyi, D.; Mueller, M.; Maldonado-Gonzalez, E.; Zejnilovic, S.; Haslacher, H.; Perkmann, T.; Strassl, R.; Anders, S.; et al. Arterial stiffness in acute COVID-19 and potential associations with clinical outcome. *J. Intern. Med.* **2021**, *290*, 437–443. [CrossRef] [PubMed]
5. Turan, T.; Özderya, A.; Şahin, S.; Konuş, A.H.; Kul, S.; Akyüz, A.R.; Kalaycıoğlu, E.; Sayın, M.R. Left ventricular global longitudinal strain in low cardiac risk outpatients who recently recovered from coronavirus disease 2019. *Int. J. Cardiovasc. Imaging* **2021**, *37*, 2979–2989. [CrossRef]
6. Hoffmann, M.; Kleine-Weber, H.; Schroeder, S.; Kruger, N.; Herrler, T.; Erichsen, S.; Schiergens, T.S.; Herrler, G.; Wu, N.H.; Nitsche, A.; et al. SARS-CoV-2 Cell Entry Depends on ACE2 and TMPRSS2 and Is Blocked by a Clinically Proven Protease Inhibitor. *Cell* **2020**, *181*, 271–280.e8. [CrossRef]
7. Lambadiari, V.; Kousathana, F.; Raptis, A.; Katogiannis, K.; Kokkinos, A.; Ikonomidis, I. Pre-Existing Cytokine and NLRP3 Inflammasome Activation and Increased Vascular Permeability in Diabetes: A Possible Fatal Link With Worst COVID-19 Infection Outcomes? *Front. Immunol.* **2020**, *11*, 557235. [CrossRef]
8. Tomasoni, D.; Italia, L.; Adamo, M.; Inciardi, R.M.; Lombardi, C.M.; Solomon, S.D.; Metra, M. COVID-19 and heart failure: From infection to inflammation and angiotensin II stimulation. Searching for evidence from a new disease. *Eur. J. Heart Fail.* **2020**, *22*, 957–966. [CrossRef]
9. Ratchford, S.M.; Stickford, J.L.; Province, V.M.; Stute, N.; Augenreich, M.A.; Koontz, L.K.; Bobo, L.K.; Stickford, A.S.L. Vascular alterations among young adults with SARS-CoV-2. *Am. J. Physiol. Heart Circ. Physiol.* **2021**, *320*, H404–H410. [CrossRef]
10. Szeghy, R.E.; Province, V.M.; Stute, N.L.; Augenreich, M.A.; Koontz, L.K.; Stickford, J.L.; Stickford, A.S.L.; Ratchford, S.M. Carotid stiffness, intima-media thickness and aortic augmentation index among adults with SARS-CoV-2. *Exp. Physiol.* **2022**, *107*, 694–707. [CrossRef]
11. Laurent, S.; Cockcroft, J.; Van Bortel, L.; Boutouyrie, P.; Giannattasio, C.; Hayoz, D.; Pannier, B.; Vlachopoulos, C.; Wilkinson, I.; Struijker-Boudier, H. Expert consensus document on arterial stiffness: Methodological issues and clinical applications. *Eur. Heart J.* **2006**, *27*, 2588–2605. [CrossRef]
12. Lacolley, P.; Regnault, V.; Nicoletti, A.; Li, Z.; Michel, J.B. The vascular smooth muscle cell in arterial pathology: A cell that can take on multiple roles. *Cardiovasc. Res.* **2012**, *95*, 194–204. [CrossRef]
13. Lacolley, P.; Regnault, V.; Segers, P.; Laurent, S.V. Vascular smooth muscle cell and arterial stiffening: Relevance in development, ageing and disease. *Phys. Rev.* **2017**, *97*, 1555–1617. [CrossRef]
14. Davies, J.I.; Struthers, A.D. Pulse wave analysis and pulse wave velocity: A critical review of their strengths and weaknesses. *J. Hypertens.* **2003**, *21*, 463–472. [CrossRef]
15. McEniery, C.M.; Cockcroft, J.R.; Roman, M.J.; Franklin, S.S.; Wilkinson, I.B. Central blood pressure: Current evidence and clinical importance. *Eur. Heart J.* **2014**, *35*, 1719–1725. [CrossRef]
16. Podrug, M.; Sunjic, B.; Bekavac, A.; Koren, P.; Dogas, V.; Mudnic, I.; Boban, M.; Jeroncic, A. The effects of experimental, meteorological, and physiological factors on short-term repeated pulse wave velocity measurements, and measurement difficulties: A randomized crossover study with two devices. *Front. Cardiovasc. Med.* **2023**, *9*, 993971. [CrossRef]
17. Podrug, M.; Šunjić, B.; Koren, P.; Đogaš, V.; Mudnić, I.; Boban, M.; Jerončić, A. What Is the Smallest Change in Pulse Wave Velocity Measurements That Can Be Attributed to Clinical Changes in Arterial Stiffness with Certainty: A Randomized Cross-Over Study. *J. Cardiovasc. Dev. Dis.* **2023**, *10*, 44. [CrossRef]
18. Butlin, M.; Qasem, A.; Battista, F.; Bozec, E.; McEniery, C.M.; Millet-Amaury, E.; Pucci, G.; Wilkinson, I.B.; Schillaci, G.; Boutouyrie, P.; et al. Carotid-femoral pulse wave velocity assessment using novel cuff-based techniques: Comparison with tonometric measurement. *J. Hypertens.* **2013**, *31*, 2237–2243, discussion 2243. [CrossRef]
19. Hwang, M.H.; Yoo, J.K.; Kim, H.K.; Hwang, C.L.; Mackay, K.; Hemstreet, O.; Nichols, W.W.; Christou, D.D. Validity and reliability of aortic pulse wave velocity and augmentation index determined by the new cuff-based SphygmoCor Xcel. *J. Hum. Hypertens.* **2014**, *28*, 475–481. [CrossRef]
20. Townsend, R.R.; Wilkinson, I.B.; Schiffrin, E.L.; Avolio, A.P.; Chirinos, J.A.; Cockcroft, J.R.; Heffernan, K.S.; Lakatta, E.G.; McEniery, C.M.; Mitchell, G.F.; et al. Recommendations for Improving and Standardizing Vascular Research on Arterial Stiffness: A Scientific Statement From the American Heart Association. *Hypertension* **2015**, *66*, 698–722. [CrossRef]
21. Cohen, J. *Statistical Power Analysis for the Behavioral Sciences*, 2nd ed.; Routledge: New York, NY, USA, 1988; p. 15, 415p.

22. Bastard, P.; Rosen, L.B.; Zhang, Q.; Michailidis, E.; Hoffmann, H.H.; Zhang, Y.; Dorgham, K.; Philippot, Q.; Rosain, J.; Beziat, V.; et al. Autoantibodies against type I IFNs in patients with life-threatening COVID-19. *Science* **2020**, *370*, eabd4585. [CrossRef]
23. Gatto, M.; Perricone, C.; Tonello, M.; Bistoni, O.; Cattelan, A.M.; Bursi, R.; Cafaro, G.; De Robertis, E.; Mencacci, A.; Bozza, S.; et al. Frequency and clinical correlates of antiphospholipid antibodies arising in patients with SARS-CoV-2 infection: Findings from a multicentre study on 122 cases. *Clin. Exp. Rheumatol.* **2020**, *38*, 754–759. [PubMed]
24. Zuo, Y.; Estes, S.K.; Ali, R.A.; Gandhi, A.A.; Yalavarthi, S.; Shi, H.; Sule, G.; Gockman, K.; Madison, J.A.; Zuo, M.; et al. Prothrombotic autoantibodies in serum from patients hospitalized with COVID-19. *Sci. Transl. Med.* **2020**, *12*, eabd3876. [CrossRef] [PubMed]
25. Douaud, G.; Lee, S.; Alfaro-Almagro, F.; Arthofer, C.; Wang, C.; McCarthy, P.; Lange, F.; Andersson, J.L.R.; Griffanti, L.; Duff, E.; et al. SARS-CoV-2 is associated with changes in brain structure in UK Biobank. *Nature* **2022**, *604*, 697–707. [CrossRef] [PubMed]
26. Proal, A.D.; VanElzakker, M.B. Long COVID or Post-acute Sequelae of COVID-19 (PASC): An Overview of Biological Factors That May Contribute to Persistent Symptoms. *Front. Microbiol.* **2021**, *12*, 698169. [CrossRef]
27. Su, Y.; Yuan, D.; Chen, D.G.; Ng, R.H.; Wang, K.; Choi, J.; Li, S.; Hong, S.; Zhang, R.; Xie, J.; et al. Multiple early factors anticipate post-acute COVID-19 sequelae. *Cell* **2022**, *185*, 881–895.e20. [CrossRef]
28. Jain, S.; Khera, R.; Corrales-Medina, V.F.; Townsend, R.R.; Chirinos, J.A. Inflammation and arterial stiffness in humans. *Atherosclerosis* **2014**, *237*, 381–390. [CrossRef]
29. Maamar, M.; Artime, A.; Pariente, E.; Fierro, P.; Ruiz, Y.; Gutierrez, S.; Tobalina, M.; Diaz-Salazar, S.; Ramos, C.; Olmos, J.M.; et al. Post-COVID-19 syndrome, low-grade inflammation and inflammatory markers: A cross-sectional study. *Curr. Med. Res. Opin.* **2022**, *38*, 901–909. [CrossRef]
30. Chang, R.; Yen-Ting Chen, T.; Wang, S.I.; Hung, Y.M.; Chen, H.Y.; Wei, C.J. Risk of autoimmune diseases in patients with COVID-19: A retrospective cohort study. *EClinicalMedicine* **2023**, *56*, 101783. [CrossRef]
31. Thiebaud, R.S.; Fahs, C.A.; Rossow, L.M.; Loenneke, J.P.; Kim, D.; Mouser, J.G.; Beck, T.W.; Bemben, D.A.; Larson, R.D.; Bemben, M.G. Effects of age on arterial stiffness and central blood pressure after an acute bout of resistance exercise. *Eur. J. Appl. Physiol.* **2016**, *116*, 39–48. [CrossRef]
32. Rosenberg, A.; Lane-Cordova, A.; Bunsawat, K.; Ouk Wee, S.; Baynard, T.; Fernhall, B. 5.3 The influence of sex and age on arterial function in response to an acute inflammatory stimulus. *Artery Res.* **2015**, *12*, 46. [CrossRef]
33. Wang, Y.; Fu, Z.; Li, X.; Liang, Y.; Pei, S.; Hao, S.; Zhu, Q.; Yu, T.; Pei, Y.; Yuan, J.; et al. Cytoplasmic DNA sensing by KU complex in aged CD4(+) T cell potentiates T cell activation and aging-related autoimmune inflammation. *Immunity* **2021**, *54*, 632–647.e639. [CrossRef]
34. Palatini, P.; Casiglia, E.; Gasowski, J.; Gluszek, J.; Jankowski, P.; Narkiewicz, K.; Saladini, F.; Stolarz-Skrzypek, K.; Tikhonoff, V.; Van Bortel, L.; et al. Arterial stiffness, central hemodynamics, and cardiovascular risk in hypertension. *Vasc. Health Risk Manag.* **2011**, *7*, 725–739. [CrossRef]
35. Martínez-Salazar, B.; Holwerda, M.; Stüdle, C.; Piragyte, I.; Mercader, N.; Engelhardt, B.; Rieben, R.; Döring, Y. COVID-19 and the Vasculature: Current Aspects and Long-Term Consequences. *Front. Cell Dev. Biol.* **2022**, *10*, 824851. [CrossRef]
36. Lambadiari, V.; Mitrakou, A.; Kountouri, A.; Thymis, J.; Katogiannis, K.; Korakas, E.; Varlamos, C.; Andreadou, I.; Tsoumani, M.; Triantafyllidi, H.; et al. Association of COVID-19 with impaired endothelial glycocalyx, vascular function and myocardial deformation 4 months after infection. *Eur. J. Heart Fail.* **2021**, *23*, 1916–1926. [CrossRef]
37. Ikonomidis, I.; Lambadiari, V.; Mitrakou, A.; Kountouri, A.; Katogiannis, K.; Thymis, J.; Korakas, E.; Pavlidis, G.; Kazakou, P.; Panagopoulos, G.; et al. Myocardial work and vascular dysfunction are partially improved at 12 months after COVID-19 infection. *Eur. J. Heart Fail.* **2022**, *24*, 727–729. [CrossRef]
38. Akpek, M. Does COVID-19 Cause Hypertension? *Angiology* **2022**, *73*, 682–687. [CrossRef]
39. Nandadeva, D.; Young, B.E.; Stephens, B.Y.; Grotle, A.K.; Skow, R.J.; Middleton, A.J.; Haseltine, F.P.; Fadel, P.J. Blunted peripheral but not cerebral vasodilator function in young otherwise healthy adults with persistent symptoms following COVID-19. *Am. J. Physiol. Heart Circ. Physiol.* **2021**, *321*, H479–H484. [CrossRef]
40. Szeghy, R.E.; Stute, N.L.; Province, V.M.; Augenreich, M.A.; Stickford, J.L.; Stickford, A.S.L.; Ratchford, S.M. Six-month longitudinal tracking of arterial stiffness and blood pressure in young adults following SARS-CoV-2 infection. *J. Appl. Physiol.* **2022**, *132*, 1297–1309. [CrossRef]
41. Stute, N.L.; Szeghy, R.E.; Stickford, J.L.; Province, V.P.; Augenreich, M.A.; Ratchford, S.M.; Stickford, A.S.L. Longitudinal observations of sympathetic neural activity and hemodynamics during 6 months recovery from SARS-CoV-2 infection. *Physiol. Rep.* **2022**, *10*, e15423. [CrossRef]
42. Grillo, A.; Salvi, P.; Furlanis, G.; Baldi, C.; Rovina, M.; Salvi, L.; Faini, A.; Bilo, G.; Fabris, B.; Carretta, R.; et al. Mean arterial pressure estimated by brachial pulse wave analysis and comparison with currently used algorithms. *J. Hypertens.* **2020**, *38*, 2161–2168. [CrossRef] [PubMed]

Disclaimer/Publisher's Note: The statements, opinions and data contained in all publications are solely those of the individual author(s) and contributor(s) and not of MDPI and/or the editor(s). MDPI and/or the editor(s) disclaim responsibility for any injury to people or property resulting from any ideas, methods, instructions or products referred to in the content.

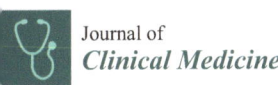

Article

Role of Chemerin and Perivascular Adipose Tissue Characteristics on Cardiovascular Risk Assessment by Arterial Stiffness Markers in Patients with Morbid Obesity

Viviana Aursulesei Onofrei [1,2,†], Ecaterina Anisie [2], Carmen Lacramioara Zamfir [1,†], Alexandr Ceasovschih [1,2,*], Mihai Constantin [1], Florin Mitu [1,3,4,5], Elena-Daniela Grigorescu [1], Antoneta Dacia Petroaie [1] and Daniel Vasile Timofte [1,2,4]

1. Department of Medical Specialties, Grigore T. Popa, University of Medicine and Pharmacy, University Street No. 16, 700115 Iasi, Romania
2. Cardiology Clinic, St. Spiridon, Clinical Emergency Hospital, Independence Boulevard No. 1, 700111 Iasi, Romania
3. Clinical Rehabilitation Hospital, Cardiovascular Rehabilitation Clinic, Pantelimon Halipa Street No. 14, 700661 Iasi, Romania
4. Academy of Medical Sciences, Ion C. Brătianu Boulevard No. 1, 030173 Bucharest, Romania
5. Romanian Academy of Scientists, Dimitrie Mangeron Boulevard No. 433, 700050 Iasi, Romania
* Correspondence: alexandr.ceasovschih@yahoo.com
† This author has the same contribution as the first author.

Abstract: Background and objective: The development of arterial stiffness (AS) in obesity is a multifactorial and complex process. The pleomorphic actions of adipokines and their local activity in perivascular adipose tissue (PVAT) are potential modulators of AS appearance and progression. We aimed to assess the correlations between two adipokines (chemerin, adiponectin), PVAT morphological changes (adipocyte size, blood vessel wall thickness) and AS parameters in the special subgroup of patients with morbid obesity. Material and methods: We enrolled 25 patients with morbid obesity and 25 non-obese patients, who were age- and gender-matched, untreated for cardiovascular risk factors, and admitted to hospital for laparoscopic surgical procedures (bariatric surgery for morbid obesity and non-inflammatory benign pathology surgery for non-obese patients). Before the surgical procedures, we evaluated demographic and anthropometric data and biochemical parameters including the studied adipokines. Arterial stiffness was evaluated using a Medexpert Arteriograph™ TL2 device. In both groups, adipocyte size and vascular wall thickness as well as local adiponectin activity were analyzed in PVAT from intraoperative biopsies. Results: In our study, adiponectin ($p = 0.0003$), chemerin ($p = 0.0001$) and their ratio ($p = 0.005$) had statistically significant higher mean values in patients with morbid obesity compared to normal-weight patients. In patients with morbid obesity there were significant correlations between chemerin and AS parameters such as aortic pulse wave velocity ($p = 0.006$) and subendocardial viability index ($p = 0.009$). In the same group adipocyte size was significantly correlated with another AS parameter, namely, aortic systolic blood pressure ($p = 0.030$). In normal-weight patients, blood vessel wall thickness positively correlated with AS parameters such as brachial ($p = 0.023$) and aortic augmentation index ($p = 0.023$). An important finding was the negative adipoR1 and adipoR2 immunoexpression in PVAT adipocytes of patients with morbid obesity. Additionally, we found significant correlations between blood vessel wall thickness and blood fasting glucose ($p < 0.05$) in both groups. Conclusions: Chemerin and adipocyte size could be predictive biomarkers for AS in patients with morbid obesity. Given the small number of patients included, our results need further validation.

Keywords: arterial stiffness; adipokines; morbid obesity; cardiovascular risk; perivascular adipose tissue

Citation: Onofrei, V.A.; Anisie, E.; Zamfir, C.L.; Ceasovschih, A.; Constantin, M.; Mitu, F.; Grigorescu, E.-D.; Petroaie, A.D.; Timofte, D.V. Role of Chemerin and Perivascular Adipose Tissue Characteristics on Cardiovascular Risk Assessment by Arterial Stiffness Markers in Patients with Morbid Obesity. *J. Clin. Med.* **2023**, *12*, 2885. https://doi.org/10.3390/jcm12082885

Academic Editors: Paolo Salvi and Andrea Grillo

Received: 12 February 2023
Revised: 9 April 2023
Accepted: 10 April 2023
Published: 14 April 2023

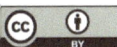

Copyright: © 2023 by the authors. Licensee MDPI, Basel, Switzerland. This article is an open access article distributed under the terms and conditions of the Creative Commons Attribution (CC BY) license (https://creativecommons.org/licenses/by/4.0/).

1. Introduction
Potential Biomarkers for Assessing Cardiovascular Risk in Morbid Obesity

Cardiovascular disease (CVD) is one of the leading causes of mortality, accounting for about a third of deaths worldwide [1–4]. The increasing prevalence of major cardiovascular risk factors and the identification of new biomolecules involved in global cardiovascular risk assessment require the development of new, easy and clinician-friendly diagnostic algorithms to adequately estimate the cardiovascular outcomes [3,5,6]. Obesity is a major risk factor in the cardiovascular continuum, deeply implicated in the development of atherosclerotic processes [7–9]. Obesity, dyslipidemia, diabetes mellitus and hypertension are also involved in the progression of arteriosclerosis defined as arterial stiffness and atherosclerosis, thus, have a prognostic role. Literature data have correlated their presence with major molecular changes in adipose tissue metabolism [10,11]. Adiposity acts as an endocrine tissue that secretes adipokines, molecules involved in altering immune response, lipid metabolism, insulin resistance and angiogenesis [12–16].

Obesity leads to increased expression of pro-inflammatory adipokines and thus, maintains a constant inflammatory status [17], which contributes to the development of atherosclerotic CVD [14,18]. Chemerin is an adipokine that modulates metabolic changes and correlates with body mass index (BMI), insulin resistance and serum triglyceride levels [5,19]. The literature highlights its role as an independent predictor of coronary artery disease and acute coronary event risk [20–22]. Chemerin also acts at the perivascular tissue level; clinical studies in the literature show an association between its high local titers and the presence of both aortic and coronary atherosclerotic lesions [22,23]. There are data about the modulatory role of chemerin in the development of arterial stiffness through its inflammatory action and interaction with the components of metabolic syndrome [24–26]. The development of arterial stiffness in patients with obesity is a multifactorial process, mainly determined by inflammation of perivascular adipose tissue (PVAT), remodeling of the extracellular matrix, alteration of the immune system and development of cellular and endothelial stiffness in vessels [27,28].

Based on the known role of cytokines and some adipokines secreted by PVAT, various current clinical studies are designed to determine its potential as a therapeutic target to lower arterial stiffness and cardiovascular risk [29]. The influence of PVAT on vascular reactivity has been investigated since the 1990s. More recently, preclinical and clinical evidence have demonstrated that PVAT characteristics are associated with arterial stiffness [30–32]. Metabolic changes produced in adipose tissue (secondary to excessive secretion of TNF-α and adiponectin) amplify the pro-inflammatory status by activating a diverse cell population in the vascular wall and modulating insulin sensitivity and lipogenesis, mechanisms that contribute to arterial stiffness [27].

The aim of this study was to evaluate the potential role of adipokines such as chemerin and adiponectin and PVAT morphological characteristics as biomarkers associated with arterial stiffness in patients with morbid obesity, given its role of independent cardiovascular risk factor.

2. Materials and Methods
2.1. Study Design and Population

We conducted a case-control study which included 25 consecutive adult patients with morbid obesity (body mass index [BMI] > 40 kg/m^2) and 25 age- and gender-matched non-obese patients who were part of the control group (BMI < 30 kg/m^2). The study period was January–May 2017. All patients were referred to the Third General Surgery Department of "St. Spiridon" Hospital for laparoscopic surgical procedures (bariatric surgery for patients with morbid obesity and non-inflammatory benign pathology for normal-weight patients). Cardiological evaluation was part of preoperative assessments. Patients with any treated cardiovascular risk factors, medical or surgical comorbidities generating inflammation, or treated with drugs interfering inflammation were excluded. Also, patients who presented with any three of the five criteria for defining metabolic syndrome [33] or had concurrent enrollment in another study were excluded. Patients included in the study had no associated cardiovascular risk factors requiring drug treatment.

2.2. Laboratory Measurements

We evaluated demographic parameters (age, gender); cardiovascular (CV) risk factors; anthropometric parameters; vital signs (systolic blood pressure (SBP, mmHg), diastolic blood pressure (DBP, mmHg)); biological parameters (both biochemical and hematological); as well as arterial stiffness (AS) parameters. Anthropometric measurements included BMI (kg/m^2), waist circumference, waist to hip circumference ratio (WHR) and index of central obesity (waist circumference to height ratio).

As we described in a previously published paper [34], all venous blood samples were collected after overnight fast and processed using specific techniques. The assessment of biochemical parameters was performed within two hours. Fasting glucose, total cholesterol and triglycerides were determined applying enzymatic colorimetric method, while HDL-cholesterol was measured using imunoturbidimetry. LDL-cholesterol levels were calculated using the Friedewald equation [35]. Fasting insulinemia and serum TNF-α were assessed using chemiluminiscence immunoassay kits (Siemens Healthcare GmbH., Erlangen, Germany) automated by an Immulite 1000 analyzer. Insulin resistance (IR) and insulin sensitivity (IS) completed the assessment of metabolic profile and were calculated applying the Homeostasis Model Assessment (HOMA) and quantitative check index (QUICKI) [36], respectively.

Serum levels of the two studied adipokines (chemerin and adiponectin) were processed after venous blood collection in vacutainer tubes without anticoagulant and centrifugation. Chemerin, known as retinoic acid receptor responder protein 2—RARRES2, is a 14 kDa protein, 131–137 amino acids long, resulting from proteolytic cleavage of the inactive molecule [37]. Serum levels of chemerin and adiponectin were assessed using quantitative specific human ELISA (enzyme-linked immunosorbent assay) kits (ab155430, ab99968, respectively) supplied by Abcam Cambridge, UK, for research use only. Chemerin/adiponectin ratio was calculated for studying the relation with AS. All biological samples were stored at $-20\ °C$ and processed after completing the enrollment of patients [37].

2.3. Arterial Stiffness Evaluation

Arterial stiffness was assessed by oscillometric method using the Medexpert ArteriographTM TL2 device. After data entry into the software (identification data, anthropometric parameters, age) and brachial blood pressure (BP) measurement, the AS parameters were generated: aortic pulse wave velocity (PWV), aortic and brachial augmentation index (Aix), systolic area under the pulse wave curve (SAI) and diastolic area below the pulse wave curve (DAI), diastolic reflection area (DRA), central BP and central pulse pressure (PP). The recommendations of the 2012 Expert consensus document [38] were followed. A complete report was produced in approximately 10 min. Subendocardial viability ratio (SEVR) was determined using the ratio of the areas of the systolic and diastolic portions below the aortic pulse wave curve and denoted as systolic area index (SAI) and diastolic area index (DAI), respectively. Knowing that SAI is calculated as the product of mean systolic LV pressure and systole duration, and DAI as the product of the difference between mean aortic diastolic pressure and mean diastolic LV pressure and diastole duration, we rewrote the calculation formula as follows:

$$SEVR = \frac{(mean\ aortic\ diastolic\ pressure - mean\ diastolic\ LV\ pressure) \times diastole\ duration}{mean\ systolic\ LV\ pressure \times systole\ duration}$$

The measurement protocol using the Arteriograph device involved the following steps: (1) recording general patient data (name, date of birth, weight, height, arm circumference and abdominal circumference, the distance between the sternal notch and the upper edge of the pubic symphysis, without following the abdominal relief); (2) locating the area of maximum pulsatility of the brachial artery and positioning the device cuff at this level; (3) the initiation of measurements, with the patient lying on his back and tracking the recording of pulse waves on the monitor to observe the morphology of the route; and (4) the interpretation of the results. In addition, before and during the recording the examination was performed in a quiet environment; avoidance of speech and mobilization during the measurement were encouraged. When white coat hypertension was suspected, an attempt was made to reassure the patient and the measurement was repeated. Smoking and coffee consumption were suppressed at least 3 h before the examination, copious meals were avoided during this period, as was the administration of nitrates. Alcohol consumption was prohibited for a period of 10 h before AS measurements [39].

2.4. Local Adipocytes and Adiponectin Expression Evaluation

During laparoscopic bariatric surgery, intraoperative biopsy of abdominal perivascular fat (PVAT) was performed. Specimens of 1 cm^3 were collected from the great/small epiploon region, including a visible small artery, for local adiponectin activity assessment

Samples from both groups were collected, fixed in 4% formaldehyde solution, embedded in paraffin, cut in 2 μm sections, stained (hematoxylin-eosin staining—H&E) and examined with a Nikon Eclipse 50i microscope. The sections were also subjected to immunohistochemical assay and treated with anti-Adiponectin Receptor 1/ADIPOR1 antibody EPR6626 (ab126611) and anti-Adiponectin Receptor 2/ADIPOR2 antibody (ab77612), according to standard protocols. Images were captured and analyzed using Zeiss Observer Z1 Tissue FAXS 4.2 Cell analysis SystemAdipocyte; size and number per field were quantified on microphotographs. Examination of the sampled sections included separate analyses of five different fields on slides obtained from the two batches. Initially, the long and short axis of the adipocytes were determined in order to make an assessment of the order of cell size in the two groups. The adipocytes detected in the center and the four extremities of each image were morphologically characterized. Subsequently, histological changes of the vascular wall layers were analyzed and the thickness of vascular wall was measured. The fields selected for analysis were chosen from the four extremities of each histopathological image so as to include vessels with the most different caliber and wall profile. We added a scale bar for all the images, to permit comparisons between control and obese groups.

2.5. Statistical Analysis

Statistical analyses were performed using SPSS statistics software (Statistical Package for the Social Science version 26, for Windows; SPSS Inc., Chicago, IL, USA). Initially, the descriptive analysis of the variables was performed for the continuous type variables, calculating the mean, median, minimum and maximum values, quartiles and standard deviation. Skewness (measuring the symmetry of the variables with respect to the mean value) and kurtosis (flattening coefficient) were determined to assess the normal distribution of continuous variables.

To compare the mean values between two groups of continuous values in order to identify statistically significant differences, the t test (independent *t* test) and ANOVA (one way analysis of variance) were used. Pearson and Spearman (r) correlation coefficients were used to assess the presence of correlations between the studied variables. A natural logarithmic transformation was performed for the variables without a normal distribution. This transformation allowed us to use the Pearson coefficient to determine if there was a linear correlation between the studied variables. Kendall's tau coefficient was used to evaluate correlations in the whole sample. For the subsequent analysis of the relationship between variables that met the threshold for statistically significant correlations, a simple linear regression was performed. After selecting several independent variables that influenced a dependent variable, a simple linear regression was extended to a multiple regression. A p-value ≤ 0.05 was considered statistically significant.

2.6. Ethics

The study protocol was approved by the local Ethics Committees of "Grigore T. Popa" University of Medicine and Pharmacy Iasi and of "St. Spiridon" Clinical Emergency

Hospital Iasi, and was conducted in accordance with the terms of the Helsinki Declaration. All participants signed an informed written consent before enrollment.

3. Results

Our study included 50 patients divided into two equal groups according to the presence of morbid obesity. Statistical analyses included several demographic, anthropometric and paraclinical parameters, which are presented in Table 1. Both groups included predominantly female patients (68% vs. 84%), with a slightly higher average age in the group of normal-weight patients ($p = 0.021$).

Table 1. Demographics, anthropometric and paraclinical parameters in the two studied groups.

	Non-Obese Patients (n = 25)	Obese Patients (n = 25)	p
Demographics and anthropometric parameters			
Age (y)	43.36 ± 13.9	39.24 ± 8.74	0.021
Female sex (%)	17 (68%)	21 (84%)	-
BMI (kg/m^2)	24.24 ± 3.15	43.9 ± 6.07	0.0001
Waist circumference (cm)	83.04 ± 8.75	125.5 ± 18.68	0.0001
WHR	0.83 ± 0.08	0.96 ± 0.10	0.0001
Index of central obesity	0.50 ± 0.06	0.75 ± 0.08	0.0001
Systolic blood pressure (mmHg)	118.04 ± 11.72	129.36 ± 13.03	0.002
Diastolic blood pressure (mmHg)	67.08 ± 7.89	75.28 ± 11.12	0.004
Pulse pressure (mmHg)	51.32 ± 9.98	59.08 ± 11.28	0.013
Biological parameters			
Total cholesterol (mg/dL)	197.80 ± 41.39	201.4 ± 27.17	0.718
HDL-cholesterol (mg/dL)	50.36 ± 14.94	50 ± 9.98	0.92
LDL-cholesteol (mg/dL)	125.44 ± 39.97	127.68 ± 23.48	0.76
VLDL-cholesterol (mg/dL)	24.50 ± 10.13	24.86 ± 14.39	0.919
Triglycerides (mg/dL)	121.24 ± 25.74	124.32 ± 17.96	0.86
Fasting glucose (mg/dL)	88.32 ± 8.80	99.28 ± 14.62	0.002
Insulinemia (µU/mL)	8.23 ± 7.98	24.47 ± 6.16	0.0004
Insulin sensitivity index *	1.82 ± 1.87	6.45 ± 3.73	0.0001
Insulin resistance (HOMA) (M/mU/L)	0.16 ± 0.12	0.13 ± 0.02	0.001
Uric acid (mg/dL)	5.29 ± 1.48	6.79 ± 2.19	0.006
TNF-α (pg/mL)	11.34 ± 11.42	7.49 ± 3.38	0.116
Adiponectine (ng/mL)	16.36 ± 1.49	18.05 ±1.155	0.0003
Chemerin (ng/mL)	9.10 ± 1.89	12.22 ± 3.80	0.0001
Adiponectin/chemerin ratio	0.55 ± 0.12	0.67 ± 0.18	0.005
Arterial stiffness parameters			
Aortic Aix (%)	35.1 ± 16.2	24.1 ± 12.1	0.090
Brachial Aix (%)	−5.5 ± 0.32	−26.7 ± 0.24	0.110
Aortic SBP (mmHg)	119.42 ± 20.18	128.74 ± 20.81	0.114
Aortic PP (mmHg)	50.66 ± 12.69	52.26 ± 10.76	0.633
DRA	45.32 ± 18.82	49.68 ± 11.38	0.321
SAI (%)	46.41 ± 6.36	48.82 ± 3.81	0.112
DAI (%)	53.61 ± 6.06	51.28 ± 3.80	0.111
SEVR	1.19 ± 0.28	1.06 ± 0.16	0.054
PWVAo (m/s)	8.92 ± 2.14	9.59 ± 2.38	0.305
Cardiovascular risk factors			
Smoking	10 (40.0%)	9 (36.0%)	-
Fasting glucose above 100 mg/dL	-	2 (8.0%)	-
Dyslipidemia	9 (36.0%)	11 (44.0%)	-
Perivascular adipose tissue parameters			
Adipocyte size (µm)	6.62 ± 1.78	9.34 ± 2.11	0.027
Blood vessel wall thickness (µm)	6.92 ± 1.48	8.79 ± 2.12	0.0001

All values are expressed as mean ± standard deviation (SD) or n (%); y: years; BMI: body mass index; WHR: waist to hip ratio; HDL: high-density lipoprotein; LDL: low-density lipoprotein; SBP: systolic blood pressure; DBP: diastolic blood pressure; MBP: mean blood pressure; PP: pulse pressure; DRA: diastolic refelction area; SAI: systolic area under the pulse wave curve; DAI: diastolic area under the pulse wave; PWVAo: aortic pulse wave velocity; AIx: augmentation index; SEVR: subendocardial viability ratio; * We used the quantitative insulin-sensitivity check index (QUICKI).

Data on risk factors were included among the data on clinical characteristics of the patients that were collected for the study. In our data, smoking was a more frequent cardiovascular risk factor in normal-weight patients, while dyslipidemia was more frequently encountered in patients with morbid obesity.

Patients with morbid obesity were associated with higher mean systolic (118.04 ± 11.72 mmHg vs. 129.36 ± 13.03 mmHg, $p = 0.002$) and diastolic blood pressure values (67.08 ± 7.89 mmHg vs. 75.28 ± 11.12 mmHg, $p = 0.004$), and pulse pressure values (51.32 ± 9.98 mmHg vs. 59.08 ± 11.28 mmHg, $p = 0.013$). Various metabolic disorders, such as changes in lipid and carbohydrate profile parameters were also observed. Although there were no statistically significant differences between the two groups, the mean serum values of total cholesterol ($p = 0.718$), LDL-cholesterol ($p = 0.76$), VLDL-cholesterol ($p = 0.919$) and triglycerides ($p = 0.86$) were higher in patients with morbid obesity. Patients with morbid obesity had statistically significant higher mean serum values of fasting glucose ($p = 0.002$) and uric acid ($p = 0.006$) as well as parameters associated with insulin metabolism (insulinemia, insulin sensitivity and insulin resistance) ($p < 0.05$). Mean serum values of adiponectin ($p = 0.0003$), chemerin ($p = 0.0001$) and their ratio ($p = 0.005$), as markers of adiposity, were also significantly different between the two groups. All patients enrolled in the study were evaluated for arterial stiffness, but there were no statistically significant differences between the two studied groups.

Among the studied arterial stiffness parameters, statistically significant correlations between serum levels of chemerin and PWVAo ($r = 0.272$, $p = 0.006$) or SEVR ($r = -0.259$, $p = 0.009$) were observed in patients with morbid obesity (Figure 1).

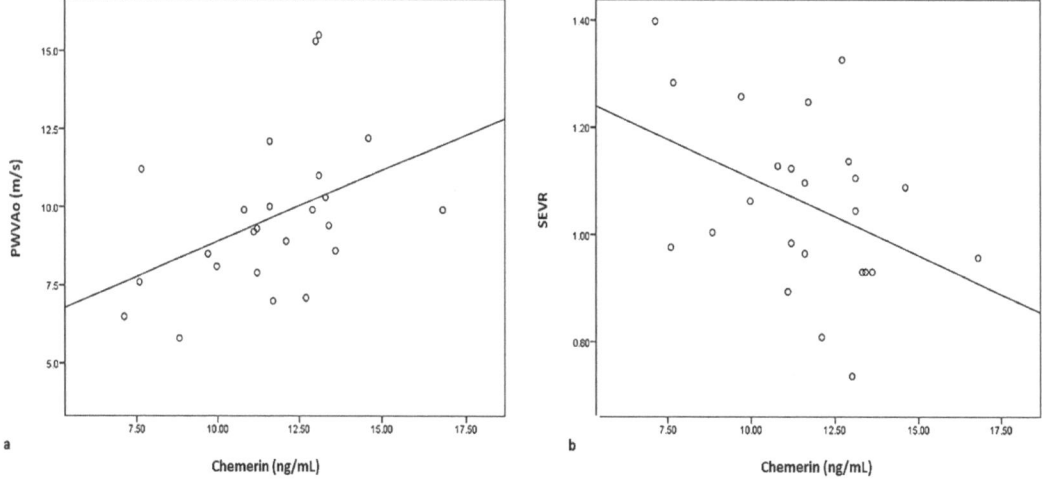

Figure 1. Correlations between serum chemerin levels and (**a**) PWVAo or (**b**) SEVR in patients with morbid obesity (PWVAo: aortic pulse wave velocity; SEVR: subendocardial viability index).

In addition to the descriptive statistical analysis presented above, a series of tests for correlation between histopathological and paraclinical parameters were performed and results are presented in Table 2.

In normal-weight patients, blood vessel wall thickness was significantly correlated with serum TNF-α levels ($p = 0.013$), fasting glucose ($p = 0.049$), age ($p = 0.020$) and with AS parameters such as brachial AIx ($p = 0.023$), aortic AIx ($p = 0.023$) and DRA ($p = 0.044$). In patients with morbid obesity, adipocyte size was correlated with serum VLDL-cholesterol ($p = 0.001$) and triglyceride levels ($p = 0.001$) as biological parameters, and with aortic SBP ($p = 0.030$) as arterial stiffness parameter. As in normal-weight patients, blood vessel wall thickness was significantly correlated with blood glucose ($p = 0.035$) in patients with morbid obesity.

Table 2. Correlations between adipocyte size and blood vessel wall thickness with demographic, clinical and paraclinical parameters.

Parameters	Non-Obese Patients				Patients with Morbid Obesity			
	Adipocyte Size		Blood Vessel Wall Thickness		Adipocyte Size		Blood Vessel Wall Thickness	
	r	p	r	p	r	p	r	p
Biochemistry								
Adiponectin	−0.220	0.123	−0.037	0.797	0.017	0.907	0.067	0.640
Chemerin	0.110	0.441	−0.189	0.190	−0.066	0.655	0.179	0.224
Chemerin/Adiponectin ratio	0.160	0.262	−0.124	0.387	−0.047	0.747	0.174	0.234
TNF-α	0.057	0.691	−0.357	0.013	0.074	0.607	0.104	0.469
Serum fibrinogen	−0.073	0.607	0.030	0.833	0.117	0.413	−0.094	0.513
HOMA	−0.093	0.513	−0.165	0.252	0.060	0.674	0.237	0.097
Insulinemia	−0.127	0.375	−0.171	0.233	0.043	0.761	0.193	0.176
Insulin sensitivity index	0.093	0.513	0.165	0.252	−0.060	0.674	−0.237	0.097
Fasting glucose	−0.034	0.815	0.287	0.049	−0.017	0.907	0.304	0.035
Total cholesterol	−0.144	0.427	0.185	0.198	0.181	0.207	−0.050	0.726
LDL-cholesterol	0.010	0.944	0.182	0.206	−0.044	0.761	0.007	0.963
HDL-cholesterol	−0.081	0.574	0.027	0.851	−0.176	0.223	0.010	0.944
VLDL-cholesterol	−0.037	0.797	0.114	0.426	0.482	0.001	−0.017	0.907
Triglycerides	0.003	0.981	0.101	0.483	0.482	0.001	−0.017	0.907
Uric acid	0.071	0.623	−0.082	0.574	−0.047	0.744	0.003	0.981
Serum creatinine	0.081	0.574	0.038	0.796	0.125	0.387	0.222	0.123
Hemodynamic parameters								
Systolic blood pressure	0.030	0.833	0.116	0.426	−0.269	0.061	0.239	0.097
Diastolic blood pressure	0.013	0.925	0.051	0.725	−0.212	0.141	0.183	0.206
Aortic pulse pressure	−0.088	0.543	0.126	0.386	−0.132	0.361	0.183	0.206
Mean blood pressure	0.020	0.888	0.132	0.361	−0.266	0.064	0.162	0.261
Demographics and anthropometric parameters								
Body mass index	0.153	0.283	−0.097	0.498	−0.124	0.387	0.093	0.513
Abdominal circumference	0.181	0.214	−0.124	0.398	0.003	0.981	0.203	0.160
Waist to hip ratio	−0.060	0.674	−0.138	0.337	0.170	0.233	0.193	0.176
Central obesity index	0.213	0.135	−0.252	0.079	−0.017	0.907	0.247	0.084
Age	−0.115	0.426	0.337	0.020	−0.249	0.087	0.061	0.673
Arterial stiffness parameters								
AIx brachial	−0.013	0.926	0.326	0.023	−0.043	0.761	0.180	0.207
SBP aortic	0.100	0.483	0.185	0.198	−0.311	0.030	0.220	0.123
PP aortic	−0.033	0.815	0.216	0.134	−0.281	0.050	0.230	0.107
AIx aortic	−0.033	0.515	0.326	0.023	−0.043	0.761	0.180	0.207
DRA	0.037	0.797	−0.292	0.044	0.261	0.071	−0.068	0.639
SAI	0.03	0.761	0.054	0.708	−0.242	0.092	0.117	0.413
DAI	−0.050	0.726	−0.094	0.512	0.259	0.072	−0.141	0.326
SEVR	−0.070	0.624	−0.067	0.640	0.248	0.084	−0.124	0.387
PWVAo	0.003	0.981	0.175	0.224	−0.151	0.293	0.054	0.708

r: Pearson Correlation; HDL: high-density lipoprotein; LDL: low-density lipoprotein; VLDL: very-low-density lipoprotein cholesterol; SBP: systolic blood pressure; DBP: diastolic blood pressure; MBP: mean blood pressure; PP: pulse pressure; DRA: diastolic reflection area; SAI: systolic area under the pulse wave curve; DAI: diastolic area under the pulse wave; PWVAo: pulse wave velocity at the central level; AIx: augmentation index; SEVR: subendocardial viability index;.

Histopathological Study

Histological and immunohistochemical evaluation of white adipose tissue samples of patients from both groups was performed.

Analyzing separately five different fields on the slides obtained from the two studied groups, we first determined the long axis of adipocytes to assess the order of size of fat cells in the two groups. Adipocytes detected in the center and at the four extremities of each image were monitored. Statistical processing of these data allowed us to reveal that adipocytes in the group with morbid obesity are more voluminous compared to those in the control group, suggesting that the abundance of adipose tissue may be the result of, not only increased adipocyte number, but also adipocyte hypertrophy.

The second parameter assessed was blood vessel wall thickness. The fields selected for analysis were chosen from the four extremities of each image so as to include vessels with the most different caliber and wall profile. After completing the database, the statistical processing of data allowed us to observe that in the group with morbid obesity the blood vessels had a larger diameter and a thicker wall compared to the control group.

Microscopic exam of samples from the control group revealed a normal morphology of white adipocytes, with a single lipid inclusion occupying almost the entire cytoplasm and a flattened nucleus compressed at one of the cell poles (Figure 2a). The histologic exam of samples from the group with morbid obesity revealed white adipocytes whose morphology did not differ significantly under light microscopy compared to that of adipocytes from the control group. However, their size was greater and in some areas the shape was slightly irregular, due to their adjacent compression (Figure 2b). A rich vascularization was mainly represented by microvascular elements; in our study, among the adipocytes, in the compact adipose tissue, small blood vessels with intact endothelium and vascular wall could be observed (Figure 3a). The vessels showed a consistent vascular wall, the tunica media was visibly thickened due to hyperplasia of smooth muscle fibers, and congestive areas were frequent. Most blood vessels were distended, with a stellate, irregular lumen and a sinuous periadipocytic course (Figure 3b).

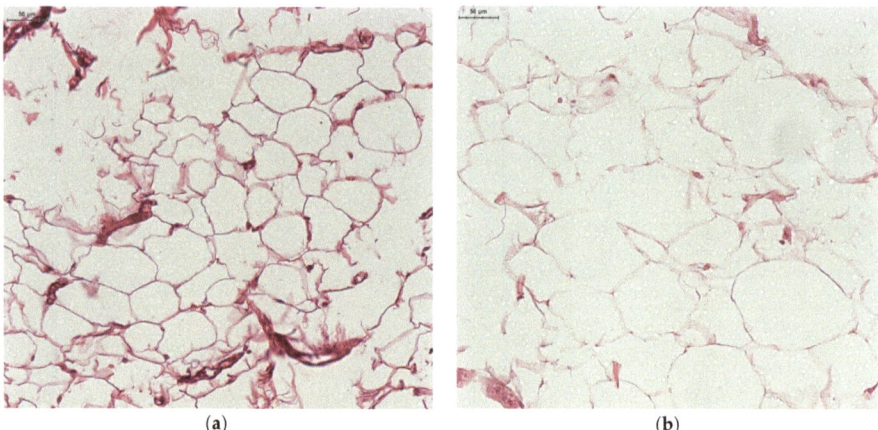

Figure 2. Adipose tissue: a control group ((**a**) non-obese patient); (**b**) Obese patient (H&E staining).

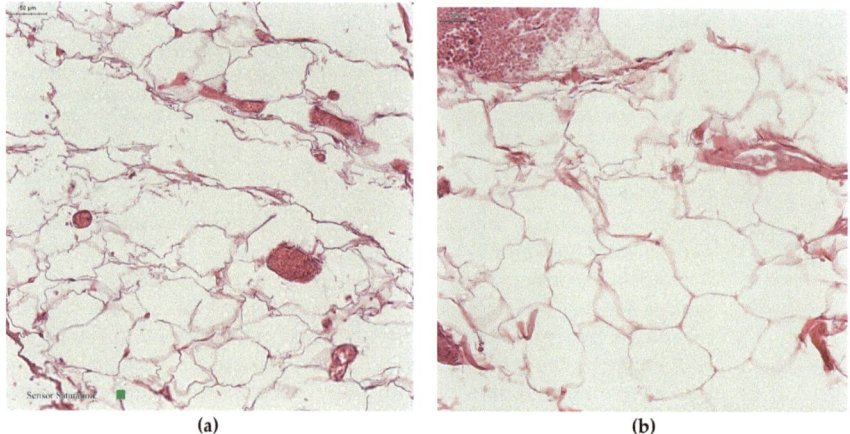

Figure 3. Histopathological images. Blood vessels, adipose tissue. (**a**) control group (non-obese patient); (**b**) obese patient (H&E staining).

Immunohistochemical evaluation of the expression of the two adiponectin receptors (R1 and R2) was performed. We observed a positive AdipoR1 immunoexpression for adipocytes from the control group and a reduced, even negative AdipoR1 immunoexpression for the adipocytes from the group with morbid obesity (Figure 4). At the same time, we observed a positive AdipoR2 immunoexpression for adipocytes from control group and a very low AdipoR2 immunoexpression for the group with morbid obesity (Figure 5).

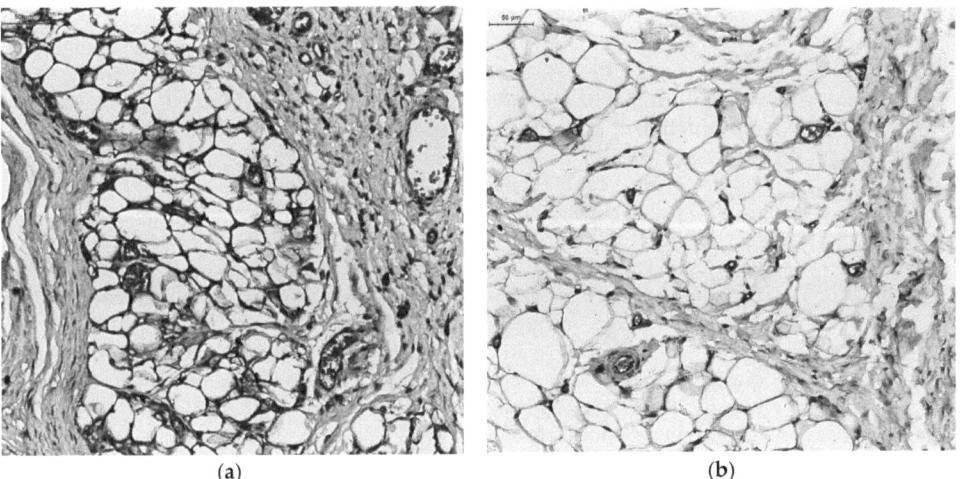

Figure 4. AdipoR1 immunoexpression (**a**) control group. AdipoR1—intense immunoexpression; (**b**) obese patient—AdipoR1 reduced immunoexpression.

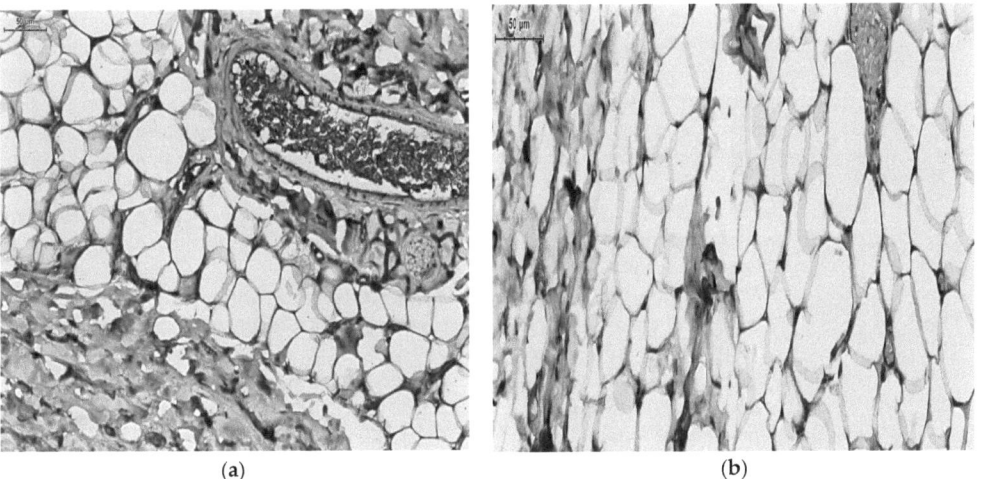

Figure 5. AdipoR2 immunoexpression (**a**) control group—AdipoR2 positive immunoexpression, (**b**) obese patient—AdipoR2 very low immunoexpression.

4. Discussion

Current data in the literature suggest that adipokines have a pleomorphic action responsible for arterial stiffness development. So, we studied the potential roles of circulating chemerin and local adiponectin activity in PVAT, as well as morphological features of abdominal PVAT in relation to arterial stiffness and with demographic, anthropometric and metabolic parameters in a special subgroup of patients with morbid obesity.

In our study, patients with morbid obesity had higher serum values of lipid and carbohydrate profile parameters ($p = 0.002$ for fasting glucose). Insulinemia ($p = 0.0004$), insulin sensitivity ($p = 0.0001$) and insulin resistance ($p = 0.001$), as well as the mean serum levels of adiponectin ($p = 0.0003$), chemerin ($p = 0.0001$) and their ratio ($p = 0.005$) were parameters with statistically significant higher mean values in this group.

In addition, our study patients with morbid obesity had higher, but normal mean blood pressure values compared to normal-weight patients. This observation is important as hypertension modulates the progression of arterial stiffness even in normal-weight patients. In this category of patients, Li et al. [39] demonstrated a significant correlation between visceral adiposity index and brachial PWV. In a similar study, Kim et al. [40] highlighted that brachial PWV correlates positively with WHR and visceral fat area, but not with BMI or abdominal circumference.

Yoo et al. [24] demonstrated that chemerin is an independent predictor for arterial stiffness, with multiple statistically significant correlations with both anthropometric and biochemical parameters. Similar correlations between chemerin and aortic PWV ($p = 0.006$) and SEVR ($p = 0.009$) were reported in our study among patients with morbid obesity. SEVR, also known as the Buckberg index, is an arterial stiffness parameter correlated with coronary flow reserve, useful in assessing coronary microvascular circulation. SEVR is a measure of cardiac oxygen supply-to-demand ratio that can be estimated by noninvasive validated methods [41], and is currently used in research and clinical practice [42]. The current data highlight the inverse relationship between decreased values of SEVR and cardiovascular risk [42]. In a recent study, Tocci et al. [43,44], demonstrated that overweight adolescent patients have reduced SEVR values compared to normal-weight patients, similar to their carotid-femoral pulse wave velocity and aortic systolic blood pressure. Other recent studies conclude that SEVR values decrease with increased number of metabolic syndrome elements ($p = 0.005$) [44] and are correlated with both IR and IS [45,46]. So, we could hypothesize that chemerin may be a biomarker for arterial stiffness and for the risk of microvascular coronary damage.

Chemerin is also a determinant of endothelial dysfunction, with high titers negatively correlated with flow-mediated dilatation (odds ratio of 1.58) and arterial stiffness (odds ratio of 3.75) in hypertensive patients [47]. Our results suggest that in morbid obesity, chemerin would indicate the development of AS before hypertension is documented. Clinical studies also report that high serum levels of chemerin are associated with enhanced carotid intima media thickness ($p = 0.035$), and are a marker of subclinical atherosclerosis in diabetic patients [48]. In our group with morbid obesity and normal values of fasting glucose, chemerin was correlated with AS, also a marker of subclinical atherosclerosis. It is worth mentioning that this group had changes of insulin metabolism which could mediate chemerin action.

In peripheral tissues, chemerin induces tissue enlargement, while stimulating inflammation and angiogenesis in adipose tissue [11,49]. Obesity is morphopathologically characterized by hyperplasia and hypertrophy of adipocytes, accompanied by macrophage infiltration of adipose tissue [50]. These aspects correlate with pro-inflammatory status [50,51], as our study also demonstrated. Unlike the data from the literature, our study could not demonstrate statistically significant correlations between chemerin, chemerin/adiponectin ratio and histopathological parameters in perivascular tissues. However, our results suggest that adipocyte size is correlated with aortic SBP ($p = 0.030$), a parameter of AS, in patients with morbid obesity. Similar to our results, Arner et al. [52] demonstrated that PWVAo correlated positively with subcutaneous adipocyte volume and negatively with fat cell count in patients with obesity. Weight loss could be associated with improvement in PWVAo but positive long-term results on arterial stiffness can only be achieved by bariatric surgery [53]. Regarding blood vessel wall thickness, no significant correlations with parameters of arterial stiffness were reported in our study. These data are supported by the results of previously published clinical studies that showed arterial stiffness assessed by PWV measurement is independent of arterial wall thickening [54].

Knowledge regarding the relationship between PVAT and arterial stiffness among those with obesity is limited, and many confounders affect the ability to infer causality [55].

White visceral fat has an essential role in the production of adipokines, while PVAT through direct contact with blood vessels has a paracrine role, modulating cardiovascular effects, independent of obesity [56]. On the other hand, obesity could cause PVAT dysfunction, an emerging paradigm, thus, highlighting its deleterious effects. PVAT dysfunction is induced by complex and not fully elucidated interactions among adipocyte hypoxia, insulin resistance, oxidative stress, vascular inflammation, and macrophage activation in the early stages of atherosclerosis [57–59]. Clinical studies in the literature to date have demonstrated that PVAT infiltration with pro-inflammatory cytokines is a morphopathological feature in patients with obesity and insulin resistance, thus, contributing to the maintenance of inflammatory status, endothelial dysfunction and further development of arterial stiffness [27,60–62].

Studying different adipokines that could regulate the atherosclerotic process might provide new opportunities for developing potential biomarkers predictive for AS, which is especially important in apparently healthy obese individuals. Clarifying the relationship between adipokines and established markers of atherosclerosis is an effective approach to refine the characterization of cardiovascular risk in patients with obesity and prevent CVD [50]. Growing evidence suggest that, in obesity, some adipokines directly mediate the process of atherosclerosis, regulating the redox state and inflammation [63–65]. Very recently it has also been shown that humans with obesity have a higher expression of vascular/perivascular TNF-α [66], in addition to NF-Kb and IL-6. In our study, there was no statistically significant difference in the serum levels of TNF-α between the two groups, possibly due to the metabolic status of patients with morbid obesity.

Compromised bioavailability of adiponectin also has been established as an independent risk factor for type 2 diabetes and cardiovascular diseases [67]. Some studies link circulating adiponectin to vascular structural changes involved in early vascular aging, while locally produced molecules modulate the contractile function of small arteries [68,69].

Mean serum adiponectin levels were significantly higher among morbidly obese patients ($p = 0.0003$), a finding which is distinct from other published data and could suggest the presence of adiponectin resistance. Histopathological studies demonstrated that serum adiponectin levels were negatively correlated with adipose tissue mass. Low adiponectin titers correlate with the development of insulin resistance, type 2 diabetes or metabolic syndrome [70–72]. Several clinical studies demonstrated that serum adiponectin level is an independent predictor of aortic or brachial PWV [73,74]. This adipokine exerts its effects via two receptors, R1 and R2, whose expression is decreased in patients with obesity induced in experimental studies [75]. A high level of AdipoR1 is found in normal adipose tissue, while in obese patients its level is significantly reduced. In our study, the AdipoR1 and adipoR2 immunoexpression was clearly positive in normal adipose tissue. The negative results in patients with morbid obesity could be interpreted as difficult to detect because of the absence, or very low level of adiponectin receptors

Our study has some limitations. Firstly, the most important one is the small number of patients included; our results could be seen as preliminary results which need further studies for validation. Secondly, it would have been preferable that patients with morbid obesity to be their own witnesses over a period of 6–12 months. Such a design involves some ethical limitations because it would be required a repeated biopsy and a longer observational period for study. Thirdly, we proposed the study of local adiponectin activity from abdominal PVAT, under the assumption that it shares similar properties with other regions of perivascular fat.

5. Conclusions

The studied adipokine chemerin and adipocyte size in abdominal PVAT could represent predictive biomarkers for arterial stiffness in patients with morbid obesity. Although our study did not demonstrate the relationship between adiponectin and parameters of AS, the negative/weak immunoexpression of its receptors in abdominal PVAT could influence this process. In addition, our results could be influenced by the metabolic status of the patients studied. Given the small size of our sample, the current results need further validation.

Author Contributions: V.A.O. wrote the paper, performed the arterial stiffness measurements and revised the final script; A.C. and M.C. performed the statistical analysis; F.M., E.-D.G. and A.D.P. helped review editing; E.A. performed the immunological tests, C.L.Z. performed histometry and immunohistochemistry interpretation, statistical analysis, selected the figures; D.V.T. performed all laparoscopic procedures and intraoperative biopsies. All authors have read and agreed to the published version of the manuscript.

Funding: This research was funded by "Grigore T. Popa" University of Medicine and Pharmacy Grant no. 31583/ 23.12.2015.

Institutional Review Board Statement: The study was conducted in accordance with the Declaration of Helsinki, and approved by the Ethics Committee of the "Grigore T. Popa" University of Medicine and Pharmacy Iași and of "St. Spiridon" Clinical Emergency Hospital (number 5/06.01.2017).

Informed Consent Statement: Informed consent was obtained from all subjects involved in the study.

Data Availability Statement: The data presented in this study are available on request from the corresponding author. The data are not publicly available due to local policies.

Conflicts of Interest: The authors declare that they have no conflict of interest.

References

1. GBD 2019 Diseases and Injuries Collaborators Global Burden of 369 Diseases and Injuries in 204 Countries and Territories, 1990–2019: A Systematic Analysis for the Global Burden of Disease Study 2019. *Lancet Lond. Engl.* **2020**, *396*, 1204–1222. [CrossRef] [PubMed]
2. Adam, C.A.; Șalaru, D.L.; Prisacariu, C.; Marcu, D.T.M.; Sascău, R.A.; Stătescu, C. Novel Biomarkers of Atherosclerotic Vascular Disease—Latest Insights in the Research Field. *Int. J. Mol. Sci.* **2022**, *23*, 4998. [CrossRef] [PubMed]
3. Anghel, R.; Adam, C.; Marcu, D.; Mitu, O.; Mitu, F. Impact of Comorbidities on the Long-Term Prognosis of Patients with Intermittent Claudication. *Intern. Med. Interna* **2021**, *18*, 7–19. [CrossRef]
4. Adam, C.A.; Anghel, R.; Marcu, D.T.M.; Mitu, O.; Roca, M.; Mitu, F. Impact of Sodium–Glucose Cotransporter 2 (SGLT2) Inhibitors on Arterial Stiffness and Vascular Aging—What Do We Know So Far? (A Narrative Review). *Life* **2022**, *12*, 803. [CrossRef] [PubMed]
5. Macvanin, M.T.; Rizzo, M.; Radovanovic, J.; Sonmez, A.; Paneni, F.; Isenovic, E.R. Role of Chemerin in Cardiovascular Diseases. *Biomedicines* **2022**, *10*, 2970. [CrossRef]
6. Anghel, R.; Adam, C.A.; Mitu, O.; Marcu, D.T.M.; Onofrei, V.; Roca, M.; Costache, A.D.; Miftode, R.S.; Tinica, G.; Mitu, F. Cardiac Rehabilitation and Mortality Risk Reduction in Peripheral Artery Disease at 6-Month Outcome. *Diagnostics* **2022**, *12*, 1500. [CrossRef]
7. Powell-Wiley, T.M.; Poirier, P.; Burke, L.E.; Després, J.-P.; Gordon-Larsen, P.; Lavie, C.J.; Lear, S.A.; Ndumele, C.E.; Neeland, I.J.; Sanders, P.; et al. Obesity and Cardiovascular Disease: A Scientific Statement From the American Heart Association. *Circulation* **2021**, *143*, e984–e1010. [CrossRef]
8. Anghel, R.; Adam, C.A.; Marcu, D.T.M.; Mitu, O.; Roca, M.; Tinica, G.; Mitu, F. Cardiac Rehabilitation in Peripheral Artery Disease in a Tertiary Center—Impact on Arterial Stiffness and Functional Status after 6 Months. *Life* **2022**, *12*, 601. [CrossRef]
9. Anghel, R.; Adam, C.A.; Marcu, D.T.M.; Mitu, O.; Mitu, F. Cardiac Rehabilitation in Patients with Peripheral Artery Disease—A Literature Review in COVID-19 Era. *J. Clin. Med.* **2022**, *11*, 416. [CrossRef]
10. Rizvi, A.A.; Stoian, A.P.; Rizzo, M. Metabolic Syndrome: From Molecular Mechanisms to Novel Therapies. *Int. J. Mol. Sci.* **2021**, *22*, 10038. [CrossRef]
11. Helfer, G.; Wu, Q.-F. Chemerin: A Multifaceted Adipokine Involved in Metabolic Disorders. *J. Endocrinol.* **2018**, *238*, R79–R94. [CrossRef] [PubMed]
12. Karastergiou, K.; Mohamed-Ali, V. The Autocrine and Paracrine Roles of Adipokines. *Mol. Cell. Endocrinol.* **2010**, *318*, 69–78. [CrossRef] [PubMed]
13. Pardo, M.; Roca-Rivada, A.; Seoane, L.M.; Casanueva, F.F. Obesidomics: Contribution of Adipose Tissue Secretome Analysis to Obesity Research. *Endocrine* **2012**, *41*, 374–383. [CrossRef] [PubMed]
14. Nakamura, K.; Fuster, J.J.; Walsh, K. Adipokines: A Link between Obesity and Cardiovascular Disease. *J. Cardiol.* **2014**, *63*, 250–259. [CrossRef] [PubMed]
15. Rizvi, A.A.; Nikolic, D.; Sallam, H.S.; Montalto, G.; Rizzo, M.; Abate, N. Adipokines and Lipoproteins: Modulation by Antihyperglycemic and Hypolipidemic Agents. *Metab. Syndr. Relat. Disord.* **2014**, *12*, 1–10. [CrossRef]

16. Kirichenko, T.V.; Markina, Y.V.; Bogatyreva, A.I.; Tolstik, T.V.; Varaeva, Y.R.; Starodubova, A.V. The Role of Adipokines in Inflammatory Mechanisms of Obesity. *Int. J. Mol. Sci.* **2022**, *23*, 14982. [CrossRef]
17. Hamjane, N.; Benyahya, F.; Nourouti, N.G.; Mechita, M.B.; Barakat, A. Cardiovascular Diseases and Metabolic Abnormalities Associated with Obesity: What Is the Role of Inflammatory Responses? A Systematic Review. *Microvasc. Res.* **2020**, *131*, 104023. [CrossRef]
18. Ouchi, N.; Parker, J.L.; Lugus, J.J.; Walsh, K. Adipokines in Inflammation and Metabolic Disease. *Nat. Rev. Immunol.* **2011**, *11*, 85–97. [CrossRef]
19. Rourke, J.L.; Dranse, H.J.; Sinal, C.J. Towards an Integrative Approach to Understanding the Role of Chemerin in Human Health and Disease. *Obes. Rev.* **2013**, *14*, 245–262. [CrossRef]
20. Yan, Q.; Zhang, Y.; Hong, J.; Gu, W.; Dai, M.; Shi, J.; Zhai, Y.; Wang, W.; Li, X.; Ning, G. The Association of Serum Chemerin Level with Risk of Coronary Artery Disease in Chinese Adults. *Endocrine* **2012**, *41*, 281–288. [CrossRef]
21. Dong, B.; Ji, W.; Zhang, Y. Elevated Serum Chemerin Levels Are Associated with the Presence of Coronary Artery Disease in Patients with Metabolic Syndrome. *Intern. Med. Tokyo Jpn.* **2011**, *50*, 1093–1097. [CrossRef] [PubMed]
22. Wang, B.; Kou, W.; Ji, S.; Shen, R.; Ji, H.; Zhuang, J.; Zhao, Y.; Li, B.; Peng, W.; Yu, X.; et al. Prognostic Value of Plasma Adipokine Chemerin in Patients with Coronary Artery Disease. *Front. Cardiovasc. Med.* **2022**, *9*, 968349. [CrossRef] [PubMed]
23. Spiroglou, S.G.; Kostopoulos, C.G.; Varakis, J.N.; Papadaki, H.H. Adipokines in Periaortic and Epicardial Adipose Tissue: Differential Expression and Relation to Atherosclerosis. *J. Atheroscler. Thromb.* **2010**, *17*, 115–130. [CrossRef] [PubMed]
24. Yoo, H.J.; Choi, H.Y.; Yang, S.J.; Kim, H.Y.; Seo, J.A.; Kim, S.G.; Kim, N.H.; Choi, K.M.; Choi, D.S.; Baik, S.H. Circulating Chemerin Level Is Independently Correlated with Arterial Stiffness. *J. Atheroscler. Thromb.* **2012**, *19*, 59–66. [CrossRef] [PubMed]
25. Molica, F.; Morel, S.; Kwak, B.R.; Rohner-Jeanrenaud, F.; Steffens, S. Adipokines at the Crossroad between Obesity and Cardiovascular Disease. *Thromb. Haemost.* **2015**, *113*, 553–566. [CrossRef]
26. Fontes, V.S.; Neves, F.S.; Cândido, A.P.C. Quemerina e fatores relacionados ao risco cardiovascular em crianças e adolescentes: Uma revisão sistemática. *Rev. Paul. Pediatr.* **2018**, *36*, 221–229. [CrossRef] [PubMed]
27. Aroor, A.R.; Jia, G.; Sowers, J.R. Cellular Mechanisms Underlying Obesity-Induced Arterial Stiffness. *Am. J. Physiol. Regul. Integr. Comp. Physiol.* **2018**, *314*, R387–R398. [CrossRef]
28. Fuster, J.J.; Ouchi, N.; Gokce, N.; Walsh, K. Obesity-Induced Changes in Adipose Tissue Microenvironment and Their Impact on Cardiovascular Disease. *Circ. Res.* **2016**, *118*, 1786–1807. [CrossRef]
29. Fleenor, B.S.; Carlini, N.A.; Ouyang, A.; Harber, M.P. Perivascular Adipose Tissue-Mediated Arterial Stiffening in Aging and Disease: An Emerging Translational Therapeutic Target? *Pharmacol. Res.* **2022**, *178*, 106150. [CrossRef]
30. DeVallance, E.; Branyan, K.W.; Lemaster, K.C.; Anderson, R.; Marshall, K.L.; Olfert, I.M.; Smith, D.M.; Kelley, E.E.; Bryner, R.W.; Frisbee, J.C.; et al. Exercise Training Prevents the Perivascular Adipose Tissue-Induced Aortic Dysfunction with Metabolic Syndrome. *Redox Biol.* **2019**, *26*, 101285. [CrossRef]
31. Ouyang, A.; Garner, T.B.; Fleenor, B.S. Hesperidin Reverses Perivascular Adipose-Mediated Aortic Stiffness with Aging. *Exp. Gerontol.* **2017**, *97*, 68–72. [CrossRef]
32. Ben-Shlomo, Y.; Spears, M.; Boustred, C.; May, M.; Anderson, S.G.; Benjamin, E.J.; Boutouyrie, P.; Cameron, J.; Chen, C.-H.; Cruickshank, J.K.; et al. Aortic Pulse Wave Velocity Improves Cardiovascular Event Prediction. *J. Am. Coll. Cardiol.* **2014**, *63*, 636–646. [CrossRef] [PubMed]
33. Rochlani, Y.; Pothineni, N.V.; Kovelamudi, S.; Mehta, J.L. Metabolic Syndrome: Pathophysiology, Management, and Modulation by Natural Compounds. *Ther. Adv. Cardiovasc. Dis.* **2017**, *11*, 215–225. [CrossRef] [PubMed]
34. Aursulesei, V.; Timofte, D.; Tarau, L.M.; Mocanu, V.; Namat, R.A.; Aursulesei, V.C.; Costache, I.I. Circulating Chemerin Levels, Anthropometric Indices and Metabolic Profile in Morbid Obesity. *Rev. Chim.* **2018**, *69*, 1419–1423. [CrossRef]
35. Friedewald, W.T.; Levy, R.I.; Fredrickson, D.S. Estimation of the Concentration of Low-Density Lipoprotein Cholesterol in Plasma, without Use of the Preparative Ultracentrifuge. *Clin. Chem.* **1972**, *18*, 499–502. [CrossRef] [PubMed]
36. Gutch, M.; Kumar, S.; Razi, S.; Gupta, K.; Gupta, A. Assessment of Insulin Sensitivity/Resistance. *Indian J. Endocrinol. Metab.* **2015**, *19*, 160. [CrossRef] [PubMed]
37. Mattern, A.; Zellmann, T.; Beck-Sickinger, A.G. Processing, Signaling, and Physiological Function of Chemerin. *IUBMB Life* **2014**, *66*, 19–26. [CrossRef]
38. Van Bortel, L.M.; Laurent, S.; Boutouyrie, P.; Chowienczyk, P.; Cruickshank, J.K.; De Backer, T.; Filipovsky, J.; Huybrechts, S.; Mattace-Raso, F.U.S.; Protogerou, A.D.; et al. Expert Consensus Document on the Measurement of Aortic Stiffness in Daily Practice Using Carotid-Femoral Pulse Wave Velocity. *J. Hypertens.* **2012**, *30*, 445–448. [CrossRef]
39. Li, J.; Zhu, J.; Tan, Z.; Yu, Y.; Luo, L.; Zhou, W.; Zhu, L.; Wang, T.; Cao, T.; Liu, L.; et al. Visceral Adiposity Index Is Associated with Arterial Stiffness in Hypertensive Adults with Normal-Weight: The China H-Type Hypertension Registry Study. *Nutr. Metab.* **2021**, *18*, 90. [CrossRef]
40. Kim, H.-L.; Ahn, D.-W.; Kim, S.H.; Lee, D.S.; Yoon, S.H.; Zo, J.-H.; Kim, M.-A.; Jeong, J.B. Association between Body Fat Parameters and Arterial Stiffness. *Sci. Rep.* **2021**, *11*, 20536. [CrossRef]
41. Salvi, P.; Baldi, C.; Scalise, F.; Grillo, A.; Salvi, L.; Tan, I.; De Censi, L.; Sorropago, A.; Moretti, F.; Sorropago, G.; et al. Comparison Between Invasive and Noninvasive Methods to Estimate Subendocardial Oxygen Supply and Demand Imbalance. *J. Am. Heart Assoc.* **2021**, *10*, e021207. [CrossRef]

42. Hoffman, J.I.E.; Buckberg, G.D. The Myocardial Oxygen Supply:Demand Index Revisited. *J. Am. Heart Assoc.* **2014**, *3*, e000285. [CrossRef]
43. Tocci, N.D.; Collier, S.R.; Meucci, M. Measures of ejection duration and subendocardial viability ratio in normal weight and overweight adolescent children. *Physiol. Rep.* **2021**, *9*, e14852. [CrossRef] [PubMed]
44. Fantin, F.; Giani, A.; Gasparini, L.; Rossi, A.P.; Zoico, E.; Mazzali, G.; Zamboni, M. Impaired subendocardial perfusion in patients with metabolic syndrome. *Diabetes Vasc. Dis. Res.* **2021**, *18*, 14791641211047135. [CrossRef]
45. Khoshdel, A.R.; Eshtiaghi, R. Assessment of Arterial Stiffness in Metabolic Syndrome Related to Insulin Resistance in Apparently Healthy Men. *Metab. Syndr. Relat. Disord.* **2019**, *17*, 90–96. [CrossRef] [PubMed]
46. Hoffman, R.P.; Copenhaver, M.M.; Zhou, D.; Yu, C.Y. Increased body fat and reduced insulin sensitivity are associated with impaired endothelial function and subendocardial viability in healthy, non-Hispanic white adolescents. *Pediatr. Diab.* **2019**, *20*, 842–848. [CrossRef] [PubMed]
47. Gu, P.; Cheng, M.; Hui, X.; Lu, B.; Jiang, W.; Shi, Z. Elevating Circulation Chemerin Level Is Associated with Endothelial Dysfunction and Early Atherosclerotic Changes in Essential Hypertensive Patients. *J. Hypertens.* **2015**, *33*, 1624–1632. [CrossRef]
48. Lu, B.; Zhao, M.; Jiang, W.; Ma, J.; Yang, C.; Shao, J.; Gu, P. Independent Association of Circulating Level of Chemerin With Functional and Early Morphological Vascular Changes in Newly Diagnosed Type 2 Diabetic Patients. *Medicine* **2015**, *94*, e1990. [CrossRef]
49. Hu, W.; Zhang, H.; Liu, Z.; Duan, Q.; Liu, J.; Dong, Q.; You, L.; Wen, X.; Zhang, D. Relationship between Adipose Tissue Distribution and Arterial Stiffness in HFpEF. *Nutrition* **2022**, *102*, 111726. [CrossRef]
50. Para, I.; Albu, A.; Porojan, M.D. Adipokines and Arterial Stiffness in Obesity. *Medicina* **2021**, *57*, 653. [CrossRef]
51. Rodríguez, A.; Ezquerro, S.; Méndez-Giménez, L.; Becerril, S.; Frühbeck, G. Revisiting the Adipocyte: A Model for Integration of Cytokine Signaling in the Regulation of Energy Metabolism. *Am. J. Physiol. Endocrinol. Metab.* **2015**, *309*, E691–E714. [CrossRef] [PubMed]
52. Arner, P.; Bäckdahl, J.; Hemmingsson, P.; Stenvinkel, P.; Eriksson-Hogling, D.; Näslund, E.; Thorell, A.; Andersson, D.P.; Caidahl, K.; Rydén, M. Regional Variations in the Relationship between Arterial Stiffness and Adipocyte Volume or Number in Obese Subjects. *Int. J. Obes. 2005* **2015**, *39*, 222–227. [CrossRef] [PubMed]
53. Bäckdahl, J.; Andersson, D.P.; Eriksson-Hogling, D.; Caidahl, K.; Thorell, A.; Mileti, E.; Daub, C.O.; Arner, P.; Rydén, M. Long-Term Improvement in Aortic Pulse Wave Velocity After Weight Loss Can Be Predicted by White Adipose Tissue Factors. *Am. J. Hypertens.* **2018**, *31*, 450–457. [CrossRef]
54. Cecelja, M.; Jiang, B.; Keehn, L.; Hussain, T.; Silva Vieira, M.; Phinikaridou, A.; Greil, G.; Spector, T.D.; Chowienczyk, P. Arterial Stiffening Is a Heritable Trait Associated with Arterial Dilation but Not Wall Thickening: A Longitudinal Study in the Twins UK Cohort. *Eur. Heart J.* **2018**, *39*, 2282–2288. [CrossRef] [PubMed]
55. Sabbatini, A.R.; Fontana, V.; Laurent, S.; Moreno, H. An Update on the Role of Adipokines in Arterial Stiffness and Hypertension. *J. Hypertens.* **2015**, *33*, 435–444. [CrossRef] [PubMed]
56. Siegel-Axel, D.I.; Häring, H.U. Perivascular Adipose Tissue: An Unique Fat Compartment Relevant for the Cardiometabolic Syndrome. *Rev. Endocr. Metab. Disord.* **2016**, *17*, 51–60. [CrossRef] [PubMed]
57. Greenstein, A.S.; Khavandi, K.; Withers, S.B.; Sonoyama, K.; Clancy, O.; Jeziorska, M.; Laing, I.; Yates, A.P.; Pemberton, P.W.; Malik, R.A.; et al. Local Inflammation and Hypoxia Abolish the Protective Anticontractile Properties of Perivascular Fat in Obese Patients. *Circulation* **2009**, *119*, 1661–1670. [CrossRef]
58. Lim, S.; Meigs, J.B. Links between Ectopic Fat and Vascular Disease in Humans. *Arterioscler. Thromb. Vasc. Biol.* **2014**, *34*, 1820–1826. [CrossRef]
59. Brown, N.K.; Zhou, Z.; Zhang, J.; Zeng, R.; Wu, J.; Eitzman, D.T.; Chen, Y.E.; Chang, L. Perivascular Adipose Tissue in Vascular Function and Disease: A Review of Current Research and Animal Models. *Arterioscler. Thromb. Vasc. Biol.* **2014**, *34*, 1621–1630. [CrossRef]
60. Nosalski, R.; Guzik, T.J. Perivascular Adipose Tissue Inflammation in Vascular Disease. *Br. J. Pharmacol.* **2017**, *174*, 3496–3513. [CrossRef]
61. Jia, G.; Aroor, A.R.; DeMarco, V.G.; Martinez-Lemus, L.A.; Meininger, G.A.; Sowers, J.R. Vascular Stiffness in Insulin Resistance and Obesity. *Front. Physiol.* **2015**, *6*, 231. [CrossRef] [PubMed]
62. Gómez-Hernández, A.; Beneit, N.; Díaz-Castroverde, S.; Escribano, Ó. Differential Role of Adipose Tissues in Obesity and Related Metabolic and Vascular Complications. *Int. J. Endocrinol.* **2016**, *2016*, 1216783. [CrossRef] [PubMed]
63. Yoo, H.J.; Choi, K.M. Adipokines as a Novel Link between Obesity and Atherosclerosis. *World J. Diabetes* **2014**, *5*, 357–363. [CrossRef] [PubMed]
64. Ntaios, G.; Gatselis, N.K.; Makaritsis, K.; Dalekos, G.N. Adipokines as Mediators of Endothelial Function and Atherosclerosis. *Atherosclerosis* **2013**, *227*, 216–221. [CrossRef]
65. Hajjar, D.P.; Gotto, A.M. Biological Relevance of Inflammation and Oxidative Stress in the Pathogenesis of Arterial Diseases. *Am. J. Pathol.* **2013**, *182*, 1474–1481. [CrossRef]
66. Virdis, A.; Duranti, E.; Rossi, C.; Dell'Agnello, U.; Santini, E.; Anselmino, M.; Chiarugi, M.; Taddei, S.; Solini, A. Tumour Necrosis Factor-Alpha Participates on the Endothelin-1/Nitric Oxide Imbalance in Small Arteries from Obese Patients: Role of Perivascular Adipose Tissue. *Eur. Heart J.* **2015**, *36*, 784–794. [CrossRef]

67. Lindberg, S.; Jensen, J.S.; Bjerre, M.; Pedersen, S.H.; Frystyk, J.; Flyvbjerg, A.; Galatius, S.; Jeppesen, J.; Mogelvang, R. Adiponectin, type 2 diabetes and cardiovascular risk. *Eur. J. Prev. Cardiol.* **2015**, *22*, 276–283. [CrossRef]
68. Ouchi, N.; Shibata, R.; Walsh, K. Cardioprotection by Adiponectin. *Trends Cardiovasc. Med.* **2006**, *16*, 141–146. [CrossRef]
69. Barandier, C.; Montani, J.-P.; Yang, Z. Mature Adipocytes and Perivascular Adipose Tissue Stimulate Vascular Smooth Muscle Cell Proliferation: Effects of Aging and Obesity. *Am. J. Physiol. Heart Circ. Physiol.* **2005**, *289*, H1807–H1813. [CrossRef]
70. Sommer, G.; Kralisch, S.; Stangl, V.; Vietzke, A.; Köhler, U.; Stepan, H.; Faber, R.; Schubert, A.; Lössner, U.; Bluher, M.; et al. Secretory Products from Human Adipocytes Stimulate Proinflammatory Cytokine Secretion from Human Endothelial Cells. *J. Cell. Biochem.* **2009**, *106*, 729–737. [CrossRef]
71. Turer, A.T.; Khera, A.; Ayers, C.R.; Turer, C.B.; Grundy, S.M.; Vega, G.L.; Scherer, P.E. Adipose Tissue Mass and Location Affect Circulating Adiponectin Levels. *Diabetologia* **2011**, *54*, 2515–2524. [CrossRef] [PubMed]
72. Galic, S.; Oakhill, J.S.; Steinberg, G.R. Adipose Tissue as an Endocrine Organ. *Mol. Cell. Endocrinol.* **2010**, *316*, 129–139. [CrossRef] [PubMed]
73. Youn, J.-C.; Kim, C.; Park, S.; Lee, S.-H.; Kang, S.-M.; Choi, D.; Son, N.H.; Shin, D.-J.; Jang, Y. Adiponectin and Progression of Arterial Stiffness in Hypertensive Patients. *Int. J. Cardiol.* **2013**, *163*, 316–319. [CrossRef]
74. Chen, M.-C.; Lee, C.-J.; Yang, C.-F.; Chen, Y.-C.; Wang, J.-H.; Hsu, B.-G. Low Serum Adiponectin Level Is Associated with Metabolic Syndrome and Is an Independent Marker of Peripheral Arterial Stiffness in Hypertensive Patients. *Diabetol. Metab. Syndr.* **2017**, *9*, 49. [CrossRef] [PubMed]
75. Yamauchi, T.; Nio, Y.; Maki, T.; Kobayashi, M.; Takazawa, T.; Iwabu, M.; Okada-Iwabu, M.; Kawamoto, S.; Kubota, N.; Kubota, T.; et al. Targeted Disruption of AdipoR1 and AdipoR2 Causes Abrogation of Adiponectin Binding and Metabolic Actions. *Nat. Med.* **2007**, *13*, 332–339. [CrossRef]

Disclaimer/Publisher's Note: The statements, opinions and data contained in all publications are solely those of the individual author(s) and contributor(s) and not of MDPI and/or the editor(s). MDPI and/or the editor(s) disclaim responsibility for any injury to people or property resulting from any ideas, methods, instructions or products referred to in the content.

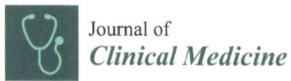

Article

Comparison of Parameters for Assessment of Carotid Stiffness and Their Association with Carotid Atherosclerosis in Rural Australian Adults: A Pilot Study

Marjana Petrova, Alex Gavino, Yujie Li and Craig S. McLachlan *

Centre for Healthy Futures, Torrens University Australia, Sydney, NSW 2010, Australia
* Correspondence: craig.mclachlan@torrens.edu.au

Abstract: Carotid stiffness has been associated with the development and progression of carotid artery disease and is an independent factor for stroke and dementia. There has also been a lack of comparison of different ultrasound-derived carotid stiffness parameters and their association with carotid atherosclerosis. This pilot study aimed to investigate the associations between carotid stiffness parameters (derived via ultrasound echo tracking) and the presence of carotid plaques in Australian rural adults. In cross-sectional analyses, we assessed forty-six subjects (68 ± 9 years; mean ± SD) who underwent carotid ultrasound examinations. Carotid stiffness was assessed by a noninvasive echo-tracking method, measuring and comparing multiple carotid stiffness parameters, including stroke change in diameter (ΔD), stroke change in lumen area (ΔA), β- stiffness index, pulse wave velocity beta (PWV-β), compliance coefficient (CC), distensibility coefficient (DC), Young's elastic modulus (YEM), Peterson elastic modulus (Ep), and strain. Carotid atherosclerosis was assessed bilaterally by the presence of plaques in the common and internal carotid arteries, while carotid stiffness was assessed at the right common carotid artery. β-stiffness index, PWV-β, and Ep were significantly higher ($p = 0.006$, $p = 0.004$, $p = 0.02$, respectively), whilst ΔD, CC, DC, and strain were lower among subjects with carotid plaques ($p = 0.036$, $p = 0.032$, $p = 0.01$, $p = 0.02$, respectively) comparing to subjects without carotid plaques. YEM and ΔA did not significantly differ among the groups. Carotid plaques were associated with age, history of stroke, coronary artery disease, and previous coronary interventions. These results suggest that unilateral carotid stiffness is associated with the presence of carotid plaques.

Keywords: carotid stiffness; carotid plaques; carotid ultrasound; echo-tracking; rural population

1. Introduction

The aging process is associated with an increased risk for vascular stiffness [1,2]. Precise noninvasive methods to measure stiffness in the carotid artery have emerged and can be conducted in clinical settings [3,4]. Several smaller and larger scale studies suggest that individuals with pre-existing cardiovascular diseases (sub-clinical or overt) have increased indices of carotid stiffness compared to individuals without established cardiovascular disease [5–7]. Carotid stiffness has also been suggested to predict cardiovascular events and all-cause mortality [8]. Greater carotid stiffness measured by beta (β) stiffness, Young's elastic modulus, distensibility coefficient, and compliance coefficient has also been associated with the incidence of stroke, independently from other covariates such as age, sex, and recognized common population cardiovascular risk factors [9].

The association between arterial stiffness and localized atherosclerosis may be explained by the natural progression of atherosclerosis or an increase in pulse pressure. In the early stages of atherosclerosis, arterial elasticity and compliance decrease due to the degradation of elastic fibers and increased collagen deposition in the arterial wall. As a result, arterial stiffness increases before any visible changes appear in the vascular wall structure [10]. Moreover, stiffening in the carotid arteries may lead to increased pulse pressure and flow pulsatility, which can induce endothelial dysfunction, a precursor to the development of atherosclerosis [11]. Hence, the noninvasive determination of arterial stiffness may be useful in the evaluation of early-stage carotid disease.

Carotid ultrasound and automated software for wall tracking [3,4] are some of the several imaging modalities that allow accurate measurement of local carotid stiffness, even though the methods and reference values of carotid stiffness parameters have not been standardized to use in routine clinical practice.

While associations between arterial stiffness and atherosclerotic disease have been explored, most studies have examined carotid stiffness on underlying atherosclerotic pathology in the same corresponding carotid site of stiffness. Hence, it remains unknown whether stiffness in one segment of the carotid can be associated with remote carotid plaque burden. Additionally, while rural populations have an increased risk for stroke, the role of arterial stiffness and risk for carotid plaques in those cohorts have been rarely reported [12]. Our study aims to evaluate the association between various carotid stiffness parameters from a wall-tracking software platform and the presence of carotid plaque in both carotid arteries among a community sample from the Ararat rural population.

2. Materials and Methods

2.1. Study Settings

The present sub-study was a cross-sectional analysis of a prospective community study conducted among rural residents of Ararat in Victoria, Australia, aged 35 and older. The participant recruitment and study design details have been described previously [13]. Between March 2022 and July 2022, forty-five subjects completed follow-up health assessments and underwent carotid ultrasound examinations, and one new participant was enrolled in the study. All study subjects included in these analyses were Caucasian and aged between 48 to 81 years.

2.2. Ethical Consideration

All subjects provided written informed consent before completing the health survey and the health assessments. The Ararat Health Study was approved by the Human Research Ethics Committee of Ballarat Health Service and St. John of God Hospital.

2.3. Health Assessments

Health assessments included anthropometric measurements, blood pressure (BP), and 12-lead electrocardiogram (ECG). Mean arterial pressure (MAP) was calculated as 2/3 diastolic blood pressure (DBP) + 1/3 systolic blood pressure (SBP).

2.4. Carotid Artery Ultrasound

In addition to the abovementioned follow-up health assessments, a carotid ultrasound examination was performed for this study. All imaging was performed using the Phillips affinity 70 ultrasound equipment and an eL18-4 ultra-broadband linear transducer with PureWave crystal technology.

Carotid artery images and cine loops were acquired using standardized protocols in accordance with the recommendations of the Manheim statements and recommendations [14].

Carotid ultrasound examinations were performed in a comfortable room with a temperature of 21–22 °C. All subjects were placed in a relaxed supine position with the neck tilted 45° opposite to the scanned side. Bilateral carotid arteries (including the common carotid, carotid bifurcation, and internal carotid arteries) were scanned in transverse and longitudinal sections.

2.5. Intima-Media Thickness and Carotid Stiffness Parameters

First, a clear longitudinal image in B-mode was obtained from the right common carotid artery. Then, 5–10 s (150–301 frames) cine loops were recorded and transferred to an ultrasound database for further offline analyses. Finally, all cine loops were reviewed to select loops that met the critical optimization criteria: precise near and far wall intima-media, clear lumen, a minimum of 3 cardiac cycles, and straight vessel.

Carotid intima-media thickness (IMT), maximum lumen diameter (Ds), and stroke change in diameter (ΔD) were measured at least 5–10 mm below the carotid bifurcation in a region free of carotid plaque using an automatic software platform for ultrasound imaging analyses (CAROLAB v5.0) [15]. Carotid IMT analyzed by CAROLAB was expressed as the mean of the maximum IMT measured in each carotid segment (in 3–6 cardiac cycles).

The following carotid stiffness parameters for subsequently calculated:
Stroke change in the lumen area (ΔA)

$$\Delta A = \pi (Ds^2 - Dd^2)/4 \ (mm^2)$$

β stiffness parameter

$$\beta = \ln (SBP/DBP)/[\Delta D/Dd] \ (unitless)$$

Cross-sectional distensibility coefficient (DC)—relative change in lumen area during systole for a given pressure change

$$DC = 2\Delta D/\Delta PDs \ (Kpa \ 10^{-3})$$

Cross-sectional compliance coefficient (CC)—absolute change in lumen area during systole for a given pressure change

$$CC = (\pi \times Ds \times \Delta D)/(2 \times \Delta P) \ (10^{-7} \ m^2 \ Kpa^{-1})$$

Peterson's elastic modulus (Ep)—the inverse of distensibility coefficient: the pressure change directing an increase in relative lumen area

$$Ep = (SBP - DBP)/[(Ds - Dd)/Dd] \ (Kpa)$$

Young's elastic modulus (YEM)—elasticity of the arterial wall material, considering the thickness of the arterial wall

$$YEM = (\Delta P \times Dd)/(\Delta D \times IMT) \ (mmHg/mm)$$

Strain

$$Strain = \Delta D/Dd \times 100 \ (\%)$$

One-point pulse wave velocity β (PWV-β)—calculated from the time delay between two adjacent distensions waveforms from the water hammer equation with the usage of β-stiffness parameter

$$PWV\text{-}\beta = \sqrt{(\beta \times Pd/2 \times \varrho)} \ (m \ s^{-1}),$$

where Ds = systolic diameter; Dd = diastolic diameter; IMT = intima-media thickness, SBP = systolic blood pressure, DBP = diastolic blood pressure; ΔP = pulse pressure; ϱ- blood density = 1050 kg/m^3

2.6. Carotid Plaque Measurement

The presence of atherosclerotic plaques in the carotid arteries was determined by evaluation of the ultrasound images of the common, internal, and bifurcation sites of the left and right carotid arteries. According to the Manheim consensus [14], plaques were defined as structures encroaching into the arterial lumen of at least 0.5 mm or 50% of the surrounding IMT value or demonstrated a thickness $\geq$ 1.5 mm as measured from the intima-lumen interface to the media-adventitia interface.

2.7. Statistical Analyses

Continuous data were expressed as means and standard deviations or as medians and interquartile ranges. Categorical data were expressed as total counts and percentages. The normality of data was assessed using the Shapiro—Wilk test. We used an independent *t*-test and Mann—Whitney U test to investigate differences among carotid stiffness parameters and risk factors in the groups with and without carotid plaques. Categorical variables were compared by Chi-square test (χ^2 test). The results were considered significant at $p < 0.05$. All data were analyzed using IBM SPSS Statistics version 28.01.

2.8. Reproducibility

Intra-observer reproducibility was assessed by two consecutive offline measurements (at different time points) of IMT, Ds, and ΔD in 15 randomly selected subjects. Intra-observer reproducibility was expressed by calculating the intraclass correlation coefficient (ICC).

3. Results

3.1. Subject Characteristics

Table 1 shows the demographic characteristics of the study subjects. The mean age was 67.91 ± 8.72 years, with 30 (65.2%) subjects falling in the 55–74 years age range. Among the 46 subjects, there were 27 females (58.7%) and 19 males (41.3%).

Table 1. Demographic characteristics of the study subjects.

Demographic Characteristics (n = 46)	Mean ± SD or n (%)
Age (years)	67.91 ± 8.72
35–54	4 (8.7)
55–74	30 (65.2)
>75	12 (26.1)
Gender	
Male	19 (41.3)
Female	27 (58.7)
Smoking	
Current	2 (4.3)
Former	17 (37)
Never smoked	27 (58.7)
Living in Ararat (years)	31.18 ± 17.88
Anthropometric characteristics	
BMI (kg/m^2)	27.4 ± 4.74
Normal	17 (37)
Overweight	20 (43.5)
Obese	9 (19.6)
Height (cm)	167.50 ± 8.58
Weight (kg)	77.08 ± 15.50
Waist circumference (cm)	
Male	96.84 ± 11.43

Table 1. Cont.

Demographic Characteristics (n = 46)	Mean ± SD or n (%)
Females	89.56 ± 12.4
Self-reported medical conditions	
Hypertension	19 (41.3)
Antihypertensive medications	15 (32.6)
Dyslipidemia	24 (52.2)
Antilipid medications (statins)	9 (19.6)
Diabetes type 2	4 (8.7)
Cardiovascular disease	7 (15.2)
Hemodynamic parameters	
SBP (mmHg)	130.13 ± 13.23
DBP (mmHg)	75.91 ± 9.21
MAP (mmHg)	93.99 ± 9.36
PP (mmHg)	54.21 ± 11.32
Resting HR (beats per min, bpm)	64.48 ± 10.60
QRS duration (ms)	102.02 ± 22.59
Carotid ultrasound parameters	
IMT (mm)	0.75 ± 0.16
Carotid plaques	15 (32.6)
Carotid plaques, unilateral (Left CCA and ICA)	4 (26.6)
Carotid plaques, unilateral (Right CCA and ICA)	3 (20)
Carotid plaques (bilateral)	8 (53.3)

CCA—common carotid artery; ICA—internal carotid artery; SBP = systolic blood pressure; DBP = diastolic blood pressure; MAP = mean arterial pressure; PP = pulse pressure

3.2. Carotid Stiffness Parameters in Subjects with and without Plaque

Patients were divided into two groups depending on the presence of plaque. Plaques were present on either left or right common and internal carotid arteries. Fifteen subjects had a carotid plaque in at least one carotid bed—eight had bilateral carotid plaques, four had plaques on the left, and three had plaques on the right (Table 1). One subject was excluded from the comparative analyses, as we were unable to perform an estimation of the stiffness parameters due to the low quality of the ultrasound cine loops. We evaluated the difference in mean or median (sd or IQR) in the following markers of carotid stiffness—ΔD (mm), ΔA (mm^2), β, PWV-β (m/s^{-1}), CC (10^{-7} m^2 Kpa^{-1}), DC (10^{-3} Kpa), YEM (mmHg/mm), Ep (Kpa), Strain (%)—as well as the systolic and diastolic carotid diameter and the IMT. Results are presented in Table 2.

In subjects with no carotid plaques, the stroke change in diameter (ΔD), distensibility coefficient (DC), and strain (%) were significantly higher compared to the group with atherosclerotic plaques, i.e., ΔD ($p < 0.036$); DC ($p = 0.01$); Strain ($p = 0.02$). The following stiffness parameters—β-index, PWV-β, and Peterson Elastic Modulus (Ep)—were significantly lower in subjects without plaque compared to subjects with atherosclerotic plaques, as follows: β ($p = 0.006$); PWV-β ($p = 0.04$); Ep ($p = 0.02$). We also found that IMT was significantly higher among subjects with carotid plaques ($p = 0.01$). In contrast, YEM did not significantly differ among the groups. Mean systolic (Ds) and diastolic (Dd) carotid diameters were higher in the plaque group; however, these differences were not statistically significant.

Table 2. Carotid stiffness parameters in subjects with or without carotid plaque.

	Plaques, No (n = 31)	Plaques, Yes (n = 14)	
	Mean ± SD	Mean ± SD	p-Value
Ds (mm)	5.93 ± 0.54	6.01 ± 0.57	0.63
Dd (mm)	5.44 ± 0.52	5.59 ± 0.53	0.41
ΔD (mm)	0.48 ± 0.91	0.41 ± 0.08	0.036 *
ΔA (mm^2)	4.33 ± 1.00	3.86 ± 1.47	0.16
β stiffness	6.09 ± 1.53	7.73 ± 2.15	0.006 *
PWV β (m/s^{-1})	5.36 ± 0.59	5.99 ± 0.71	0.004 *
CC (mm^2 Kpa^{-1})	6.59 ± 1.58	5.76 ± 7.97	0.032 *
DC (10^{-3} Kpa)	23.80 ± 7.91	19.94 ± 0.94	0.01 *
YEM (mmHg/mm)	883.97 ± 284.51	963.49 ± 333.31	0.53
Ep (Kpa)	(613.97, 155.24) **	(749.01, 239.39) **	0.02 *
Strain, %	8.82 ± 1.84	7.56 ± 1.49	0.02 *
IMT (mm)	0.71 ± 0.13	0.84 ± 0.19	0.01 *

Legend: Ds = systolic diameter; Dd = diastolic diameter; ΔD = stroke change in diameter; ΔA = stroke change in lumen area; CC = compliance coefficient; DC = distensibility coefficient; YEM = Young's elastic modulus; Ep = Peterson's Elastic modulus, * $p < 0.05$, ** median (IQR).

3.3. Carotid Plaque and Traditional Risk Factors

Subjects in the carotid plaque group were significantly older compared to the group without carotid plaque ($p < 0.01$). Both groups were comparable in gender, SBP, DBP, PP, BMI, waist circumference, hypertension, and lipid status. In subjects with carotid plaque, the percentage of stroke, myocardial infarction (MI), and coronary intervention were higher compared to the group without plaque ($p = 0.01$, $p = 0.03$, and $p = 0.003$, respectively). Detailed characteristics of cardiovascular risk factors are presented in Table 3.

Table 3. Cardiovascular risk factors among subjects with and without carotid plaque.

	Plaques, No (n = 31)	Plaques, Yes (n = 15)	
	Mean ± SD or n (%)	Mean ± SD or n (%)	p-Value
Age	65.71 ± 8.69	72.47 ± 7.029	0.01 *
Sex, males	9 (32.3)	10 (60.0)	0.73
SBP	130.84 ± 13.16	133.93 ± 15.87	0.5
DBP	80.23 ± 8.40	77.27 ± 7.06	0.12
PP	50.71 ± 11.93	56.67 ± 12.34	0.12
MAP	96.16 ± 8.50	96.20 ± 8.98	0.9
BMI	27.55 ± 5.23	27.08 ± 3.66	0.75
Waist circumference	91.90 ± 13.48	93.93 ± 10.13	0.61
Self-reported conditions			
Hypertension	9 (29.0)	6 (40.0)	0.45
Dyslipidemia	15 (62.5)	9 (37.5)	0.46
Diabetes	2 (6.5)	2 (13.3)	0.43
Stroke	0 (0)	3 (27.9)	0.01 *
Myocardial infarction	0 (0)	2 (13.3)	0.03 *
Coronary intervention	0 (0)	4 (26.7)	0.003 *

* $p < 0.05$; SBP = systolic blood pressure; DBP = diastolic blood pressure; MAP = mean arterial pressure; PP = pulse pressure

3.4. Intra-Observer Reproducibility

Intra-observer reliability was excellent for IMT (Reading 1 (0.82 ± 0.19, mean ± SD); Reading 2 (0.88 ± 1.19, mean ± SD); ICC = 0.94); good for Ds (Reading 1 (6.25 ± 0.58, mean ± SD); Reading 2 (6.68 ± 0.82), ICC = 0.78); and good for ΔD (Reading 1 (0.52 ± 0.11, mean ± SD); Reading 2 (0.55 ± 0.14., mean ± SD), ICC = 0.76).

4. Discussion

Our study demonstrates, for the first time, an ability to comprehensively compare carotid ultrasound parameters using various validated formulae of stiffness and their association with the presence of carotid plaques. Stiffness parameters that we included were absolute distensibility (ΔD), stroke change in absolute diameter (ΔA), cross-sectional compliance coefficient (CC), distensibility coefficient (DC), β stiffness index, βPWV, Peterson elastic modulus (Ep), and strain. Of these stiffness parameters, we found β, PWV-β, and Ep were significantly higher, whilst absolute distensibility, distensibility coefficient, and strain were lower among subjects with carotid plaques. These results are consistent with individual studies examining carotid distensibility, compliance, and stiffness indices in atherosclerotic patients [16–18]. Studies show that carotid distensibility is significantly associated with the presence and severity of atherosclerosis [19,20]. The carotid distensibility coefficient and Young's elastic modulus were related to symptomatic carotid disease [21,22], and these correlate with the degree of atherosclerosis [23]. Giannattasio et al. [16] found that arterial distensibility was markedly lower in the stenotic internal carotid artery compared to the plaque-free contralateral internal carotid artery. However, it was also found to be lower in the ipsilateral common carotid artery, indicating the effect of stiffness beyond the actual plaque site. It is essential to highlight that in our study, we measured the stiffness in the right common carotid artery; however, the presence of plaque was determined across both the left and right common and internal carotid arteries.

The presence of atherosclerotic plaques has been associated with arterial stiffness in studies investigating different vascular beds. For example, atherosclerotic plaques in the aorta were associated with decreased aortic distensibility [24]. The augmentation index of the aorta was also found to be significantly associated with peripheral artery disease [25].

A few possibilities for the determined association between carotid stiffness and carotid atherosclerosis can be hypothesized. One possibility is that the atherosclerotic process leads to an increase in arterial stiffness by triggering hemodynamic changes and vascular cell dysfunction, promoting atherosclerosis [26]. An alternative possibility is that the increased arterial stiffness precedes the damage of the vascular wall and then causes atherosclerosis. Without the buffering capacity, stiff arterial walls may be exposed to increased intraluminal stress related to increased pulse pressure [27]. A third possibility is that both mechanisms are valid. Atherosclerosis may be a result of increased stiffness, but then it may further increase arterial stiffness in advanced stages. Finally, another possibility is that these processes may be independently processed but may happen simultaneously in the arterial wall without a specific temporal or causational relationship.

Despite the availability of accurate imaging modalities for evaluating carotid stiffness, there are no current standardized methods and parameters for evaluating carotid stiffness, and their application in clinical practice is limited [28].

In our study, the presence of carotid plaques was associated with older age and a history of previous stroke, myocardial infarction, and previous coronary interventions. Age is a common risk factor for atherosclerotic disease, and a close relationship between coronary and carotid atherosclerosis has been examined in symptomatic and asymptomatic patients [29,30]. Johnses et al. [31] reported that carotid plaque is a strong risk factor and predictor of myocardial infarction, while Novo et al. [32] reported a high presence of asymptomatic plaques in patients with three-vessel disease. Such evidence, along with our study findings, aligns with the hypothesis that atherosclerosis is a systemic disease and is often not limited to one single vascular bed.

To the best of our knowledge, our study is the first to simultaneously investigate multiple carotid stiffness ultrasound parameters published in the literature and their associations with carotid atherosclerosis.

Populations living in rural areas have an increased burden of carotid plaque coronary artery disease and cardiovascular risk factors compared to urban populations [33,34]. However, there is a paucity of data to estimate the global burden of carotid atherosclerosis among rural populations [21]. Increased intima-media thickness and carotid plaques are well-established parameters for diagnosing subclinical and clinical carotid artery disease; however, screening in the general population is still under debate [35,36]. Other ultrasound imaging modalities, such as the assessment of carotid plaque burden using 3D ultrasound imaging, have been useful for the assessment of carotid plaque burden, progression, risk stratification, and evaluation of new risk factors [37]. However, despite the significant prognostic implications and high accuracy, 3D modality remains a niche area, mainly due to the high cost of the probes and the need for specialized vascular laboratories.

While we can hypothesize that carotid stiffness may be associated with plaque risk in the other vascular territory, such as the right common carotid, we, however, could not measure stiffness in the contralateral or other vascular beds. Hence, we can say that when we find stiffness in one carotid artery with non-plaque deposits, it is possible to observe plaques in the opposite carotid artery. This may be explained by remote signaling, or in fact, the other bed may also be stiff; if the latter is the case, we currently do not have a plausible explanation. Finally, as our study was cross-sectional by design, causality cannot be inferred.

Our study has a few perceived limitations that warrant discussion. Firstly, our study has a moderate number of participants. On the other hand, this study was pre-planned as a pilot study to assess methodological assessment on the basis of which stiffness parameter is best associated with carotid plaque burden. Thus, the study had a sufficient sample size to explore these associations. The second perceived limitation is that this study focused on plaque burden and not stenosis. The study was not pre-designed to consider variances in carotid artery stenosis, apart from high-grade stenosis. Indeed, increased aortic stiffness has been associated with the presence of higher-grade carotid stenosis > 50% [38]. It should be noted that none of our participants had high-grade carotid stenosis.

Our study shows that carotid distensibility and stiffness indices are associated with the presence of carotid atherosclerosis. Future studies with more standardized methods of measurement and validation of carotid stiffness may contribute to greater clinical implementation of ultrasound imaging parameters into clinical practice and assessment of early carotid atherosclerosis. The assessment of carotid stiffness was dependent on the type of ultrasound parameter used to reliably reflect sub-clinical carotid atherosclerosis.

Author Contributions: Conceptualization: M.P. and C.S.M.; Data curation: M.P. and Y.L.; Formal analysis: M.P. and Y.L.; Investigation: M.P.; Methodology: M.P. and A.G.; Project administration: M.P. and A.G.; Supervision: C.S.M.; Roles/Writing—original draft: M.P and C.S.M.; Writing—review and editing: M.P., A.G. and C.S.M. All authors have read and agreed to the published version of the manuscript.

Funding: This research received no external funding.

Institutional Review Board Statement: The study was conducted in accordance with the Declaration of Helsinki, and approved by the Ballarat Health Services and St John of God Healthcare Human Research Ethics Committee. Approval number HREC/15/BHSSJOG/97 from 10 November 2015. Review Reference AM/29700/BHSSJOG-2021-249013(v3) from 23 February 2021.

Informed Consent Statement: Informed consent was obtained from all subjects involved in the study.

Data Availability Statement: Sharing of data is unavailable due to privacy or ethical restrictions.

Acknowledgments: This research was supported by the East Grampians Health Service, Ararat, Victoria, Australia.

Conflicts of Interest: The authors declare no conflict of interest.

References

1. Mitchell, G.F. Arterial Stiffness in Aging: Does It Have a Place in Clinical Practice? *Hypertension* **2021**, *77*, 768–780. [CrossRef] [PubMed]
2. Mikael, L.D.R.; de Paiva, A.M.G.; Gomes, M.M.; Sousa, A.L.L.; Jardim, P.C.B.V.; Vitorino, P.V.D.O.; Euzebio, M.B.; de Moura Sousa, W.; Barroso, W.K.S. Vascular Aging and Arterial Stiffness. *Arq. Bras. Cardiol.* **2017**, *109*, 253–258. [CrossRef] [PubMed]
3. Pewowaruk, R.J.; Korcarz, C.; Tedla, Y.; Burke, G.; Greenland, P.; Wu, C.; Gepner, A.D. Carotid Artery Stiffness Mechanisms Associated With Cardiovascular Disease Events and Incident Hypertension: The Multi-Ethnic Study of Atherosclerosis (MESA). *Hypertension* **2022**, *79*, 659–666. [CrossRef] [PubMed]
4. Gu, W.; Wu, J.; Pei, Y.; Ji, J.; Wu, H.; Wu, J. Evaluation of Common Carotid Stiffness via Echo Tracking in Hypertensive Patients Complicated by Acute Aortic Dissection. *J. Ultrasound Med.* **2021**, *40*, 929–936. [CrossRef] [PubMed]
5. Irie, Y.; Sakamoto, K.; Kubo, F.; Okusu, T.; Katura, T.; Yamamoto, Y.; Umayahara, Y.; Katakami, N.; Kaneto, H.; Kashiyama, T.; et al. Association of coronary artery stenosis with carotid atherosclerosis in asymptomatic type 2 diabetic patients. *J. Atheroscler. Thromb.* **2011**, *18*, 337–344. [CrossRef]
6. Kablak-Ziembicka, A.; Przewlocki, T.; Tracz, W.; Pieniazek, P.; Musialek, P.; Sokolowski, A. Gender Differences in Carotid Intima-Media Thickness in Patients With Suspected Coronary Artery Disease. *Am. J. Cardiol.* **2005**, *96*, 1217–1222. [CrossRef]
7. Lee, E.; Emoto, M.; Teramura, M.; Tsuchikura, S.; Ueno, H.; Shinohara, K.; Morioka, T.; Mori, K.; Koyama, H.; Shoji, T.; et al. The combination of IMT and stiffness parameter beta is highly associated with concurrent coronary artery disease in type 2 diabetes. *J. Atheroscler. Thromb.* **2009**, *16*, 33–39. [CrossRef]
8. Vlachopoulos, C.; Aznaouridis, K.; Stefanadis, C. Prediction of Cardiovascular Events and All-Cause Mortality With Arterial Stiffness: A Systematic Review and Meta-Analysis. *J. Am. Coll. Cardiol.* **2010**, *55*, 1318–1327. [CrossRef]
9. Van Sloten, T.T.; Sedaghat, S.; Laurent, S.; London, G.M.; Pannier, B.; Ikram, M.A.; Kavousi, M.; Mattace-Raso, F.; Franco, O.H.; Boutouyrie, P.; et al. Carotid Stiffness Is Associated with Incident Stroke A Systematic Review and Individual Participant Data Meta-Analysis. *J. Am. Coll. Cardiol.* **2015**, *66*, 2116–2125. [CrossRef]
10. Bonetti, P.O.; Lerman, L.O.; Lerman, A. Endothelial dysfunction: A marker of atherosclerotic risk. *Arterioscl. Thromb. Vasc. Biol.* **2003**, *23*, 168–175.
11. Steppan, J.; Barodka, V.; Berkowitz, D.E.; Nyhan, D. Vascular Stiffness and Increased Pulse Pressure in the Aging Cardiovascular System. *Cardiol. Res. Pract.* **2011**, *2011*, 263585. [CrossRef] [PubMed]
12. Petrova, M.; Kiat, H.; Gavino, A.; McLachlan, C.S. Carotid ultrasound screening programs in rural communities: A systematic review. *J. Pers. Med.* **2021**, *11*, 897. [CrossRef] [PubMed]
13. Gavino, A.I. Studies on Atrial Fibrillation and Associated Risk Factors in a Rural Australian Population. Ph.D. Thesis, UNSW Sydney, Kensington, Australia, 2019; p. 237.
14. Touboul, P.J.; Hennerici, M.G.; Meairs, S.; Adams, H.; Amarenco, P.; Bornstein, N.; Csiba, L.; Desvarieux, M.; Ebrahim, S.; Hernandez Hernandez, R.; et al. Mannheim Carotid Intima-Media Thickness and Plaque Consensus (2004–2006–2011): An Update on Behalf of the Advisory Board of the 3rd and 4th Watching the Risk Symposium 13th and 15th European Stroke Conferences, Mannheim, Germany, 2004, and Brussels, Belgium, 2006. *Cerebrovasc. Dis.* **2012**, *34*, 290–296. [PubMed]
15. Zahnd, G.; Orkisz, M.; Serrano, E.E.; Vray, D. CAROLAB—A platform to analyze carotid ultrasound data. In *IEEE Ultrasonics Symposium*; IEEE: Glasgow, Scotland, 2019.
16. Giannattasio, C.; Failla, M.; Emanuelli, G.; Grappiolo, A.; Boffi, L.; Corsi, D.; Manica, G. Local Effects of Atherosclerotic Plaque on Arterial Distensibility. *Hypertension* **2001**, *38*, 1177–1180. [CrossRef]
17. Boesen, M.E.; Singh, D.; Menon, B.K.; Frayne, R. A systematic literature review of the effect of carotid atherosclerosis on local vessel stiffness and elasticity. *Atherosclerosis* **2015**, *243*, 211–222. [CrossRef]
18. Santelices, L.C.; Rutman, S.J.; Prantil-Baun, R.; Vorp, D.A.; Aheam, J.M. Relative Contributions of Age and Atherosclerosis to Vascular Stiffness. *Clin. Transl. Sci.* **2008**, *1*, 62–66. [CrossRef]
19. Lind, L.; Andersson, J.; Hansen, T.; Johansson, L.; Ahlström, H. Atherosclerosis measured by whole body magnetic resonance angiography and carotid artery ultrasound is related to arterial compliance, but not to endothelium-dependent vasodilation—The Prospective Investigation of the Vasculature in Uppsala Seniors (PIVUS) study. *Clin. Physiol. Funct. Imaging* **2009**, *29*, 321–329.
20. Imanaga, I.; Hara, H.; Koyanagi, S.; Tanaka, K. Correlation between Wave Components of the Second Derivative of Plethysmogram and Arterial Distensibility. *Jpn. Heart J.* **1998**, *39*, 775–784. [CrossRef]
21. Huang, X.Z.; Wang, Z.Y.; Dai, X.H.; Yun-Zhang Zhang, M. Velocity Vector Imaging of Longitudinal Mechanical Properties of Upstream and Downstream Shoulders and Fibrous Cap Tops of Human Carotid Atherosclerotic Plaque. *Echocardiography* **2013**, *30*, 211–218. [CrossRef]
22. Sadat, U.; Usman, A.; Howarth, S.P.S.; Tang, T.Y.; Alam, F.; Graves, M.J.; Gillard, J.H. Carotid artery stiffness in patients with symptomatic carotid artery disease with contralateral asymptomatic carotid artery disease and in patients with bilateral asymptomatic carotid artery disease: A cine phase-contrast carotid MR study. *J. Stroke Cerebrovasc. Dis.* **2014**, *23*, 743–748. [CrossRef]
23. Beaussier, H.; Naggara, O.; Calvet, D.; Joannides, R.; Guegan-Massardier, E.; Gerardin, E.; Iacob, M.; Laloux, B.; Bozec, E.; Bellien, J.; et al. Mechanical and structural characteristics of carotid plaques by combined analysis with echotracking system and MR imaging. *JACC Cardiovasc. Imaging* **2011**, *4*, 468–477. [CrossRef] [PubMed]

24. Siegel, E.; Thai, W.E.; Techasith, T.; Major, G.; Szymonifka, J.; Tawakol, A.; Nagurney, J.T.; Hoffman, U.; Truong, Q.A. Aortic distensibility and its relationship to coronary and thoracic atherosclerosis plaque and morphology by MDCT: Insights from the ROMICAT Trial. *Int. J. Cardiol.* **2014**, *167*, 1616–1621. [CrossRef] [PubMed]
25. Zahner, G.J.; Gruendl, M.A.; Spaulding, K.A.; Schaller, M.S.; Hills, N.K.; Gasper, W.J.; Grenon, S.M. Association between arterial stiffness and peripheral artery disease as measured by radial artery tonometry. *J. Vasc. Surg.* **2017**, *66*, 1518–1526. [CrossRef] [PubMed]
26. Palombo, C.; Kozakova, M. Arterial stiffness, atherosclerosis and cardiovascular risk: Pathophysiologic mechanisms and emerging clinical indications. *Vasc. Pharmacol.* **2016**, *77*, 1–7. [CrossRef]
27. Jankowski, P.; Czarnecka, D. Pulse Pressure, Blood Flow, and Atherosclerosis. *Am. J. Hypertens.* **2012**, *25*, 1040–1041. [CrossRef]
28. Baradaran, H.; Gupta, A. Carotid Artery Stiffness: Imaging Techniques and Impact on Cerebrovascular Disease. *Front. Cardiovasc. Med.* **2022**, *9*, 852173. [CrossRef]
29. Sirimarco, G.; Amarenco, P.; Labreuche, J.; Touboul, P.J.; Alberts, M.; Goto, S.; Rother, J.; Mas, J.-L.; Bhatt, D.L.; Steg, P.G. REACH Registry Investigators Carotid atherosclerosis and risk of subsequent coronary event in outpatients with atherothrombosis. *Stroke* **2013**, *44*, 373–379. [CrossRef]
30. Seo, W.K.; Yong, H.S.; Koh, S.B.; Suh, S.I.; Kim, J.H.; Yu, S.W.; Lee, J.-Y. Correlation of coronary artery atherosclerosis with atherosclerosis of the intracranial cerebral artery and the extracranial carotid artery. *Eur. Neurol.* **2008**, *59*, 292–298. [CrossRef]
31. Johnsen, S.H.; Mathiesen, E.B.; Joakimsen, O.; Stensland, E.; Wilsgaard, T.; Løchen, M.L.; Njølstad, I.; Arnesen, E. Carotid Atherosclerosis Is a Stronger Predictor of Myocardial Infarction in Women Than in Men. *Stroke* **2007**, *38*, 2873–2880. [CrossRef]
32. Novo, S.; Corrado, E.; Novo, G.; Dell'Oglio, S. Association of carotid atherosclerosis with coronary artery disease: Comparison between carotid ultrasonography and coronary angiography in patients with chest pain. *G. Ital. Cardiol.* **2012**, *13*, 118–123.
33. Alston, L.; Allender, S.; Peterson, K.; Jacobs, J.; Nichols, M. Rural Inequalities in the Australian Burden of Ischaemic Heart Disease: A Systematic Review. *Heart Lung Circ.* **2017**, *26*, 122–133. [CrossRef] [PubMed]
34. Kapral, M.K.; Austin, P.C.; Jeyakumar, G.; Hall, R.; Chu, A.; Khan, A.M.; Jin, A.Y.; Matin, C.; Manuel, D.; Silver, F.L.; et al. Rural-Urban Differences In Stroke Risk Factors, Incidence, And Mortality In People With And Without Prior Stroke. *Circ. Cardiovasc. Qual. Outcomes* **2019**, *12*, e004973. [CrossRef] [PubMed]
35. Urbina, E.M.; Williams, R.V.; Alpert, B.S.; Collins, R.T.; Daniels, S.R.; Hayman, L.; Jacobson, M.; Mahoney, L.; Mietus-Snyder, M.; Rocchini, A.; et al. Noninvasive assessment of subclinical atherosclerosis in children and adolescents: Recommendations for standard assessment for clinical research: A scientific statement from the American Heart Association. *Hypertension* **2009**, *54*, 919–950. [CrossRef] [PubMed]
36. Song, P.; Fang, Z.; Wang, H.; Cai, Y.; Rahimi, K.; Zhu, Y.; Fowkes, F.G.R.; Fowkes, F.J.I.; Rudan, I. Global and regional prevalence, burden, and risk factors for carotid atherosclerosis: A systematic review, meta-analysis, and modelling study. *Lancet Glob. Health* **2020**, *8*, e721–e729. [CrossRef]
37. López-Melgar, B.; Varona, J.F.; Ortiz-Regalón, R.; Sánchez-Vera, I.; Díaz, B.; Castellano, J.M.; Parra Jiménez, F.J.; Fer-nández-Friera, L. Carotid Plaque Burden by 3-Dimensional Vascular Ultrasound as a Risk Marker for Patients with Met-abolic Syndrome. *J. Cardiovasc. Transl. Res.* **2021**, *14*, 1030–1039. [CrossRef]
38. Kadoglou, N.P.E.; Moulakakis, K.G.; Mantas, G.; Kakisis, J.D.; Mylonas, S.N.; Valsami, G.; Liapis, C.D. The As-sociation of Arterial Stiffness With Significant Carotid Atherosclerosis and Carotid Plaque Vulnerability. *Angiology* **2022**, *73*, 668–674. [CrossRef]

Disclaimer/Publisher's Note: The statements, opinions and data contained in all publications are solely those of the individual author(s) and contributor(s) and not of MDPI and/or the editor(s). MDPI and/or the editor(s) disclaim responsibility for any injury to people or property resulting from any ideas, methods, instructions or products referred to in the content.

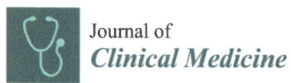

Article

Cardio-Ankle Vascular Index and Aging: Differences between CAVI and CAVI0

Anna Giani [1], Rocco Micciolo [2], Elena Zoico [3], Gloria Mazzali [3], Mauro Zamboni [1] and Francesco Fantin [3,*]

[1] Section of Geriatric Medicine, Department of Surgery, Dentistry, Pediatric and Gynecology, University of Verona, 37100 Verona, Italy; anna.giani@univr.it (A.G.); mauro.zamboni@univr.it (M.Z.)
[2] Centre for Medical Sciences and Department of Psychology and Cognitive Sciences, University of Trento, 38123 Trento, Italy; rocco.micciolo@unitn.it
[3] Section of Geriatric Medicine, Department of Medicine, University of Verona, 37100 Verona, Italy; elena.zoico@univr.it (E.Z.); gloria.mazzali@univr.it (G.M.)
* Correspondence: francesco.fantin@univr.it; Tel.: +39-045-8122537; Fax: +39-045-8122043

Abstract: Background: Cardio-ankle vascular index (CAVI) and CAVI0 (a mathematical expression derived from CAVI, supposed to be less dependent on blood pressure), can describe arterial stiffness, considering a wide proportion of the arterial tree. The aim of this study was to examine the relationship between CAVI, CAVI0 and aging, looking at the differences between the two arterial stiffness indexes. Methods: A total of 191 patients (68 male, mean age 68.3 ± 14.4 years) referred to the Geriatric Ward and Outpatient Clinic at Verona University Hospital were included and underwent a comprehensive clinical evaluation. CAVI and CAVI0 were obtained for each. Results: CAVI0 steeply rises in the elderly age strata, widening the gap between CAVI and CAVI0. An inverse relationship is evident between CAVI0 and DBP in older patients, and CAVI0 is shown to be dependent on age, DBP and age-DBP interaction ($R^2 = 0.508$). Age modifies the effect of DBP on CAVI0, but not on CAVI. Conclusions: The real new findings of our study are that the association between CAVI0 and diastolic blood pressure (DBP) is modified by age, whereas the association between CAVI and DBP is not modified by age. From a clinical point of view, these are very important findings, as DBP decreases with aging, affecting in elderly populations the reliability of CAVI0, which strictly depends on DBP in the formula to calculate it. To monitor the effect of CV therapies, progression of CV diseases and to evaluate clinical outcomes in elderly populations, we suggest using CAVI and not CAVI0.

Keywords: arterial stiffness; arterial aging; CAVI; CAVI0; older adults

1. Introduction

Arterial wall stiffness plays a key role in the pathophysiological mechanism of vascular aging [1] and its evaluation is of paramount importance to characterize the cardiovascular risk [2]. Several parameters have recently been described, yet less is known about which of them are more appropriate in the geriatric settings. In addition to the well-known tonometric pulse wave velocity (PWV), which is also considered the gold standard under the latest European guidelines [3], the cardio-ankle vascular index (CAVI) can provide an interesting description of arterial stiffness, aimed to include the whole arterial tree and to reduce the dependence on blood pressure [4]. First described by Shirai and colleagues [4], CAVI adjusts the PWV (calculated from aortic valve orifice to the ankle) considering both arterial wall compliance and elastic properties, and blood viscosity, providing a global evaluation of stiffness, from the aorta to the tibial arteries. Later in 2016, Spronck and colleagues suggested a new formula [5] to define CAVI0, in order to reduce the dependence of CAVI on arterial blood pressure (BP) at the time of measuring, introducing a reference pressure of 100 mmHg. Consolidated knowledge demonstrated the association between CAVI and CAVI0 [6,7]; nevertheless, the choice of CAVI instead of CAVI0 has been widely debated [5,8,9], and the real independence of CAVI0 from BP is yet to be clearly demonstrated [6,7,10,11]. Thus, there is a fair uncertainty regarding CAVI0, which might not be accurate in any subsets, and its suitability in older adults should be further examined.

What is acknowledged is that older adults display increased arterial stiffness, and accordingly, CAVI and CAVI0 are shown to be increased [6,8]. As a matter of fact, CAVI increases with age; the increasing trend is quite controversial: a 0.5 increase in CAVI every 10 years has been described [12], but other studies outlined a differential increase in different age strata, due to a nonlinear relation [13]. So far, less is known about CAVI0.

It should be noted that several cardiovascular disorders and risk factors, broadly common in older age, are known to be associated with higher CAVI: namely arterial hypertension [14,15], diabetes [12], dyslipidemia [16], coronary artery disease [17] and carotid artery plaques [18].

The aim of the present study was to compare CAVI and CAVI0 in a wide population of adults, to examine the relationship between CAVI, CAVI0 and aging, looking at the differences between the two arterial stiffness indexes.

2. Materials and Methods

A total of 191 subjects (119 female and 64 male), mean age 67.5 ± 14.3 years, hospitalized at the Geriatric Clinic of Verona University Hospital or referred to the outpatient clinic (medical nutrition or arterial hypertension) formed the study population. Exclusion criteria were: (I) limb amputation or history of surgical treatment of the aorta or carotid or femoral arteries; (II) severe peripheral arterial disease or proximal arterial stenosis; (III) atrial fibrillation or other major arrhythmias. A comprehensive clinical evaluation was performed, including clinical history collection.

The study was approved by the Ethical Committee of the University of Verona. All participants gave informed consent to be involved in the research study.

2.1. Anthropometric Variables

Body weight (Salus scale, Milan, Italy) and height were recorded (Salus stadiometer, Milan, Italy), with the subject barefoot and wearing light indoor clothing. Whenever patients could not assume the erect position, the last anamnestic height was recoded. BMI was calculated as body weight adjusted by stature (kg/m^2).

2.2. Biochemical Analyses

All patients received venous blood sampling, after overnight fasting. Plasma glucose was measured with a glucose analyzer (Roche Cobas 8000, Monza, Italy). Cholesterol and triacylglycerol concentrations were determined with spectrophotometric method (Roche Cobas 8000, Monza, Italy). High-density-lipoprotein (HDL) cholesterol was measured by using the method of Warnick and Albers. LDL cholesterol was calculated using the Friedwald formula. Creatinine was measured by a modular analyzer (Roche Cobas 8000, Monza, Italy).

2.3. Blood Pressure and Arterial Stiffness Measurements

As we previously described [19], VaSera-1500 (Fukuda-Denshi Company, Ltd., Tokyo, Japan) was used to obtain CAVI, blood pressure and heart rate; the same device provides mean arterial pressure (MAP) and pulse pressure (PP). BP cuffs were placed simultaneously on the four limbs and inflated two by two (right and left side) to increase the accuracy of measurements. ECG was obtained by two electrodes placed on both arms; to obtain phonocardiography, a microphone was placed on the sternum (second rib space). CAVI derives from the Bramwell-Hill Formula [20,21], which is based on heart-ankle PWV, obtained by the following equation:

$$\text{CAVI} = a * \left(\ln \frac{\text{SBP}}{\text{DBP}} * \frac{\text{PWV}^2 * 2\rho}{\text{SBP} - \text{DBP}} \right) + b \qquad (1)$$

where a and b are constants, and ρ is considered the blood density. The device can directly provide heart-ankle PWV (haPWV) as the ratio between aortic valve to ankle length and the time T, where T stands for tb + tba, taken by pulse wave to run this distance (tb: time from the second heart sound to the dicrotic notch at the brachial pulse wave form, tba: time from brachial to ankle pulse waves) [22]. A brachial-ankle PWV (baPWV) can be eventually derived [23]. CAVI0 was derived by proper electronic calculator [24] following the formula

$$CAVI0 = \frac{CAVI - b}{a} * \frac{\frac{SBP}{DBP} - 1}{\ln\left(\frac{SBP}{DBP}\right)} - \ln\left(\frac{SBP}{P_{ref}}\right) \quad (2)$$

and considering P_{ref} as a standard pressure of 100 mmHg.

2.4. Statistical Analyses

The results are shown as mean value ± standard deviation (SD). Pearson correlation coefficient was used to estimate associations between variables. Linear multiple regression analysis was employed to evaluate the effect of age and DBP on CAVI and CAVI0, taking into account the effect of other selected variables (SBP, sex and BMI). Analysis of variance (ANOVA) was performed to evaluate the effect of independent variables included in regression models. Among the considered variables, CAVI0, CAVI, height and SBP showed a normal quantile plot giving some evidence for a difference from the normal distribution. However, the same result was found when logarithmic, square root and reciprocal transformations were employed. Furthermore, computer simulations showed that sample means based on samples of about 100 observations (like those presented in this study) can be considered normally distributed. However, when comparing mean values from two samples of subjects, in addition to the standard Student's *t* test for unpaired data, the non-parametric Mann-Whitney U test was employed.

A significance threshold level of 0.05 was used throughout the study. All statistical analyses were performed using R (version 4.2.2, R Core Team (2022)), a language and environment for statistical computing (R Foundation for Statistical Computing, Vienna, Austria; https://www.R-project.org/).

Residuals of regression analyses were visually checked for normality employing a normal quantile plot. Although the tails of the distribution points did not lie close to a straight line, the pattern was symmetric. The significance of the results was also checked employing a distribution free permutation test for regression models implemented in the R package "lmPerm" (Wheeler, B.; Torchiano, M. lmPerm: Permutation Tests for Linear Models; R package version 2.1.0, 2016; https://CRAN.R-project.org/package=lmPerm (accessed on 18 October 2023)).

3. Results

Data were considered for a total of 191 patients (68, 35.6%, male). Their ages ranged between 40 and 96 years (mean age 68.3 ± 14.4 years; median age 69 years). DBP ranged between 55 and 109 mmHg (mean DBP 81.2 ± 10.7 mmHg; median DBP 81 mmHg). The main characteristics of the population, subdivided using an age threshold of 70 years (100 subjects < 70 years, 91 subjects ≥ 70 years), are listed in Table 1. All the mean values (except height, SBP, glucose levels and tryglicerides) of these two samples showed highly significant differences both when the Student's *t*-test for unpaired data and the non-parametric Mann-Whitney U test were employed.

As compared to the younger subgroup, older patients (≥70 years) had significantly lower DBP (mean 76.51 ± 10.21 mmHg vs. 85.4 ± 9.35 mmHg $p < 0.001$) and MAP (97.2 ± 13.71 mmHg vs. 105.4 ± 10.64 mmHg, $p < 0.001$). Higher CAVI (10.25 ± 2.15 vs. 7.78 ± 1.21, $p < 0.001$) and CAVI0 (18.9 ± 6.64 vs. 11.49 ± 2.64, $p < 0.001$) were described in the oldest subgroup. As concerns the anthropometric variables, older subjects had both lower BMI (25.84 ± 5.68 kg/m^2 vs. 31.38 ± 4.82 kg/m^2 $p < 0.001$) and lower waist circumference (97.18 ± 15.19 cm vs. 103.6 ± 13.88 cm, $p = 0.006$) than younger patients.

Table 1. Characteristics of the study population, divided by age strata.

	<70 Years (n = 100)					≥70 Years (n = 91)						
	Mean	SD	Median	1st q.le	3rd q.le	Mean	SD	Median	1st q.le	3rd q.le	p	p*
Age (years)	56.86	8.53	58.00	51.00	64.00	80.79	7.49	79.00	74.00	87.00	<0.001	<0.001
DBP (mmHg)	85.40	9.35	86.00	79.00	92.00	76.51	10.21	76.00	70.00	84.00	<0.001	<0.001
SBP (mmHg)	141.81	16.36	139.50	130.00	153.00	137.07	20.17	136.00	126.00	148.00	0.075	0.086
MAP (mmHg)	105.4	10.64	106.00	98.75	114.33	97.2	13.71	96.7	89.33	97.21	<0.001	<0.001
PP (mmHg)	54.9	13.18	53.00	46.75	60.00	60.07	14.53	59.00	50.50	67.00	0.011	0.004
CAVI0	11.49	2.64	10.91	9.58	13.44	18.90	6.64	17.00	14.09	21.83	<0.001	<0.001
CAVI	7.78	1.21	7.75	7.00	8.80	10.25	2.15	9.80	8.90	11.20	<0.001	<0.001
Weight (Kg)	83.2	15.6	81.55	73.40	93.50	68.27	15.68	65.90	57.10	80.00	<0.001	<0.001
Height (cm)	162.63	9.51	162.00	155.00	168.00	162.36	8.41	161.00	156.00	169.00	0.084	0.758
BMI (kg/m^2)	31.38	4.82	31.15	28.20	34.60	25.84	5.68	25.40	21.50	30.30	<0.001	<0.001
Waist circumference (cm)	103.6	13.88	103.00	94.25	113.75	97.18	15.19	98.00	87.00	105.00	0.006	0.007
Glicemia (mg/dL)	99.5	23.34	93.00	86.00	106.00	103.6	38.68	93.00	82.75	109.50	0.396	0.980
Total cholesterol (mg/dL)	202.8	41.42	207.5	177.20	231.00	150.4	38.31	151.00	122.00	179.00	<0.001	<0.001
LDL cholesterol (mg/dL)	123.2	35.54	123.5	97.50	151.00	70.8	35.16	78.5	57.50	104.75	<0.001	<0.001
HDL cholesterol (mg/dL)	55.5	15.42	53.5	44.00	64.75	45.5	17.15	44.00	34.00	59.00	<0.001	<0.001
Triglycerides (mg/dL)	132.9	68.69	122.00	81.00	160.00	128.9	64.17	118.00	79.75	151.75	0.680	0.853
Creatinine (mg/dL)	0.86	0.19	0.84	0.72	0.98	1.05	0.58	0.92	0.73	1.14	0.005	0.078
	n	%				n	%				Chi-Square p	
Male sex	28	28				40	44				0.031	
Smoke	24	24				32	35				0.120	
Hypertension	62	62				71	78				0.024	
Diabetes	21	21				27	29				0.225	
Dyslipidemia	74	74				53	58				0.031	

p: p-value of the Student's t-test; p*: p-value of the Mann-Whitney U test; SD: standard deviation, DBP: diastolic blood pressure; SBP: systolic blood pressure; CAVI: cardio-ankle vascular index; BMI: body mass index.

No significant difference was detected in glucose and triglycerides levels between groups; on the other hand, older patients had reduced total cholesterol (150.4 ± 3831 mg/dL vs. 202.8 ± 41.42 mg/dL, $p < 0.001$), LDL cholesterol (70.8 ± 35.16 mg/dL vs. 123.2 ± 35.54 mg/dL, $p < 0.001$) and HDL cholesterol (45.5 ± 17.15 mg/dL vs. 55.5 ± 15.42 mg/dL, $p < 0.001$).

Cardiovascular risk factors have also been considered: arterial hypertension was significantly more prevalent in older subjects ($p = 0.02$), whereas dyslipidemia was significantly more prevalent in younger patients ($p = 0.031$). Any significant difference was detected when looking at smoking habits and diabetes prevalence.

A significant negative association was found between DBP and age (R = −0.464, $p < 0.001$). CAVI and CAVI0 progressively increased through consecutive age strata (Figure 1), with a significant trend even after adjustment for DBP. Noteworthily, CAVI0 steeply increased after the age threshold of 70 years, therefore increasing the gap between CAVI and CAVI0.

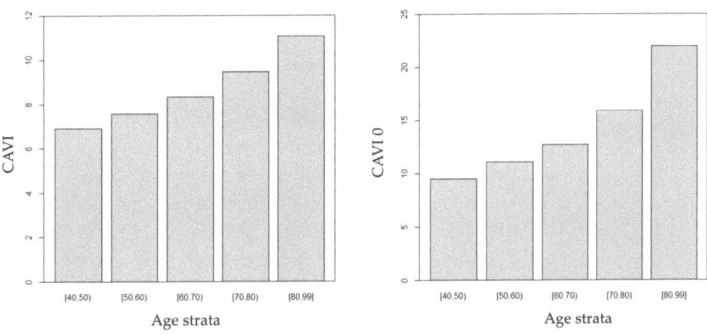

Figure 1. CAVI and CAVI0 increased through consecutive age strata.

CAVI0 was significantly associated both with age (R = 0.703; $p < 0.001$) and, negatively, with DBP (−0.360; $p < 0.001$). Noteworthily, when CAVI0 was considered as the dependent variable in a regression model, a significant interaction between age and DBP was found ($p = 0.027$), revealing that the relationship between CAVI0 and DBP was modified by age. Figure 2 shows predicted CAVI0 values in relation to DBP for selected ages. Predicted values were calculated employing the estimates of the regression coefficients shown in Table 2.

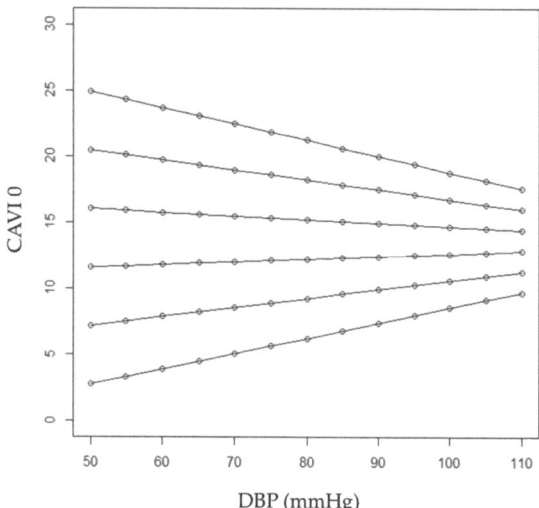

Figure 2. Predicted CAVI0 values in relation to DBP for selected ages (from bottom to top: 40, 50, 60, 70, 80 and 90 years).

Table 2. Regression model considering CAVI0 as dependent variable, and age, DBP and the interaction between them as independent variables.

	Estimate	S.E.	t	p	p*
Intercept	−30.301	12.841	−2.360	0.019	0.012
Age	0.682	0.176	3.876	<0.001	<0.001
DBP	0.306	0.152	2.013	0.046	0.033
Interaction (age × DBP)	−0.005	0.002	−2.233	0.027	0.010

SE: standard error, DBP: diastolic blood pressure; p*: p-value of the permutation test.

In younger ages (40 and 50 years, the first three lines from bottom in the figure), subjects with higher DBP were expected to have higher CAVI0 values. On the other hand, in older patients, an inverse relationship between CAVI0 and DBP was expected (see the first two lines from the top in the figure, referring to patients aged 90 and 80). Expected CAVI0 values for 60-year-old patients range from 11.6 to 12.8 when DBP values varied between 50 and 110 mmHg, respectively. On the other hand, expected CAVI0 values for 70-year-old patients ranged from 16.0 to 14.4 when DBP values varied between 50 and 110 mmHg, respectively. At the age of (about) 64 years, CAVI0 was expected to be constant (i.e., independent from DBP) at the value of 13.5.

The regression model, which included age, DBP and the interaction between age and DBP, showed a multiple R^2 of 0.508 (R = 0.713). Table 2 shows the estimated regression coefficients for this model, together with the corresponding standard errors.

Residuals of these two regression analyses were visually checked for normality employing a normal quantile plot, which showed a symmetric pattern of the points even if in the tails of the distribution they did not lie close to a straight line. The significance of the results was also checked employing a distribution-free permutation test for regression models implemented in the R package "lmPerm".

When SBP, sex and BMI were included as independent variables in the regression model, the interaction between age and DBP maintained the statistical significance ($p = 0.025$). In addition, when this model was considered, the effects of SBP and BMI were also statistically significant (with a negative association for BMI); the R^2 of this model was 0.530 ($R = 0.728$). Table 3 shows the estimated regression coefficients for this model, together with the corresponding standard errors.

Table 3. Regression model considering CAVI0 as dependent variable, and age, DBP, the interaction between them, sex and BMI as independent variables.

	Estimate	S.E.	t	p	p*
Intercept	−25.947	13.041	−1.990	0.048	0.032
Age	0.631	0.176	3.579	<0.001	<0.001
DBP	0.255	0.153	1.664	0.098	0.109
Interaction (age × DBP)	−0.005	0.002	−2.184	0.030	0.021
SBP	0.045	0.022	2.070	0.040	0.011
Male sex	0.712	0.685	1.039	0.300	0.473
BMI	−0.133	0.064	−2.084	0.039	0.032

SE: standard error, DBP: diastolic blood pressure; SBP: systolic blood pressure; BMI: body mass index; *p**: *p*-value of the permutation test.

CAVI was significantly associated both with age ($R = 0.683$; $p < 0.001$) and, negatively, with DBP (-0.266; $p < 0.001$). However, when CAVI was considered the dependent variable in a multiple regression model, only age was significantly associated with the response ($p = 0.01$), while DBP as well as the interaction between age and DBP were not significant ($p = 0.181$ and $p = 0.259$, respectively). Table 4 shows the estimated regression coefficients for this model, together with the corresponding standard errors.

Table 4. Regression model considering CAVI as dependent variable, and age, DBP and the interaction between them as independent variables.

	Estimate	S.E.	t	p	p*
Intercept	−4.16	4.55	−0.914	0.362	0.253
Age	0.175	0.062	2.803	0.006	0.001
DBP	0.072	0.054	1.344	0.181	0.227
Interaction (age × DBP)	−0.001	0.001	−1.132	0.259	0.289

SD: standard error, DBP: diastolic blood pressure; *p**: *p*-value of the permutation test.

A similar result was found when the interaction term was removed from the previous model. Therefore, when the effect of age was accounted for, the correlation between CAVI and DBP was no longer significant and only age remained significantly associated with CAVI.

When SBP, sex and BMI were included as independent variables in the regression model, the interaction between age and DBP confirmed it was not a significant result ($p = 0.246$). Furthermore, when this model was considered, DBP ($p = 0.265$) and SBP ($p = 0.633$) were not significantly associated with CAVI, while a significant effect of both BMI ($p = 0.005$) and sex ($p = 0.019$) was found. The R^2 of this model was 0.511 ($R = 0.715$). Table 5 shows the estimated regression coefficients for this model, together with the corresponding standard errors.

Residuals of these two regression analyses were visually checked for normality employing a normal quantile plot, which showed a symmetric pattern of the points even if in the tails of the distribution they did not lie close to a straight line. The significance of the results was also checked employing a distribution-free permutation test for regression models implemented in the R package "lmPerm" (version 2.1.0, 2016).

Table 5. Regression model considering CAVI as dependent variable, and age, DBP, the interaction between them, SBP, sex and BMI as independent variables.

	Estimate	S.E.	t	p	p*
Intercept	−0.332	4.552	−0.073	0.942	0.572
Age	0.138	0.062	2.243	0.026	0.024
DBP	0.054	0.053	1.004	0.317	0.172
Interaction (age × DBP)	−0.001	0.001	−0.808	0.420	0.368
SBP	0.003	0.008	0.395	0.693	0.941
Male sex	0.533	0.239	2.228	0.027	0.012
BMI	−0.063	0.022	−2.828	0.005	0.018

SE: standard error, DBP: diastolic blood pressure; SBP: systolic blood pressure; BMI: body mass index; p*: p-value of the permutation test.

Therefore, when considering CAVI0 and CAVI as dependent variables, two different results were found. The main difference was that age modified the effect of DBP on CAVI0, but not on CAVI. Furthermore, BMI appeared to have a significant (and negative) effect on both CAVI0 and CAVI, while sex was significant only for CAVI (with higher values for males).

4. Discussion

The present study, of 191 adults ranging from 40 to 96 years, shed light on the significant association between aging and arterial stiffness, measured by CAVI and CAVI0; however, our data suggest that age modifies the effect of DBP on CAVI0, but not on CAVI, opening significant perspectives on the choice of CAVI rather than CAVI0 when examining arterial stiffening in older adults.

Our study moves from the assumption that CAVI is a valid estimate of arterial stiffening in older ages [25]. Although guidelines endorse the use of cfPWV as the gold standard for arterial stiffness evaluation [3], there has been increasing interest in CAVI and CAVI0 [26]. As compared to cfPWV, which is a particular measurement of the central aortic segments, CAVI is known to be representative of a wider proportion of the arterial tree, including both central and peripheral segments [13]. Owing to this intrinsic property of the technique, in older adults, CAVI rather than cfPWV might be considered more effective in highlighting the hallmarks of aging-related pathophysiological changings; we previously demonstrated [19] a significant relationship between arterial stiffness indexes and age, showing that the strength of the association is higher for CAVI and CAVI0, as compared to cfPVW.

CAVI0 derives from CAVI with the main aim of relieving the residual pressure dependency that was still found in CAVI [27]. In Shirai's equation [4], in fact, CAVI relies on a stiffness parameter β, which depends on the arterial pressure and on the vessel diameter, following the equation:

$$\beta = \ln\frac{SBP}{DBP} * \frac{D}{\Delta D} \quad (3)$$

where D stands for the vessel diameter and ΔD stands for its changing; thus, β is not a pressure-normalized index. On the other hand, due to the introduction of a unique P_{ref} (proposed to be equal to 100 mmHg) [24,27], CAVI0 is based on a $\beta 0$ parameter, and it is considered to be pressure normalized:

$$\beta 0 = \beta - \ln\frac{DBP}{P_{ref}} \quad (4)$$

Several features are common to CAVI and CAVI0, namely the included arterial segments (the entire arterial tree from the origin of the aorta to the ankle), the BP measurement site at the upper brachial artery and the baPWV, which accounts for the total measured artery [27,28]. Nonetheless, a major difference is pinpointed when looking at the formulas: it should be noted that CAVI depends on a mid-pressure (the arithmetic mean between

DBP and SBP, see Equation (1)), whereas CAVI0 depends on DBP [29] following an inverse relation [5]:

$$\text{CAVI0} = 2\rho * \frac{\text{PWV}^2}{\text{DBP}} - \frac{\text{DBP}}{P_{\text{ref}}} \quad (5)$$

This consideration is a trivial point to interpret the relationship connecting age, CAVI and CAVI0.

We observed that in younger ages, subjects with higher DBP were expected to have higher CAVI0 values, which is in line with previous findings by Webb and colleagues [30], who demonstrated that midlife DBP is a significant predictor of arterial stiffness and progression of arterial stiffness. Authors provided evidence that higher DBP during midlife is associated with an earlier transition from a rising to a falling DBP [30], reflecting a well-known mechanism of arterial aging which results in greater arterial stiffness and lower DBP at older ages [31]. As a matter of fact, impaired arterial compliance, due to arterial aging, is also responsible for reduced DBP among older adults. Consolidated knowledge describes isolated systolic hypertension as the most frequent phenotype in subjects aged over 50 years [32], also identifying in lower DBP a relevant risk factor for all-cause mortality [33]. Consequently, older adults are more likely to have low DBP and, mathematically, greater CAVI0.

In line with these considerations, we outlined an inverse relationship between CAVI0 and DBP in older subjects. In particular, our data showed that CAVI0 steeply increases after the age threshold of 70 years, while this was not true for CAVI.

We compared the predictors of CAVI and CAVI0, observing CAVI0 results to be strongly dependent on age, DBP and on the interaction between age and DBP. In other words, age modifies the effect of DBP on CAVI0, but not on CAVI.

Including older adults in our analyses, our results complement previous evidence, since CAVI0 has been applied in younger age sets, such as the pediatric [34] and adolescent [35] ages. So far, most of the studies led on CAVI0 compared heathy individuals versus subjects with cardiovascular disorders [6], normal weight versus overweight patients [35] and different subsets of hypertensive patients [36,37]; however, to the best of our knowledge, the possible changing of CAVI0 during aging has never been investigated.

There is a rather limited number of studies comparing CAVI and CAVI0, even taking into account the quite recent introduction of CAVI0 in research practice. Previous evidence suggested the superiority of CAVI over CAVI0 in the predictive role on atherosclerotic plaque formation [38]. Furthermore, CAVI, but not CAVI0, has been shown to be accurate in reflecting not only organic structural stiffness but also functional stiffness [12,38] and hemodynamic changes [39]. CAVI0 is deemed to underestimate arterial stiffness in subjects with high DBP [6]. In a longitudinal study of Japanese subjects, Nagayama and colleagues recently demonstrated the superior predictability of CAVI compared to PWV and CAVI0 for renal function decline [40]. However, the comparison between CAVI and CAVI0 in older adults has never been explored.

Thus, besides the agreement of both CAVI and CAVI0 in describing increased arterial stiffness among aged subjects, the suitability of CAVI0 in older age strata might be prevented by a lower DBP, which unavoidably leads to higher CAVI0.

In line with previous findings, our data suggest that BMI might have a significant and negative effect on both CAVI0 and CAVI, while sex is significant only for CAVI (with higher values for males). Previous studies demonstrated that CAVI was negatively correlated with BMI, and also with waist circumference; the result might appear counterintuitive, since higher arterial stiffness is expected in patients with obesity [41,42]. However, a recent study led by Nagayama and colleagues showed that a body shape index, instead of BMI, as proxy for visceral adiposity, was associated with CAVI increase [43].

The strengths and limitations of the present study should be recognized. This is the first study focusing on CAVI0 measurement in older adults, and its changings across aging, analyzing a heterogeneous range of age strata. On the other hand, our population was not made up of healthy subjects, and the concomitant inclusion of both inpatients and outpatients, with different clinical conditions (although all the patients were examined after achieving clinical stability), might have brought heterogeneity into the stiffness measurements. Moreover, our study was predominantly performed on female patients, and given the increased prevalence of cardiovascular diseases in the male population, associated with higher CAVI values, testing our hypothesis in a more representative male population would be beneficial.

5. Conclusions

In conclusion, our study, on a relatively wide and heterogeneous cohort of patients, outlines a strong association between arterial stiffness indexes and age, showing that the association between CAVI0 and diastolic blood pressure is modified by age, whereas the association between CAVI and DBP is not modified by age.

From a clinical point of view, this is a very important finding, as DBP decreases with aging, affecting in elderly populations the reliability of CAVI0, which strictly depends on DBP in the formula to calculate it.

In other words, for these reasons, in clinical practice we suggest that to monitor the effect of CV therapies, progression of CV diseases and to evaluate clinical outcomes, CAVI and not CAVI0 should be used in elderly populations.

Author Contributions: Conceptualization, A.G., F.F. and M.Z.; methodology, F.F. and R.M.; formal analysis, R.M.; investigation, A.G., E.Z. and G.M.; data curation, A.G., F.F., E.Z. and G.M.; writing—original draft preparation, A.G. and F.F.; writing—review and editing, A.G., M.Z. and F.F. All authors have read and agreed to the published version of the manuscript.

Funding: This research received no external funding.

Institutional Review Board Statement: The study was conducted in accordance with the Declaration of Helsinki and approved by the Ethics Committee of Verona University Hospital (protocol code 191CESC, approval date: 11 February 2015).

Informed Consent Statement: Informed consent was obtained from all subjects involved in the study.

Data Availability Statement: The data presented in this study are available on request from the corresponding author.

Conflicts of Interest: The authors declare no conflict of interest.

References

1. Mitchell, G.F.; Parise, H.; Benjamin, E.J.; Larson, M.G.; Keyes, M.J.; Vita, J.A.; Vasan, R.S.; Levy, D. Changes in Arterial Stiffness and Wave Reflection With Advancing Age in Healthy Men and Women. *Hypertension* **2004**, *43*, 1239–1245. [CrossRef] [PubMed]
2. Miyoshi, T.; Ito, H.; Shirai, K.; Horinaka, S.; Higaki, J.; Yamamura, S.; Saiki, A.; Takahashi, M.; Masaki, M.; Okura, T.; et al. Predictive Value of the Cardio-Ankle Vascular Index for Cardiovascular Events in Patients at Cardiovascular Risk. *J. Am. Heart Assoc.* **2021**, *10*, e020103. [CrossRef]
3. Williams, B.; Mancia, G.; Spiering, W.; Rosei, E.A.; Azizi, M.; Burnier, M.; Clement, D.L.; Coca, A.; De Simone, G.; Dominiczak, A.; et al. 2018 ESC/ESH Guidelines for Themanagement of Arterial Hypertension. *Eur. Heart J.* **2018**, *77*, 71–159.
4. Shirai, K.; Utino, J.; Otsuka, K.; Takata, M. A Novel Blood Pressure-Independent Arterial Wall Stiffness Parameter; Cardio-Ankle Vascular Index (CAVI). *J. Atheroscler. Thromb.* **2006**, *13*, 101–107. [CrossRef]
5. Spronck, B.; Avolio, A.P.; Tan, I.; Butlin, M.; Reesink, K.D.; Delhaas, T. Arterial Stiffness Index Beta and Cardio-Ankle Vascular Index Inherently Depend on Blood Pressure but Can Be Readily Corrected. *J. Hypertens.* **2017**, *35*, 98–104. [CrossRef] [PubMed]
6. Shirai, K.; Suzuki, K.; Tsuda, S.; Shimizu, K.; Takata, M.; Yamamoto, T.; Maruyama, M.; Takahashi, K. Comparison of Cardio-Ankle Vascular Index (CAVI) and CAVI0 in Large Healthy and Hypertensive Populations. *J. Atheroscler. Thromb.* **2019**, *26*, 603–615. [CrossRef]
7. Saiki, A.; Ohira, M.; Yamaguchi, T.; Nagayama, D.; Shimizu, N.; Shirai, K.; Tatsuno, I. New Horizons of Arterial Stiffness Developed Using Cardio-Ankle Vascular Index (CAVI). *J. Atheroscler. Thromb.* **2020**, *27*, 732–748. [CrossRef]
8. Spronck, B.; Mestanik, M.; Tonhajzerova, I.; Jurko, A.; Jurko, T.; Avolio, A.P.; Butlin, M. Direct Means of Obtaining CAVI 0—A Corrected Cardio-Ankle Vascular Stiffness Index (CAVI)—From Conventional CAVI Measurements or Their Underlying Variables. *Physiol. Meas.* **2017**, *38*, N128–N137. [CrossRef] [PubMed]
9. Shirai, K.; Song, M.; Suzuki, J.; Kurosu, T.; Oyama, T.; Nagayama, D.; Miyashita, Y.; Yamamura, S.; Takahashi, M. Contradictory Effects of B1- and A1- Aderenergic Receptor Blockers on Cardio-Ankle Vascular Stiffness Index (CAVI). *J. Atheroscler. Thromb.* **2011**, *18*, 49–55. [CrossRef]

10. Shirai, K.; Shimizu, K.; Takata, M.; Suzuki, K. Independency of the Cardio-Ankle Vascular Index from Blood Pressure at the Time of Measurement. *J. Hypertens.* **2017**, *35*, 1521–1523. [CrossRef]
11. Ibata, J.; Sasaki, H.; Kakimoto, T.; Matsuno, S.; Nakatani, M.; Kobayashi, M.; Tatsumi, K.; Nakano, Y.; Wakasaki, H.; Furuta, H.; et al. Cardio-Ankle Vascular Index Measures Arterial Wall Stiffness Independent of Blood Pressure. *Diabetes Res. Clin. Pract.* **2008**, *80*, 265–270. [CrossRef]
12. Namekata, T.; Suzuki, K.; Ishizuka, N.; Shirai, K. Establishing Baseline Criteria of Cardio-Ankle Vascular Index as a New Indicator of Arteriosclerosis: A Cross-Sectional Study. *BMC Cardiovasc. Disord.* **2011**, *11*, 51. [CrossRef]
13. Shirai, K. Analysis of Vascular Function Using the Cardio–Ankle Vascular Index (CAVI). *Hypertens. Res.* **2011**, *34*, 684–685. [CrossRef] [PubMed]
14. Kiuchi, S.; Kawasaki, M.; Hirashima, O.; Hisatake, S.; Kabuki, T.; Yamazaki, J.; Ikeda, T. Addition of a Renin-Angiotensin-Aldosterone System Inhibitor to a Calcium Channel Blocker Ameliorates Arterial Stiffness. *Clin. Pharmacol.* **2015**, *7*, 97. [CrossRef] [PubMed]
15. Nagayama, D.; Watanabe, Y.; Saiki, A.; Shirai, K.; Tatsuno, I. Difference in Positive Relation between Cardio-Ankle Vascular Index (CAVI) and Each of Four Blood Pressure Indices in Real-World Japanese Population. *J. Hum. Hypertens.* **2019**, *33*, 210–217. [CrossRef]
16. Dobsak, P.; Soska, V.; Sochor, O.; Jarkovsky, J.; Novakova, M.; Homolka, M.; Soucek, M.; Palanova, P.; Lopez-Jimenez, F.; Shirai, K. Increased Cardio-Ankle Vascular Index in Hyperlipidemic Patients without Diabetes or Hypertension. *J. Atheroscler. Thromb.* **2015**, *22*, 272–283. [CrossRef]
17. Nakamura, K.; Tomaru, T.; Yamamura, S.; Miyashita, Y.; Shirai, K.; Noike, H. Cardio-Ankle Vascular Index Is a Candidate Predictor of Coronary Atherosclerosis. *Circ. J.* **2007**, *72*, 598–604. [CrossRef] [PubMed]
18. Kim, K.J.; Lee, B.-W.; Kim, H.; Shin, J.Y.; Kang, E.S.; Cha, B.S.; Lee, E.J.; Lim, S.-K.; Lee, H.C. Associations Between Cardio-Ankle Vascular Index and Microvascular Complications in Type 2 Diabetes Mellitus Patients. *J. Atheroscler. Thromb.* **2011**, *18*, 328–336. [CrossRef] [PubMed]
19. Fantin, F.; Giani, A.; Trentin, M.; Rossi, A.P.; Zoico, E.; Mazzali, G.; Micciolo, R.; Zamboni, M. The Correlation of Arterial Stiffness Parameters with Aging and Comorbidity Burden. *J. Clin. Med.* **2022**, *11*, 5761. [CrossRef]
20. Bramwell, J.C.; Hill, A.V. Velocity of transmission of the pulse-wave. *Lancet* **1922**, *199*, 891–892. [CrossRef]
21. Saiki, A.; Sato, Y.; Watanabe, R.; Watanabe, Y.; Imamura, H.; Yamaguchi, T.; Ban, N.; Kawana, H.; Nagumo, A.; Nagayama, D.; et al. The Role of a Novel Arterial Stiffness Parameter, Cardio-Ankle Vascular Index (CAVI), as a Surrogate Marker for Cardiovascular Diseases. *J. Atheroscler. Thromb.* **2016**, *23*, 155–168. [CrossRef]
22. Hayashi, K.; Yamamoto, T.; Takahara, A.; Shirai, K. Clinical Assessment of Arterial Stiffness with Cardio-Ankle Vascular Index. *J. Hypertens.* **2015**, *33*, 1742–1757. [CrossRef]
23. Yamashina, A.; Tomiyama, H.; Takeda, K.; Tsuda, H.; Arai, T.; Hirose, K.; Koji, Y.; Hori, S.; Yamamoto, Y. Validity, Reproducibility, and Clinical Significance of Noninvasive Brachial-Ankle Pulse Wave Velocity Measurement. *Hypertens. Res.* **2002**, *25*, 359–364. [CrossRef] [PubMed]
24. Spronck, B.; Mestanik, M.; Tonhajzerova, I.; Jurko, A.; Tan, I.; Butlin, M.; Avolio, A.P. Easy Conversion of Cardio-Ankle Vascular Index into CAVI0. *J. Hypertens.* **2019**, *37*, 1913–1914. [CrossRef] [PubMed]
25. Kirkham, F.A.; Mills, C.; Fantin, F.; Tatsuno, I.; Nagayama, D.; Giani, A.; Zamboni, M.; Shirai, K.; Cruickshank, J.K.; Rajkumar, C. Are You as Old as Your Arteries? Comparing Arterial Aging in Japanese and European Patient Groups Using Cardio-Ankle Vascular Index. *J. Hypertens.* **2022**, *40*, 1758–1767. [CrossRef]
26. Spronck, B.; Obeid, M.J.; Paravathaneni, M.; Gadela, N.V.; Singh, G.; Magro, C.A.; Kulkarni, V.; Kondaveety, S.; Gade, K.C.; Bhuva, R.; et al. Predictive Ability of Pressure-Corrected Arterial Stiffness Indices: Comparison of Pulse Wave Velocity, Cardio-Ankle Vascular Index (CAVI), and CAVI0. *Am. J. Hypertens.* **2022**, *35*, 272–280. [CrossRef] [PubMed]
27. Giudici, A.; Khir, A.W.; Reesink, K.D.; Delhaas, T.; Spronck, B. Five Years of Cardio-Ankle Vascular Index (CAVI) and CAVI0: How Close Are We to a Pressure-Independent Index of Arterial Stiffness? *J. Hypertens.* **2021**, *39*, 2128–2138. [CrossRef] [PubMed]
28. Hung, T.-J.; Hsieh, N.-C.; Alizargar, E.; Bai, C.-H.; Wang, K.-W.K.; Hatefi, S.; Alizargar, J. Association of Blood Pressure Indices with Right and Left Cardio-Ankle Vascular Index (CAVI) and Its Mathematically Corrected Form (CAVI0) for the Evaluation of Atherosclerosis. *J. Pers. Med.* **2022**, *12*, 1386. [CrossRef]
29. Takahashi, K.; Yamamoto, T.; Tsuda, S.; Maruyama, M.; Shirai, K. The Background of Calculating CAVI: Lesson from the Discrepancy Between CAVI and CAVI$_0$. *Vasc. Health Risk Manag.* **2020**, *16*, 193–201. [CrossRef]
30. Webb, A.J.S. Progression of Arterial Stiffness Is Associated With Midlife Diastolic Blood Pressure and Transition to Late-Life Hypertensive Phenotypes. *J. Am. Heart Assoc.* **2020**, *9*, e014547. [CrossRef] [PubMed]
31. Franklin, S.S.; Gustin, W.; Wong, N.D.; Larson, M.G.; Weber, M.A.; Kannel, W.B.; Levy, D. Hemodynamic Patterns of Age-Related Changes in Blood Pressure. *Circulation* **1997**, *96*, 308–315. [CrossRef]
32. Liu, X.; Rodriguez, C.J.; Wang, K. Prevalence and Trends of Isolated Systolic Hypertension among Untreated Adults in the United States. *J. Am. Soc. Hypertens.* **2015**, *9*, 197–205. [CrossRef] [PubMed]
33. Koracevic, G.; Stojanovic, M.; Kostic, T.; Lovic, D.; Tomasevic, M.; Jankovic-Tomasevic, R. Unsolved Problem: (Isolated) Systolic Hypertension with Diastolic Blood Pressure below the Safety Margin. *Med. Princ. Pract.* **2020**, *29*, 301–309. [CrossRef]

34. Jurko, T.; Mestanik, M.; Jurko, A.; Spronck, B.; Avolio, A.; Mestanikova, A.; Sekaninova, N.; Tonhajzerova, I. Pediatric Reference Values for Arterial Stiffness Parameters Cardio-Ankle Vascular Index and CAVI0. *J. Am. Soc. Hypertens.* **2018**, *12*, e35–e43. [CrossRef] [PubMed]
35. Mestanik, M.; Jurko, A.; Spronck, B.; Avolio, A.P.; Butlin, M.; Jurko, T.; Visnovcova, Z.; Mestanikova, A.; Langer, P.; Tonhajzerova, I. Improved Assessment of Arterial Stiffness Using Corrected Cardio-Ankle Vascular Index (CAVI$_0$) in Overweight Adolescents with White-Coat and Essential Hypertension. *Scand. J. Clin. Lab. Investig.* **2017**, *77*, 665–672. [CrossRef] [PubMed]
36. Mills, C.E.; Govoni, V.; Faconti, L.; Casagrande, M.; Morant, S.V.; Crickmore, H.; Iqbal, F.; Maskell, P.; Masani, A.; Nanino, E.; et al. A Randomised, Factorial Trial to Reduce Arterial Stiffness Independently of Blood Pressure: Proof of Concept? The VaSera Trial Testing Dietary Nitrate and Spironolactone. *Br. J. Clin. Pharmacol.* **2020**, *86*, 891–902. [CrossRef] [PubMed]
37. Mills, C.E.; Govoni, V.; Faconti, L.; Casagrande, M.-L.; Morant, S.V.; Webb, A.J.; Cruickshank, J.K. Reducing Arterial Stiffness Independently of Blood Pressure. *J. Am. Coll. Cardiol.* **2017**, *70*, 1683–1684. [CrossRef] [PubMed]
38. Nagayama, D.; Fujishiro, K.; Suzuki, K.; Shirai, K. Comparison of Predictive Ability of Arterial Stiffness Parameters Including Cardio-Ankle Vascular Index, Pulse Wave Velocity and Cardio-Ankle Vascular Index0. *Vasc. Health Risk Manag.* **2022**, *18*, 735–745. [CrossRef]
39. Plunde, O.; Franco-Cereceda, A.; Bäck, M. Cardiovascular Risk Factors and Hemodynamic Measures as Determinants of Increased Arterial Stiffness Following Surgical Aortic Valve Replacement. *Front. Cardiovasc. Med.* **2021**, *8*, 754371. [CrossRef] [PubMed]
40. Nagayama, D.; Fujishiro, K.; Miyoshi, T.; Horinaka, S.; Suzuki, K.; Shimizu, K.; Saiki, A.; Shirai, K. Predictive Ability of Arterial Stiffness Parameters for Renal Function Decline: A Retrospective Cohort Study Comparing Cardio-Ankle Vascular Index, Pulse Wave Velocity and Cardio-Ankle Vascular Index0. *J. Hypertens.* **2022**, *40*, 1294–1302. [CrossRef] [PubMed]
41. Fantin, F.; Giani, A.; Gasparini, L.; Rossi, A.P.; Zoico, E.; Mazzali, G.; Zamboni, M. Impaired Subendocardial Perfusion in Patients with Metabolic Syndrome. *Diabetes Vasc. Dis. Res.* **2021**, *18*, 147916412110471. [CrossRef] [PubMed]
42. Topouchian, J.; Labat, C.; Gautier, S.; Bäck, M.; Achimastos, A.; Blacher, J.; Cwynar, M.; De La Sierra, A.; Pall, D.; Fantin, F.; et al. Effects of Metabolic Syndrome on Arterial Function in Different Age Groups: The Advanced Approach to Arterial Stiffness Study. *J. Hypertens.* **2018**, *36*, 824–833. [CrossRef] [PubMed]
43. Nagayama, D.; Sugiura, T.; Choi, S.-Y.; Shirai, K. Various Obesity Indices and Arterial Function Evaluated with CAVI—Is Waist Circumference Adequate to Define Metabolic Syndrome? *Vasc. Health Risk Manag.* **2022**, *18*, 721–733. [CrossRef]

Disclaimer/Publisher's Note: The statements, opinions and data contained in all publications are solely those of the individual author(s) and contributor(s) and not of MDPI and/or the editor(s). MDPI and/or the editor(s) disclaim responsibility for any injury to people or property resulting from any ideas, methods, instructions or products referred to in the content.

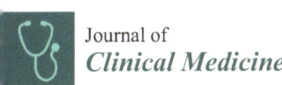

Journal of
Clinical Medicine

Article

Wall Properties of Elastic and Muscular Arteries in Children and Adolescents at Increased Cardiovascular Risk

Simonetta Genovesi [1,2], Elena Tassistro [2], Giulia Lieti [2], Ilenia Patti [2], Marco Giussani [1], Laura Antolini [2], Antonina Orlando [1], Paolo Salvi [1,*] and Gianfranco Parati [1,2]

1 Department of Cardiology, Istituto Auxologico Italiano, IRCCS, 20100 Milan, Italy
2 School of Medicine and Surgery, University of Milano-Bicocca, 20100 Milan, Italy
* Correspondence: psalvi.md@gmail.com

Citation: Genovesi, S.; Tassistro, E.; Lieti, G.; Patti, I.; Giussani, M.; Antolini, L.; Orlando, A.; Salvi, P.; Parati, G. Wall Properties of Elastic and Muscular Arteries in Children and Adolescents at Increased Cardiovascular Risk. *J. Clin. Med.* **2023**, *12*, 6919. https://doi.org/10.3390/jcm12216919

Academic Editor: Pasquale Ambrosino

Received: 15 September 2023
Revised: 23 October 2023
Accepted: 31 October 2023
Published: 3 November 2023

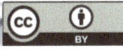

Copyright: © 2023 by the authors. Licensee MDPI, Basel, Switzerland. This article is an open access article distributed under the terms and conditions of the Creative Commons Attribution (CC BY) license (https://creativecommons.org/licenses/by/4.0/).

Abstract: Background: Pulse wave velocity (PWV) assessment represents a simple method to estimate arterial distensibility. At present, carotid-femoral PWV (cf-PWV) is considered the gold standard method in the non-invasive evaluation of the elastic properties of the aorta. On the other hand, the mechanical properties of muscular arteries can be evaluated on the axillo-brachial-radia axis by estimating the carotid-radial PWV (cr-PWV). While a number of studies have addressed these issues in adults, limited information is available on the respective features of cf-PWV and cr-PWV and on their modulating factors in children and adolescents at increased cardiovascular risk. Methods: The mechanical properties of the predominantly elastic (aorta) and muscular (axillo–brachial–radial axis) arteries were evaluated in a pediatric population characterized by either elevated blood pressure (BP) or excess body weight, and the main factors affecting cf-PWV and cr-PWV values in these individuals were investigated. Results: 443 children and adolescents (median age 11.5 years, 43.3% females) were enrolled; 25% had BP values >90th percentile and 81% were excess weight. The cf-PWV values were significantly lower than the cr-PWV values: median (Q1–Q3) = 4.8 m/s (4.3–5.5) and 5.8 m/s (5.0–6.5), respectively ($p < 0.001$). The pubertal development ($p < 0.03$), systolic BP and diastolic BP z-scores ($p = 0.002$), heart rate ($p < 0.001$), and waist-to-height ratio ($p < 0.005$) were significantly associated with cf-PWV values. No significant association was found between BMI z-score and cf-PWV. Predictors of high cf-PWV (>95th percentile) were the heart rate (OR 1.07, 95%CI 1.04–1.10, $p < 0.001$) and waist-to-height ratio (OR 1.06, 95%CI 1.0–1.13, $p = 0.04$). The variables significantly related with cr-PWV values were diastolic BP z-score ($p = 0.001$), heart rate ($p < 0.01$), and HOMA index ($p < 0.02$). No significant association was found between the cr-PWV and BMI z-score or waist-to-height ratio. Conclusions: Systolic and diastolic BP values and central obesity are associated with aortic stiffness in a population of children and adolescents at increased cardiovascular risk. In contrast, diastolic BP, heart rate, and levels of insulin resistance appear to be related to distensibility of the upper limb vascular district.

Keywords: adolescent; arterial stiffness; blood pressure; body mass index; carotid-femoral pulse wave velocity; carotid-radial pulse wave velocity; children; HOMA index; waist-to-height ratio

1. Introduction

Measurement of pulse wave velocity (PWV) represents a simple way to measure the stiffness of a specific arterial segment [1]. The pulse wave is transmitted through the arterial vessels, and its speed is inversely related to the viscoelastic properties of the wall itself; the higher the velocity, the less elastic the wall [2]. Carotid-femoral PWV (cf-PWV) investigates the viscoelastic properties of the aorta and is considered the non-invasive gold standard for estimating the degree of aortosclerosis in daily clinical practice [3,4]. In adults, high cf-PWV values represent an independent risk factor for cardiovascular events, as well as an important prognostic factor for cardiovascular mortality [3,5]. PWV can be modified both by structural and functional elements of the arterial wall [2].

Regarding the structural elements, the viscoelastic properties of the arterial wall in large arteries are guaranteed by the ratio between the elastin fibers and the collagen fibers in the tunica media [6–8]. This relationship can be altered by an increase in collagen fibers (as observed in arterial hypertension), as well as by a reduction in elastic fibers (as observed with aging) [4,9,10]. The aging process causes histological alterations in the arterial wall. Reduced elastin synthesis and increased elastase activity cause thinning and breakage of elastin fibers, and the result is a decrease in the elastin and collagen ratio. Starting from the first decades of life, there is a slow but progressive increase in aortic PWV values, with a rapid and exponential increase in adults and in the elderly population [11]. If the maintenance of the structural characteristics of the arterial wall represents an important element to guarantee the viscoelastic properties of the aorta and of the large elastic arteries, on the other hand the elastin–collagen ratio in the wall has a negligible impact on the mechanical properties of the muscular arteries.

Muscular arteries are mainly affected by functional factors, mostly related to the activity of the sympathetic nervous system [2,9]. Enhanced sympathetic activity results in an increase in heart rate, ventricular contractility, and peripheral vascular resistance, leading to a rise in mean arterial pressure. Concerning arterial vessels, the sympathetic system modulates the activity and the tone of the smooth muscle cells of the arterial wall. On the other hand, the impact of the sympathetic nervous system on the distensibility properties of the aorta is weak and it has been shown that the mechanical properties of the human aorta remain largely unaffected during sympathetic stimulation. The mechanical properties of predominantly muscular peripheral arteries can be assessed in the peripheral arterial districts of the lower limbs and upper limbs, by measuring the femoral-tibial PWV and carotid-radial PWV (cr-PWV), respectively. The latter provides an estimate of the viscoelastic properties of the axillo–brachial–radial arterial district. Several studies performed on the adult population have shown that elevated femoro-tibial and cr-PWV values have no prognostic or clinical significance [12,13]. Furthermore, while cf-PWV increases significantly with aging, cr-PWV does not change significantly with age [2]. Overall, PWV assessed at the upper limb likely reflects a functional condition of the arterial tree, which is closely related to the activation of the sympathetic system.

The relationship between PWV in the aorta and in upper limb muscular arteries has not yet been investigated in childhood and adolescence, and it is unclear what factors affect cf-PWV and cr-PWV at this age in the presence of cardiovascular risk factors. Thus, the aim of our study was to evaluate the main factors associated with cf-PWV and cr-PWV values in a pediatric population at increased cardiovascular risk.

2. Materials and Methods

2.1. Participants

We studied a cohort of children and adolescents, consecutively referred from May 2008 to September 2022 to the Unit for Cardiovascular Risk Assessment in Children of Istituto Auxologico Italiano, IRCCS (Milan, Italy) by their primary care pediatricians, for the clinical finding of excess weight or elevated blood pressure (BP) values.

Children and adolescents with diabetes mellitus, secondary hypertension, hypertension under drug treatment, congenital cardiovascular disease, and kidney disease were excluded from the study. The presence of chronic disease involving habitual therapy was considered an exclusion criterion from the study.

The study protocol was approved by the local institutional ethics committee and conformed to the ethical guidelines of the 1975 Declaration of Helsinki. Informed consent was obtained from parents or legal representatives before the enrolment in the study.

2.2. Clinical Parameters

Height, weight, and waist circumference were measured. Waist circumference was measured by means of a flexible tape in a standing position. Body mass index (BMI) was calculated as weight/height^2 (Kg/m^2). The waist-to-height ratio (WtHr) was obtained dividing waist circumference by height, and expressed as percentage [14,15]. BMI z-scores were derived from the Centre for Disease and Control prevention charts [16]. All study participants were classified as normal weight, overweight, or obese according to the International Obesity Task Force classification [17]. The pubertal stage was assessed and children were divided into two categories, pre-pubertal and pubertal, according to Tanner [18,19], considering pre-pubertal boys with gonadal stage 1 and girls with breast stage 1.

2.3. Blood Pressure Measurement

BP measurements were performed after at least 5 min of rest, in a sitting position, using an oscillometric device validated in children (Omron 705IT; Omron Co., Kyoto, Japan) with an appropriate cuff for the upper-arm size. The BP measurement was performed 3 times (at intervals of 3 min) and the average of the last two measurements was considered. Systolic BP and diastolic BP percentiles and z-scores were calculated according to the nomograms of the National High Blood Pressure Education Program Working Group on High Blood Pressure in Children and Adolescents [20,21]. The children were classified as normotensive if both systolic and diastolic BP percentiles were <90th; high-normal if systolic BP and/or diastolic BP percentiles were ≥90th but <95th; and hypertensive if systolic BP and/or diastolic BP percentiles were ≥95th.

2.4. Biochemical Dosages

Fasting blood samples were taken in all study participants to measure serum glucose, insulin, uric acid, and creatinine. Commercial kits were employed for all analyses: enzymatic method with hexokinase Glucose HK Gen.3 Cobas Roche (F. Hoffmann-La Roche AG, Basel, Switzerland), for glucose assay; ElectroChemiLuminescence Elecsys Insulin Cobas Roche immunoassay was used for the insulin assay; colorimetric enzymatic test Uric Acid 2 Cobas Roche for the serum uric acid assay; and colorimetric kinetic test based on the Jaffé method Creatinine Jaffé Gen.2 Cobas Roche for creatinine assay. The homeostatic model assessment (HOMA) index was obtained by dividing the product of the serum insulin (mU/L) and serum glucose (mmol/L) by 22.5 [22]. The glomerular filtration rate was estimated (eGFR) using the Schwartz formula [23].

2.5. Arterial Stiffness Assessment

Measurements of arterial distensibility were obtained at a stable room temperature after 10 min of rest, by a validated ETT PulsePen tonometer [24] (DiaTecne srl, San Donato Milanese, Italy), as described in detail previously [25–27]. Briefly, PulsePen consists of a pocket size, high-fidelity applanation tonometer, and an integrated ECG unit. Aortic PWV was measured by recording carotid and femoral waveforms in rapid succession. cf-PWV was defined as 80% of the distance between the measuring sites divided by the time delay between the distal (femoral) pulse wave from the proximal (carotid) pulse wave, using the R wave of the ECG trace as the reference [11]. The R−R interval on the ECG recording was used to define the heart rate. The use of the PulsePen device in children had been validated in a previous study, which provided reference values according to gender and age for cf-PWV in children and adolescents [28].

2.6. Statistical Analysis

The characteristics of the cohort, overall and stratified according to sex, were described by median and interquartile range (Q1–Q3) if the variables were continuous and by frequencies and percentages if they were categorical. Univariate analyses to compare the characteristics of the two groups of children were conducted using the Mann−Whitney test in case of continuous variables, and through the Chi-Square test in case of categorical variables.

The univariate associations between cf-PWV (or cr-PWV) and systolic BP, diastolic BP and BMI z-score values, WtHr, uric acid, and HOMA index are represented in scatterplots, where 95% confidence interval on the Pearson correlation test and the *p*-value are displayed.

Multiple linear regression models were used to assess the impact of sex, pubertal status, systolic BP (or diastolic BP) z-score, BMI z-score (or WtHr), heart rate (detected at the time of measurement of cf-PWV), uric acid, HOMA index, and eGFR on cf-PWV. Multiple linear regression models were used to assess the impact of sex, pubertal status, systolic BP (or diastolic BP) z-score, BMI z-score (or WtHr), heart rate (detected at the time of measurement of cf-PWV), uric acid, HOMA index, and eGFR on cr-PWV. Multiple logistic regression models were used to assess the impact of sex, pubertal status, systolic BP (or diastolic BP) z-score, BMI z-score (or WtHr), heart rate, uric acid, HOMA index, and eGFR on having cf-PWV values equal to or greater than the 95th percentile according to gender and age [28]. As there were no reference nomograms for cr-PWV, only the multiple linear regression model was performed for this variable. Statistical analyses were performed with R (R Fundation for Statistical Computing, Vienna, Austria) 4.1.2 version (http://www.R-project.org) accessed on 1 November 2023. All p-values were 2-sided, with p-values < 0.05 considered to be statistically significant.

3. Results

3.1. Population

The study involved 443 children and adolescents referred to our clinic. Table 1 shows the characteristics of the population enrolled in the study. The median age was 11.5 years; 43.3% of children were female and 54% were prepubescent. Here, 25.5% (n = 113) had BP values greater than or equal to the 90th percentile. Furthermore, 80.8% (n = 358) were of excess weight, and 67.5% (n = 295) had WtHr >50%. The median cf-PWV value was 4.8 m/s, and 11.4% (n = 50) of the children had cf-PWV values equal to or greater than the 95th percentile [28]. The cr-PWV values were significantly higher (median value 5.8 m/s) than the cf-PWV values (p < 0.001), without differences between males and females.

Table 1. Anthropometric and clinical characteristics according to sex.

Parameter	Overall	Females	Males	p-Value
Participants, n (%)	443	192 (43.3)	251 (56.7)	
Age, years	11.5 (9.3–13.2)	10.9 (8.7–13.0)	11.7 (9.9–13.5)	0.005
Birth weight, g	3280 (2900–3640)	3200 (2800–3530)	3300 (3000–3800)	0.004
Puberty, n (%)	201 (46.0)	91 (47.6)	110 (44.7)	0.608
Heart rate, beats/min	76 (69–85)	80 (72–87)	73 (66–82)	<0.001
Systolic BP, mmHg	111 (103–121)	109 (101–119)	112 (104–123)	0.010
Systolic BP z-score	0.58 (−0.12–1.21)	0.66 (−0.16–1.18)	0.53 (−0.09–1.27)	0.999
Diastolic BP, mmHg	65 (59–71)	65 (58–71)	64 (60–71)	0.685
Diastolic BP z-score	0.21 (−0.25–0.81)	0.31 (−0.23–0.85)	0.17 (−0.25–0.76)	0.372
BP category:				0.752
- Normotension, n (%)	330 (74.5)	144 (75.0)	186 (74.1)	
- High-normal, n (%)	42 (9.5)	16 (8.3)	26 (10.4)	
- Hypertension, n (%)	71 (16.0)	32 (16.7)	39 (15.5)	
Weight class:				0.771
- Normal weight, n (%)	85 (19.2)	39 (20.3)	46 (18.3)	
- Overweight, n (%)	141 (31.8)	58 (30.2)	83 (33.1)	
- Obese, n (%)	217 (49.0)	95 (49.5)	122 (48.6)	
BMI, Kg/m^2	24.6 (21.8–27.7)	24.2 (20.9–26.9)	25.1 (22.5–28.1)	0.010
BMI z-score	1.78 (1.20–2.11)	1.76 (1.10–2.04)	1.81 (1.32–2.17)	0.087
Waist-to-height ratio, %	53.3 (48.3–57.8)	52.4 (47.3–57.3)	54.0 (49.4–57.9)	0.021
Waist-to-height ratio >50%, %	295 (67.5)	119 (63.3)	176 (70.7)	0.126
Serum uric acid, mg/dl	4.5 (3.7–5.3)	4.4 (3.7–4.9)	4.7 (3.7–5.6)	0.003
Glucose, mg/dl	86 (81–89)	85 (80–89)	86 (82–89)	0.072
Insulin, mM/L	13.0 (9.0–18.6)	12.9 (9.2–18.4)	13.0 (9.0–18.7)	0.866
HOMA index, mmol/L × mU/L	2.6 (1.9–4.0)	2.6 (1.9–3.9)	2.7 (1.9–4.1)	0.944
Creatinine, mg/dl	0.54 (0.48–0.63)	0.52 (0.45–0.60)	0.57 (0.50–0.66)	0.003
eGFR, ml/min	149 (132–164)	151 (134–171)	147 (129–161)	0.046
cf-PWV, m/s	4.8 (4.3–5.5)	4.8 (4.3–5.5)	4.8 (4.3–5.5)	0.752
cf-PWV ≥ 95th percentile, n (%)	50 (11.4)	22 (11.6)	28 (11.3)	0.999
cr-PWV, m/s	5.8 (5.0–6.5)	5.8 (5.3–6.5)	5.6 (4.9–6.4)	0.069

Data are shown as median (interquartile range) or number (%). BMI, body mass index; BP, blood pressure; cf-PWV, carotid-femoral pulse wave velocity; cr-PWV, carotid-radial pulse wave velocity; eGFR, estimated glomerular filtration rate; HOMA, homeostatic model assessment.

3.2. Factors Affecting Arterial Stiffness

Figure 1 shows the linear regression between cf-PWV/cr-PWV values and systolic BP, diastolic BP and BMI z-scores, and WtHr. The systolic BP z-score was significantly correlated with both cf-PWV ($p < 0.01$) and cr-PWV values ($p < 0.01$). The same was true for the correlation of diastolic BP z-scores with both cf-PWV ($p < 0.001$) and cr-PWV ($p < 0.001$) values. BMI z-score and WtHr were associated with cf-PWV values ($p = 0.041$ and $p = 0.007$, respectively), but not with cr-PWV values. Both serum uric acid and HOMA index values were correlated with cf-PWV ($p < 0.001$), while only HOMA index but not serum uric acid was associated with cr-PWV ($p = 0.005$) (Figure 2).

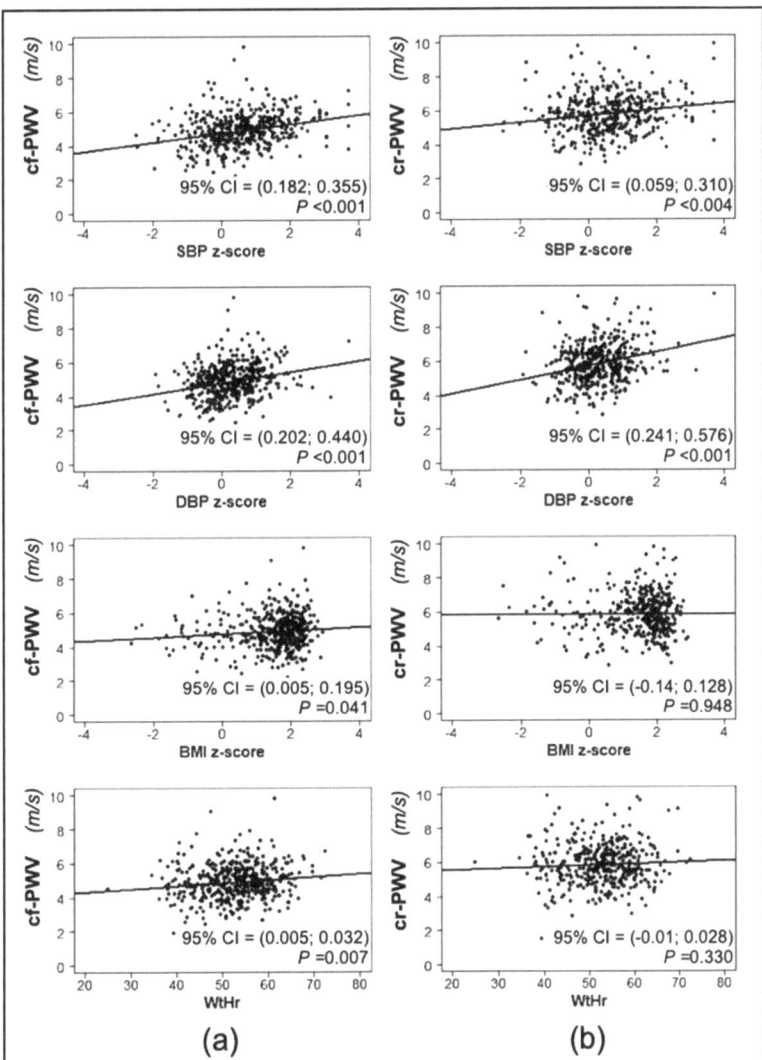

Figure 1. Linear regression between carotid-femoral pulse wave velocity (cf-PWV) (**a**) and carotid-radial pulse wave velocity (cr-PWV) (**b**) and systolic (SBP), diastolic blood pressure (DBP) z-score, body mass index (BMI) z-score, and waist-to-height ratio (WtHr).

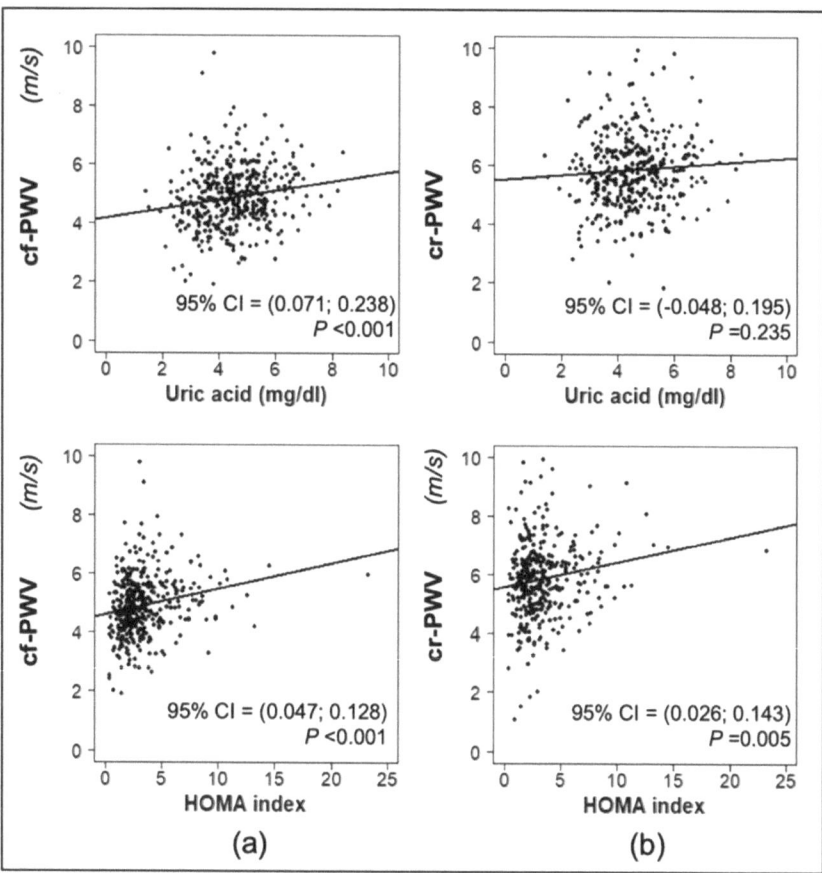

Figure 2. Linear regression between carotid-femoral pulse wave velocity (cf-PWV) (**a**) and carotid-radial pulse wave velocity (cr-PWV) (**b**) and serum uric acid and homeostatic model assessment (HOMA) index.

Multiple linear regression analysis (Table 2) showed that the variables significantly associated with cf-PWV values were the presence of pubertal development ($p < 0.03$), systolic BP and diastolic BP z-scores ($p = 0.002$), and heart rate ($p < 0.001$). A correlation between HOMA index and cf-PWV was evident when the model was adjusted for diastolic BP z-score ($p = 0.039$). The estimated glomerular filtration rate (eGFR) was inversely related with cf-PWV ($p = 0.020$). No significant association was evident between BMI z-score and cf-PWV. In contrast, when WtHr was entered into the model instead of BMI z-score, a significant correlation was shown between WtHr and cf-PWV ($p < 0.05$). All of the results of the previous model were confirmed, except for the HOMA index, which was no longer associated with cf-PWV. If the HOMA index was removed from the regressors, the association between WtHr and cf-PWV became stronger ($p < 0.01$), while the other results remained unchanged.

Table 2. Results of multiple linear regression analysis with carotid-femoral pulse wave velocity (m/s) as dependent variables in the entire sample.

	Dependent Variable: Carotid-Femoral Pulse Wave Velocity					
I Analysis						
Variable	Model A			Model B		
	β	(95% CI)	p	β	(95% CI)	p
Intercept	3.772	(2.767; 4.778)	<0.001	3.795	(2.788; 4.801)	<0.001
Sex (males)	0.066	(−0.135; 0.268)	0.517	0.076	(−0.125; 0.278)	0.456
Puberty	0.263	(0.038; 0.487)	0.022	0.312	(0.091; 0.533)	0.006
Systolic BP z-score	0.161	(0.059; 0.262)	0.002	-	-	-
Diastolic BP z-score	-	-	-	0.219	(0.084; 0.355)	0.002
BMI z-score	0.081	(−0.033; 0.195)	0.163	0.081	(−0.033; 0.195)	0.162
Heart rate, beats/min	0.018	(0.010; 0.026)	<0.001	0.017	(0.009; 0.026)	<0.001
Serum uric acid, mg/dL	−0.005	(−0.106; 0.096)	0.925	−0.003	(−0.105; 0.098)	0.947
HOMA index	0.044	(−0.001; 0.090)	0.057	0.048	(0.002; 0.093)	0.039
eGFR, mL/min	−0.005	(−0.009; −0.001)	0.020	−0.005	(−0.009; −0.001)	0.021
II Analysis						
Variable	Model A			Model B		
	β	(95% CI)	p	β	(95% CI)	p
Intercept	3.018	(1.839; 4.198)	<0.001	3.085	(1.898; 4.273)	<0.001
Sex (males)	0.052	(−0.152; 0.256)	0.616	0.061	(−0.143; 0.265)	0.557
Puberty	0.307	(0.074; 0.541)	0.010	0.350	(0.120; 0.581)	0.003
Systolic BP z-score	0.161	(0.059; 0.262)	0.002	-	-	-
Diastolic BP z-score	-	-	-	0.213	(0.075; 0.351)	0.003
WtHr	0.019	(0.003; 0.036)	0.022	0.018	(0.002; 0.035)	0.032
Heart rate, beats/min	0.018	(0.009; 0.026)	<0.001	0.017	(0.008; 0.025)	<0.001
Serum uric acid, mg/dL	−0.015	(−0.117; 0.086)	0.771	−0.011	(−0.112; 0.091)	0.836
HOMA index	0.035	(−0.013; 0.082)	0.150	0.039	(−0.008; 0.086)	0.102
eGFR, mL/min	−0.005	(−0.010; −0.001)	0.015	−0.005	(−0.010; −0.001)	0.016

In Model A and Model B, systolic blood pressure or diastolic blood pressure were considered, respectively. In Analysis I and Analysis II, body mass index (z-score) or waist-to-height ratio were considered, respectively. Coefficient β provides a measure of the relative strength of the association independent of the units of measurement. BMI, body mass index; BP, blood pressure; CI, confidence interval; eGFR, estimated glomerular filtration rate; HOMA, homeostatic model assessment; WtHr, waist-to-height ratio.

The multiple logistic regression model exploring factors significantly associated with the presence of cf-PWV values equal to or greater than the 95th percentile for sex and age, adjusted for systolic BP z-score (Table 3), showed a direct association with heart rate (OR 1.07 95%CI 1.04–1.10, $p < 001$) and an inverse association with eGFR (OR 0.98 95% CI 0.97–0.99, $p = 0.025$) (Table 4). The results were similar when the diastolic BP z-score was included in the model. When the BMI z-score was substituted for WtHr in the model adjusted for systolic BP z-score, the OR was 1.07 (95%CI 1.04–1.10, $p < 0.001$) for heart rate and 0.98 (95%CI 0.97–0.99, $p = 0.018$) for eGFR. Interestingly, in the latter model, WtHr was also significantly associated with the presence of cf-PWV values equal to or greater than the 95th percentile (OR 1.06 95%CI 1.0–1.13, $p = 0.040$). Similar results were obtained for the model adjusted for diastolic BP z-score. The results did not change when the HOMA index was removed from the model.

Table 3. Results of multiple regression model with carotid-femoral pulse wave velocity values equal to or greater than the 95th percentile as dependent variables.

	Dependent Variable: Carotid-Femoral Pulse Wave Velocity Equal to or Greater than the 95th Percentile					
I Analysis						
Variable	Model A			Model B		
	β	(95% CI)	p	β	(95% CI)	p
Sex (males)	1.448	(0.746; 2.866)	0.279	1.489	(0.765; 2.962)	0.247
Puberty	0.732	(0.342; 1.532)	0.413	0.690	(0.326; 1.425)	0.322
Systolic BP z-score	0.898	(0.632; 1.268)	0.545	-	-	-
Diastolic BP z-score	-	-	-	1.283	(0.825; 1.981)	0.262
BMI z-score	1.289	(0.884; 1.959)	0.206	1.244	(0.853; 1.891)	0.277
Heart rate, beats/min	1.068	(1.039; 1.099)	<0.001	1.065	(1.036; 1.096)	<0.001
Serum uric acid, mg/dL	0.774	(0.541; 1.095)	0.153	0.756	(0.530; 1.067)	0.116
HOMA index	0.964	(0.793; 1.137)	0.689	0.937	(0.771; 1.107)	0.482
eGFR, mL/min	0.982	(0.967; 0.997)	0.018	0.983	(0.967; 0.997)	0.025
II Analysis						
Variable	Model A			Model B		
	β	(95% CI)	p	β	(95% CI)	p
Sex (males)	1.489	(0.758; 2.996)	0.254	1.500	(0.762; 3.025)	0.247
Puberty	0.936	(0.420; 2.059)	0.870	0.872	(0.395; 1.893)	0.730
Systolic BP z-score	0.867	(0.604; 1.235)	0.431	-	-	-
Diastolic BP z-score	-	-	-	1.225	(0.773; 1.916)	0.379
WtHr	1.064	(1.004; 1.130)	0.040	1.060	(1.001; 1.126)	0.050
Heart rate, beats/min	1.069	(1.039; 1.100)	<0.001	1.066	(1.036; 1.097)	<0.001
Serum uric acid, mg/dL	0.711	(0.488; 1.020)	0.070	0.697	(0.480; 0.995)	0.051
HOMA index	0.941	(0.764; 1.123)	0.538	0.910	(0.739; 1.089)	0.340
eGFR, mL/min	0.982	(0.966; 0.996)	0.018	0.982	(0.967; 0.997)	0.022

In Model A and Model B, systolic blood pressure or diastolic blood pressure were considered, respectively. In Analysis I and Analysis II, body mass index (z-score) or waist-to-height ratio were considered, respectively. BMI, body mass index; BP, blood pressure; CI, confidence interval; eGFR, estimated glomerular filtration rate; HOMA, homeostatic model assessment; OR, odds ratio; WtHr, waist-to-height ratio.

Table 4. Results of multiple linear regression analysis with carotid-radial pulse wave velocity (m/s) as dependent variables in the entire sample.

	Dependent Variable: Carotid-Radial Pulse Wave Velocity					
I Analysis						
Variable	Model A			Model B		
	β	(95% CI)	p	β	(95% CI)	p
Intercept	5.035	(3.463; 6.607)	<0.001	5.240	(3.688; 6.791)	<0.001
Sex (males)	−0.164	(−0.467; 0.139)	0.288	−0.138	(−0.438; 0.161)	0.365
Puberty	0.017	(−0.318; 0.351)	0.922	0.033	(−0.292; 0.358)	0.842
Systolic BP z-score	0.076	(−0.077; 0.230)	0.327	-	-	-
Diastolic BP z-score	-	-	-	0.332	(0.131; 0.533)	0.001
BMI z-score	−0.066	(−0.234; 0.103)	0.444	−0.094	(−0.260; 0.073)	0.269
Heart rate, beats/min	0.022	(0.009; 0.035)	0.001	0.019	(0.006; 0.032)	0.004
Serum uric acid, mg/dL	0.015	(−0.137; 0.167)	0.845	−0.001	(−0.152; 0.149)	0.985
HOMA index	0.087	(0.019; 0.155)	0.012	0.080	(0.013; 0.146)	0.019
eGFR, mL/min	−0.007	(−0.014; −0.001)	0.022	−0.007	(−0.013; 0.000)	0.035

Table 4. Cont.

	Dependent Variable: Carotid-Radial Pulse Wave Velocity					
II Analysis						
Variable	Model A			Model B		
	β	(95% CI)	p	β	(95% CI)	p
Intercept	4.980	(3.157; 6.802)	<0.001	5.385	(3.579; 7.190)	<0.001
Sex (males)	−0.186	(−0.494; 0.121)	0.235	−0.166	(−0.470; 0.138)	0.283
Puberty	0.042	(−0.308; 0.393)	0.813	0.045	(−0.296; 0.386)	0.796
Systolic BP z-score	0.071	(−0.083; 0.225)	0.364	-	-	-
Diastolic BP z-score	-	-	-	0.329	(0.125; 0.534)	0.002
WtHr	0.004	(−0.020; 0.029)	0.728	0.000	(−0.024; 0.025)	0.992
Heart rate, beats/min	0.021	(0.008; 0.034)	0.002	0.018	(0.005; 0.031)	0.008
Serum uric acid, mg/dL	0.001	(−0.152; 0.154)	0.993	−0.015	(−0.166; 0.136)	0.844
HOMA index	0.076	(0.005; 0.147)	0.037	0.068	(−0.001; 0.138)	0.055
eGFR, mL/min	−0.008	(−0.014; −0.001)	0.016	−0.007	(−0.014; −0.001)	0.025

In Model A and Model B, systolic blood pressure or diastolic blood pressure were considered, respectively. In Analysis I and Analysis II, body mass index (z-score) or waist-to-height ratio were considered, respectively. The coefficient β provides a measure of the relative strength of the association independent of the units of measurement. BMI, body mass index; BP, blood pressure; CI, confidence interval; eGFR, estimated glomerular filtration rate; HOMA, homeostatic model assessment; WtHr, waist-to-height ratio.

Variables significantly related to cr-PWV were heart rate ($p < 0.01$) and HOMA index ($p < 0.02$), diastolic BP z-score ($p = 0.001$), but not systolic BP z-score. There was an inverse correlation between cr-PWV and eGFR ($p = 0.035$). No significant association was evident between BMI z-score and cr-PWV. When WtHr was included in the model instead of BMI z-score, the results were essentially unchanged and WtHr was not associated with cr-PWV (Table 4). The results did not change when the HOMA index was removed from the model.

4. Discussion

To our knowledge, this is the first study comparing parameters estimating the viscoelastic properties of the aorta and upper limb muscular arteries in a pediatric cohort with cardiovascular risk factors. As a main and innovative contribution, the present study highlights how, in this population, the factors significantly associated with upper limb arterial distensibility (estimated by cr-PWV) are somewhat different from those associated with aortic distensibility (estimated by cf-PWV). If the viscoelastic properties of muscular arteries in the upper limbs appear to be mediated by tonic levels of sympathetic activity, aortic distensibility appears, instead, to be more affected by blood pressure, heart rate, and WtHr. Interesting, a significant and inverse correlation with eGFR was found with both cf-PWV and cr-PWV values.

4.1. Aortic Pulse Wave Velocity

Aortic PWV depends on structural elements and transient functional changes in the arterial wall. The structural factors are stable and closely related to the relationship between elastin and collagen fibers in the tunica media of the arterial wall. The tunica media of the aorta has a typical lamellar arrangement, characterized by an orderly arrangement and interrelationship between elastic fibers and collagen fibers. Elastic fibers are characterized by an accentuated viscoelastic property and collagen fibers are mainly responsible for a structural containment function.

The characteristically different adult patterns of elastin and collagen composition of thoracic and abdominal aortic segments are already present to some degree at birth [6]. The number of lamellar units present at birth remains almost constant in the first decade of life, then increases progressively in adulthood, doubling in the thoracic aorta (from 25–30 units to approximately 56 units in the adult), while it increases less (from 15–20 units to approximately 28 units in the adult) in the abdominal aorta [29]. BP level may be an important mechanical factor influencing the relative degree of lamellar growth during the first years of life and in childhood [29,30]. Collagen is continuously degraded and deposited in a process of homeostatic regulation [31]. An increase in BP, directly or indirectly, provides the stimulus for the elaboration of fibrous collagen proteins in the arterial wall [29], in order to counterbalance the resulting transmural pressure increase [2]. The higher synthesis of collagen fibers induced by high BP values, therefore, causes an imbalance in the elastin−collagen ratio of the arterial wall, determining a condition of aortic stiffening. This action of BP on the viscoelastic properties of the aorta explains how, in our population of children and adolescents with cardiovascular risk factors, the indexed values (z-scores) of systolic and diastolic BP and heart rate were independently associated with aortic stiffness, confirming what is already widely known in the youth [32,33] and in adult population [3,11].

A condition of aortic stiffness has been described even in metabolic diseases such as diabetes [34], fatty liver disease [35–37], kidney failure [12,38,39], and alterations in calcium metabolism [40,41]. Some metabolic disorders can be accompanied by an increase in oxidative stress, arterial medial calcifications, and by inflammation of the arterial wall [42]. Inflammation causes both arterial stiffening and endothelial dysfunction [43]. There is no agreement in the literature regarding the relationship between BMI and vascular stiffness in children and adolescents. Some data suggest that there is no influence of excess weight on cf-PWV [33,44], while others go in the opposite direction [45,46]. Some authors have also suggested that in obese adolescents, there is an inverse correlation between cf-PWV and BMI values. On the other hand, several studies show a close relationship between insulin resistance and arterial stiffness in children and adolescents [44,47–49], and this suggests that excess weight and visceral fat (related to insulin resistance) may be associated with different effects on arterial viscoelasticity, although not all authors agree on this point [50]. Our study did not show an association between cf-PWV and BMI. However, we found a significant relationship between cf-PWV and WtHr. This result is interesting, because it suggests that, for the same weight class, a greater quantity of visceral fat could lead to a more severe clinical picture, presumably related to the production of cytokines, which would induce endothelial dysfunction through an increase in oxidative stress and trigger an inflammatory process that would lead to early vascular damage [51,52]. As there is a strong relationship between central obesity and insulin resistance already in childhood [53] and the cytokines produced by visceral fat can influence BP values in children [54], it is difficult to distinguish the role of insulin resistance and/or visceral obesity when determining the viscoelastic properties of the aorta.

4.2. Upper Limb Pulse Wave Velocity

Along the arterial tree there is a functional diversification that corresponds to a progressive change in the composition of the arterial wall. The aorta and large elastic arteries have the characteristic lamellar structure with layers of elastin interdigitated by layers of collagen and vascular smooth muscle. These arteries contribute to the buffering function and ensure the Windkessel effect. Progressing towards the periphery of the vascular system, the arteries lose their lamellar elastic structure and evolve into muscular-type arteries with a decrease in elastin and a predominance of smooth muscle cells.

This distinction between elastic and muscular vessels is particularly important from a clinical point of view, as, if high cf-PWV values are correlated with a high cardiovascular risk, no relationship between cr-PWV and the incidence of cardiovascular disease has been demonstrated [12,13].

In healthy young subjects, the autonomic nervous system does not have a pressure-independent role in the regulation of the large elastic central arteries [55], which are little or not at all innervated by the sympathetic system [56]. On the contrary, the distal segments of the arterial tree ("muscular" arteries) are more muscular [57] and densely innervated [58,59], thus being particularly sensitive to the activity of the sympathetic system [60]. Thus, the stiffness of muscular arteries appears to be mediated by tonic levels of sympathetic activity [61]. The results of our study are in agreement with these pathophysiological premises, as upper limb PWV was independently associated with z-score of diastolic BP and heart rate, resulting from a condition of sympathetic activation.

In agreement with other studies in humans [62,63], the HOMA index (indicative of insulin resistance) also had a significant association with cr-PWV. Given the condition of sympathetic activation associated with insulin resistance, this finding also appears likely to be induced by sympathetic activity. The interpretation of data on the relationship between insulin resistance and PWV in the two vascular districts is complex. From our results, it would appear that insulin resistance has a greater role in determining carotid-radial stiffness than carotid-femoral stiffness, which, conversely, would be more influenced by central obesity. However, these findings should be interpreted with due caution and would need to be confirmed by additional studies.

4.3. Arterial Stiffness and Glomerular Filtration Rate

Arterial stiffness is increased in children with chronic kidney disease [64]. All children and adolescents in our study population had normal renal function. However, there was a strong inverse association between eGFR values and both cf-PWV and cr-PWV. This finding may suggest that, despite the absence of renal disease, a higher filtration rate leads to better vascular compliance. We can only speculate on the possible mechanisms behind these findings. One possibility could be that children with a higher eGFR have a smaller intravascular volume and that this may contribute to an increased vascular stiffness. Further studies are needed to test this hypothesis.

4.4. Study Limitations and Strenghts

While our results are supported by the consistent number of children and adolescents at increased cardiovascular risk that we were able to include in our paper, we have to acknowledge a limitation of our study, related to the fact that we were able to collect only cross-sectional data. Indeed, our hypotheses on the mechanisms behind our findings would need longitudinal data to be tested and confirmed. However, we believe that our results are, nevertheless, important, because they pave the way for such future longitudinal evaluations.

5. Conclusions

PWVs of the aorta and upper limb have different regulatory mechanisms and clinical significance. If the viscoelastic properties of the aorta are linked to blood pressure, heart rate and visceral fat, on the other hand the distensibility of the muscular arteries of the upper limbs seems to be mainly influenced by the sympathetic system in our population of children at increased cardiovascular risk.

Further longitudinal studies are needed to clarify the prognostic significance of elevated cf-PWV and cr-PWV values in childhood and adolescence, as well as their possible role in the pathogenesis of arterial hypertension.

Author Contributions: Conceptualization, S.G. and P.S.; methodology, S.G. and P.S.; data collection, G.L., A.O., M.G. and I.P.; data analysis, E.T., L.A., S.G., P.S. and G.P.; formal analysis, E.T. and L.A.; investigation, G.L., A.O., M.G. and I.P; writing—original draft preparation, S.G., P.S. and G.P.; writing—review and editing, S.G., P.S. and G.P.; supervision, S.G., P.S. and G.P. All authors have read and agreed to the published version of the manuscript.

Funding: This research was funded by the Italian Ministry of Health ("Ricerca corrente").

Institutional Review Board Statement: The study was conducted in accordance with the Declaration of Helsinki and was approved by the Local Institutional Ethics Committee (CPP Est III 15 December 2006).

Informed Consent Statement: Informed consent was obtained from all subjects involved in the study.

Data Availability Statement: The data presented in this study are available upon reasonable request from the corresponding author. The data are not publicly available due to privacy concerns.

Conflicts of Interest: P.S. has been involved as a consultant and expert witness in DiaTecne S.R.L. The other authors declare no conflict of interest.

References

1. Bramwell, J.C.; Hill, A.V. Velocity of transmission of the pulse-wave and elasticity of the arteries. *Lancet* **1922**, *1*, 891–892. [CrossRef]
2. Salvi, P. Pulse waves. In *How Vascular Hemodynamics Affects Blood Pressure*, 2nd ed.; Springer Nature: Berlin/Heidelberg, Germany, 2017.
3. Townsend, R.R.; Wilkinson, I.B.; Schiffrin, E.L.; Avolio, A.P.; Chirinos, J.A.; Cockcroft, J.R.; Heffernan, K.S.; Lakatta, E.G.; McEniery, C.M.; Mitchell, G.F.; et al. Recommendations for Improving and Standardizing Vascular Research on Arterial Stiffness: A Scientific Statement From the American Heart Association. *Hypertension* **2015**, *66*, 698–722. [CrossRef] [PubMed]
4. Segers, P.; Chirinos, J.A. Arterial wall stiffness: Basic principles and methods of measurement in vivo. In *Textbook of Arterial Stiffness and Pulsatile Hemodynamics in Health and Disease*; Chirinos, J.A., Ed.; Academic Press: London, UK, 2022; Volume 1, pp. 111–124.
5. Chirinos, J.A.; Segers, P.; Hughes, T.; Townsend, R. Large-Artery Stiffness in Health and Disease: JACC State-of-the-Art Review. *J. Am. Coll. Cardiol.* **2019**, *74*, 1237–1263. [CrossRef] [PubMed]
6. Wahart, A.; Bennasroune, A.; Schmelzer, C.E.H.; Laffargue, M.; Blaise, S.; Romier-Crouzet, B.; Sartelet, H.; Martiny, L.; Gillery, P.; Jaisson, S.; et al. Role of elastin and elastin-derived peptides in arterial stiffness: From synthesis to potential therapeutic interventions. In *Hemodynamic Determinants of Myocardial Oxygen Demand and Supply*; Chirinos, J.A., Ed.; Elsevier: Amsterdam, The Netherlands; Academic Press: London, UK, 2022; Volume 1, pp. 299–314.
7. Giudici, A.; Wilkinson, I.B.; Khir, A.W. Review of the Techniques Used for Investigating the Role Elastin and Collagen Play in Arterial Wall Mechanics. *IEEE Rev. Biomed. Eng.* **2021**, *14*, 256–269. [CrossRef] [PubMed]
8. Cocciolone, A.J.; Hawes, J.Z.; Staiculescu, M.C.; Johnson, E.O.; Murshed, M.; Wagenseil, J.E. Elastin, arterial mechanics, and cardiovascular disease. *Am. J. Physiol. Heart Circ. Physiol.* **2018**, *315*, H189–H205. [CrossRef] [PubMed]
9. Nichols, W.W.; O'Rourke, M.; Edelman, E.R.; Vlachopoulos, C. *McDonald's Blood Flow in Arteries: Theoretical, Experimental and Clinical Principles*, 7th ed.; CRC Press: Boca Raton, FL, USA, 2022.
10. Wahart, A.; Hocine, T.; Albrecht, C.; Henry, A.; Sarazin, T.; Martiny, L.; El Btaouri, H.; Maurice, P.; Bennasroune, A.; Romier-Crouzet, B.; et al. Role of elastin peptides and elastin receptor complex in metabolic and cardiovascular diseases. *FEBS J.* **2019**, *286*, 2980–2993. [CrossRef] [PubMed]
11. Reference Values for Arterial Stiffness, C. Determinants of pulse wave velocity in healthy people and in the presence of cardiovascular risk factors: 'establishing normal and reference values'. *Eur. Heart J.* **2010**, *31*, 2338–2350. [CrossRef]
12. Pannier, B.; Guerin, A.P.; Marchais, S.J.; Safar, M.E.; London, G.M. Stiffness of capacitive and conduit arteries: Prognostic significance for end-stage renal disease patients. *Hypertension* **2005**, *45*, 592–596. [CrossRef]
13. Van Sloten, T.T.; Schram, M.T.; van den Hurk, K.; Dekker, J.M.; Nijpels, G.; Henry, R.M.; Stehouwer, C.D. Local stiffness of the carotid and femoral artery is associated with incident cardiovascular events and all-cause mortality: The Hoorn study. *J. Am. Coll. Cardiol.* **2014**, *63*, 1739–1747. [CrossRef]
14. Ashwell, M.; Gibson, S. Waist-to-height ratio as an indicator of 'early health risk': Simpler and more predictive than using a 'matrix' based on BMI and waist circumference. *BMJ Open* **2016**, *6*, e010159. [CrossRef]
15. Peterson, K.; Savoie Roskos, M. Weight Bias: A Narrative Review of the Evidence, Assumptions, Assessment, and Recommendations for Weight Bias in Health Care. *Health Educ. Behav.* **2023**, *50*, 517–528. [CrossRef] [PubMed]
16. CDC. Centers for Disease Control and Prevention. Clinical Growth Charts. Available online: https://www.cdc.gov/growthcharts/clinical_charts.htm (accessed on 20 June 2023).
17. Cole, T.J.; Lobstein, T. Extended international (IOTF) body mass index cut-offs for thinness, overweight and obesity. *Pediatr. Obes.* **2012**, *7*, 284–294. [CrossRef] [PubMed]
18. Marshall, W.A.; Tanner, J.M. Variations in the pattern of pubertal changes in boys. *Arch. Dis. Child.* **1970**, *45*, 13–23. [CrossRef] [PubMed]
19. Marshall, W.A.; Tanner, J.M. Variations in pattern of pubertal changes in girls. *Arch. Dis. Child.* **1969**, *44*, 291–303. [CrossRef] [PubMed]
20. National High Blood Pressure Education Program Working Group on High Blood Pressure in, C. Adolescents. The fourth report on the diagnosis, evaluation, and treatment of high blood pressure in children and adolescents. *Pediatrics* **2004**, *114*, 555–576. [CrossRef]
21. Lurbe, E.; Agabiti-Rosei, E.; Cruickshank, J.K.; Dominiczak, A.; Erdine, S.; Hirth, A.; Invitti, C.; Litwin, M.; Mancia, G.; Pall, D.; et al. 2016 European Society of Hypertension guidelines for the management of high blood pressure in children and adolescents. *J. Hypertens.* **2016**, *34*, 1887–1920. [CrossRef] [PubMed]
22. Matthews, D.R.; Hosker, J.P.; Rudenski, A.S.; Naylor, B.A.; Treacher, D.F.; Turner, R.C. Homeostasis model assessment: Insulin resistance and beta-cell function from fasting plasma glucose and insulin concentrations in man. *Diabetologia* **1985**, *28*, 412–419. [CrossRef]
23. Schwartz, G.J.; Haycock, G.B.; Edelmann, C.M., Jr.; Spitzer, A. A simple estimate of glomerular filtration rate in children derived from body length and plasma creatinine. *Pediatrics* **1976**, *58*, 259–263. [CrossRef]

24. Salvi, P.; Safar, M.E.; Parati, G. Arterial applanation tonometry: Technical aspects relevant for its daily clinical use. *J. Hypertens.* **2013**, *31*, 469–471. [CrossRef]
25. Salvi, P.; Lio, G.; Labat, C.; Ricci, E.; Pannier, B.; Benetos, A. Validation of a new non-invasive portable tonometer for determining arterial pressure wave and pulse wave velocity: The PulsePen device. *J. Hypertens.* **2004**, *22*, 2285–2293. [CrossRef]
26. Salvi, P.; Scalise, F.; Rovina, M.; Moretti, F.; Salvi, L.; Grillo, A.; Gao, L.; Baldi, C.; Faini, A.; Furlanis, G.; et al. Noninvasive Estimation of Aortic Stiffness Through Different Approaches. *Hypertension* **2019**, *74*, 117–129. [CrossRef] [PubMed]
27. Joly, L.; Perret-Guillaume, C.; Kearney-Schwartz, A.; Salvi, P.; Mandry, D.; Marie, P.Y.; Karcher, G.; Rossignol, P.; Zannad, F.; Benetos, A. Pulse wave velocity assessment by external noninvasive devices and phase-contrast magnetic resonance imaging in the obese. *Hypertension* **2009**, *54*, 421–426. [CrossRef] [PubMed]
28. Reusz, G.S.; Cseprekal, O.; Temmar, M.; Kis, E.; Cherif, A.B.; Thaleb, A.; Fekete, A.; Szabo, A.J.; Benetos, A.; Salvi, P. Reference values of pulse wave velocity in healthy children and teenagers. *Hypertension* **2010**, *56*, 217–224. [CrossRef] [PubMed]
29. Wolinsky, H. Comparison of medial growth of human thoracic and abdominal aortas. *Circ. Res.* **1970**, *27*, 531–538. [CrossRef] [PubMed]
30. Naeye, R.L. Arterial changes during the perinatal period. *Arch. Pathol.* **1961**, *71*, 121–128. [PubMed]
31. Humphrey, J.D. Vascular adaptation and mechanical homeostasis at tissue, cellular, and sub-cellular levels. *Cell. Biochem. Biophys.* **2008**, *50*, 53–78. [CrossRef] [PubMed]
32. Lurbe, E.; Torro, I.; Garcia-Vicent, C.; Alvarez, J.; Fernandez-Fornoso, J.A.; Redon, J. Blood pressure and obesity exert independent influences on pulse wave velocity in youth. *Hypertension* **2012**, *60*, 550–555. [CrossRef] [PubMed]
33. Genovesi, S.; Salvi, P.; Nava, E.; Tassistro, E.; Giussani, M.; Desimone, I.; Orlando, A.; Battaglino, M.; Lieti, G.; Montemerlo, M.; et al. Blood Pressure and Body Weight Have Different Effects on Pulse Wave Velocity and Cardiac Mass in Children. *J. Clin. Med.* **2020**, *9*, 2954. [CrossRef]
34. Christoforidis, A.; Georeli, I.; Dimitriadou, M.; Galli-Tsinopoulou, A.; Stabouli, S. Arterial stiffness indices in children and adolescents with type 1 diabetes mellitus: A meta-analysis. *Diabetes Metab. Res. Rev.* **2022**, *38*, e3555. [CrossRef]
35. Salvi, P.; Ruffini, R.; Agnoletti, D.; Magnani, E.; Pagliarani, G.; Comandini, G.; Pratico, A.; Borghi, C.; Benetos, A.; Pazzi, P. Increased arterial stiffness in nonalcoholic fatty liver disease: The Cardio-GOOSE study. *J. Hypertens* **2010**, *28*, 1699–1707. [CrossRef]
36. Jaruvongvanich, V.; Chenbhanich, J.; Sanguankeo, A.; Rattanawong, P.; Wijarnpreecha, K.; Upala, S. Increased arterial stiffness in nonalcoholic fatty liver disease: A systematic review and meta-analysis. *Eur. J. Gastroenterol. Hepatol.* **2017**, *29*, e28–e35. [CrossRef] [PubMed]
37. Sunbul, M.; Agirbasli, M.; Durmus, E.; Kivrak, T.; Akin, H.; Aydin, Y.; Ergelen, R.; Yilmaz, Y. Arterial stiffness in patients with non-alcoholic fatty liver disease is related to fibrosis stage and epicardial adipose tissue thickness. *Atherosclerosis* **2014**, *237*, 490–493. [CrossRef] [PubMed]
38. Kouis, P.; Kousios, A.; Kanari, A.; Kleopa, D.; Papatheodorou, S.I.; Panayiotou, A.G. Association of non-invasive measures of subclinical atherosclerosis and arterial stiffness with mortality and major cardiovascular events in chronic kidney disease: Systematic review and meta-analysis of cohort studies. *Clin. Kidney J.* **2020**, *13*, 842–854. [CrossRef] [PubMed]
39. Townsend, R.R.; Anderson, A.H.; Chirinos, J.A.; Feldman, H.I.; Grunwald, J.E.; Nessel, L.; Roy, J.; Weir, M.R.; Wright, J.T., Jr.; Bansal, N.; et al. Association of Pulse Wave Velocity with Chronic Kidney Disease Progression and Mortality: Findings from the CRIC Study (Chronic Renal Insufficiency Cohort). *Hypertension* **2018**, *71*, 1101–1107. [CrossRef] [PubMed]
40. Bellasi, A.; Raggi, P. Vascular calcification in chronic kidney disease: Usefulness of a marker of vascular damage. *J. Nephrol.* **2011**, *24* (Suppl. 18), S11–S15. [CrossRef] [PubMed]
41. Raggi, P.; Bellasi, A.; Ferramosca, E.; Islam, T.; Muntner, P.; Block, G.A. Association of pulse wave velocity with vascular and valvular calcification in hemodialysis patients. *Kidney Int.* **2007**, *71*, 802–807. [CrossRef] [PubMed]
42. Sequi-Dominguez, I.; Cavero-Redondo, I.; Alvarez-Bueno, C.; Saz-Lara, A.; Mesas, A.E.; Martinez-Vizcaino, V. Association between arterial stiffness and the clustering of metabolic syndrome risk factors: A systematic review and meta-analysis. *J. Hypertens.* **2021**, *39*, 1051–1059. [CrossRef] [PubMed]
43. Bruno, R.M.; Reesink, K.D.; Ghiadoni, L. Advances in the non-invasive assessment of vascular dysfunction in metabolic syndrome and diabetes: Focus on endothelium, carotid mechanics and renal vessels. *Nutr. Metab. Cardiovasc. Dis.* **2017**, *27*, 121–128. [CrossRef]
44. Pucci, G.; Martina, M.R.; Bianchini, E.; D'Abbondanza, M.; Curcio, R.; Battista, F.; Anastasio, F.; Crapa, M.E.; Sanesi, L.; Gemignani, V.; et al. Relationship between measures of adiposity, blood pressure and arterial stiffness in adolescents. The MACISTE study. *J. Hypertens.* **2023**, *41*, 1100–1107. [CrossRef]
45. Urbina, E.M.; Kimball, T.R.; Khoury, P.R.; Daniels, S.R.; Dolan, L.M. Increased arterial stiffness is found in adolescents with obesity or obesity-related type 2 diabetes mellitus. *J. Hypertens* **2010**, *28*, 1692–1698. [CrossRef]
46. Koopman, L.P.; McCrindle, B.W.; Slorach, C.; Chahal, N.; Hui, W.; Sarkola, T.; Manlhiot, C.; Jaeggi, E.T.; Bradley, T.J.; Mertens, L. Interaction between myocardial and vascular changes in obese children: A pilot study. *J. Am. Soc. Echocardiogr. Off. Publ. Am. Soc. Echocardiogr.* **2012**, *25*, 401–410.e401. [CrossRef]
47. Correia-Costa, A.; Correia-Costa, L.; Caldas Afonso, A.; Schaefer, F.; Guerra, A.; Moura, C.; Mota, C.; Barros, H.; Areias, J.C.; Azevedo, A. Determinants of carotid-femoral pulse wave velocity in prepubertal children. *Int. J. Cardiol.* **2016**, *218*, 37–42. [CrossRef] [PubMed]

48. Ruiz-Moreno, M.I.; Vilches-Perez, A.; Gallardo-Escribano, C.; Vargas-Candela, A.; Lopez-Carmona, M.D.; Perez-Belmonte, L.M.; Ruiz-Moreno, A.; Gomez-Huelgas, R.; Bernal-Lopez, M.R. Metabolically Healthy Obesity: Presence of Arterial Stiffness in the Prepubescent Population. *Int. J. Environ. Res. Public Health* **2020**, *17*, 96995. [CrossRef] [PubMed]
49. Genovesi, S.; Montelisciani, L.; Viazzi, F.; Giussani, M.; Lieti, G.; Patti, I.; Orlando, A.; Antolini, L.; Salvi, P.; Parati, G. Uric acid and arterial stiffness in children and adolescents: Role of insulin resistance and blood pressure. *Front. Cardiovasc. Med.* **2022**, *9*, 978366. [CrossRef] [PubMed]
50. Hvidt, K.N.; Olsen, M.H.; Holm, J.C.; Ibsen, H. Obese children and adolescents have elevated nighttime blood pressure independent of insulin resistance and arterial stiffness. *Am. J. Hypertens.* **2014**, *27*, 1408–1415. [CrossRef] [PubMed]
51. Lorincz, H.; Somodi, S.; Ratku, B.; Harangi, M.; Paragh, G. Crucial Regulatory Role of Organokines in Relation to Metabolic Changes in Non-Diabetic Obesity. *Metabolites* **2023**, *13*, 270. [CrossRef] [PubMed]
52. Dangardt, F.; Charakida, M.; Georgiopoulos, G.; Chiesa, S.T.; Rapala, A.; Wade, K.H.; Hughes, A.D.; Timpson, N.J.; Pateras, K.; Finer, N.; et al. Association between fat mass through adolescence and arterial stiffness: A population-based study from The Avon Longitudinal Study of Parents and Children. *Lancet Child. Adolesc. Health* **2019**, *3*, 474–481. [CrossRef] [PubMed]
53. Genovesi, S.; Brambilla, P.; Giussani, M.; Galbiati, S.; Mastriani, S.; Pieruzzi, F.; Stella, A.; Valsecchi, M.G.; Antolini, L. Insulin resistance, prehypertension, hypertension and blood pressure values in paediatric age. *J. Hypertens* **2012**, *30*, 327–335. [CrossRef] [PubMed]
54. Brambilla, P.; Antolini, L.; Street, M.E.; Giussani, M.; Galbiati, S.; Valsecchi, M.G.; Stella, A.; Zuccotti, G.V.; Bernasconi, S.; Genovesi, S. Adiponectin and hypertension in normal-weight and obese children. *Am. J. Hypertens.* **2013**, *26*, 257–264. [CrossRef]
55. Maki-Petaja, K.M.; Barrett, S.M.; Evans, S.V.; Cheriyan, J.; McEniery, C.M.; Wilkinson, I.B. The Role of the Autonomic Nervous System in the Regulation of Aortic Stiffness. *Hypertension* **2016**, *68*, 1290–1297. [CrossRef]
56. Grassi, G.; Giannattasio, C.; Failla, M.; Pesenti, A.; Peretti, G.; Marinoni, E.; Fraschini, N.; Vailati, S.; Mancia, G. Sympathetic modulation of radial artery compliance in congestive heart failure. *Hypertension* **1995**, *26*, 348–354. [CrossRef] [PubMed]
57. Shadwick, R.E. Mechanical design in arteries. *J. Exp. Biol.* **1999**, *202*, 3305–3313. [CrossRef] [PubMed]
58. Kienecker, E.W.; Knoche, H. Sympathetic innervation of the pulmonary artery, ascending aorta, and coronar glomera of the rabbit. A fluorescence microscopic study. *Cell Tissue Res.* **1978**, *188*, 329–333. [CrossRef] [PubMed]
59. Tebbs, B.T. The Sympathetic Innervation of the Aorta and Intercostal Arteries. *J. Anat. Physiol.* **1898**, *32*, 308–311. [PubMed]
60. Peterson, L.H. Regulation of blood vessels. *Circulation* **1960**, *21*, 749–759. [CrossRef] [PubMed]
61. Failla, M.; Grappiolo, A.; Emanuelli, G.; Vitale, G.; Fraschini, N.; Bigoni, M.; Grieco, N.; Denti, M.; Giannattasio, C.; Mancia, G. Sympathetic tone restrains arterial distensibility of healthy and atherosclerotic subjects. *J. Hypertens* **1999**, *17*, 1117–1123. [CrossRef] [PubMed]
62. Webb, D.R.; Khunti, K.; Silverman, R.; Gray, L.J.; Srinivasan, B.; Lacy, P.S.; Williams, B.; Davies, M.J. Impact of metabolic indices on central artery stiffness: Independent association of insulin resistance and glucose with aortic pulse wave velocity. *Diabetologia* **2010**, *53*, 1190–1198. [CrossRef]
63. Emoto, M.; Nishizawa, Y.; Kawagishi, T.; Maekawa, K.; Hiura, Y.; Kanda, H.; Izumotani, K.; Shoji, T.; Ishimura, E.; Inaba, M.; et al. Stiffness indexes beta of the common carotid and femoral arteries are associated with insulin resistance in NIDDM. *Diabetes Care* **1998**, *21*, 1178–1182. [CrossRef]
64. Azukaitis, K.; Kirchner, M.; Doyon, A.; Litwin, M.; Bayazit, A.; Duzova, A.; Canpolat, N.; Jankauskiene, A.; Shroff, R.; Melk, A.; et al. Arterial Stiffness and Chronic Kidney Disease Progression in Children. *Clin. J. Am. Soc. Nephrol.* **2022**, *17*, 1467–1476. [CrossRef]

Disclaimer/Publisher's Note: The statements, opinions and data contained in all publications are solely those of the individual author(s) and contributor(s) and not of MDPI and/or the editor(s). MDPI and/or the editor(s) disclaim responsibility for any injury to people or property resulting from any ideas, methods, instructions or products referred to in the content.

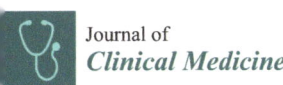

Review

Changes in Arterial Stiffness in Response to Blood Flow Restriction Resistance Training: A Narrative Review

Ioana Mădălina Zota [1], Cristina Mihaela Ghiciuc [2,*], Doina Clementina Cojocaru [1,*], Corina Lucia Dima-Cozma [1], Maria Magdalena Leon [1], Radu Sebastian Gavril [1], Mihai Roca [1], Alexandru Dan Costache [1], Alexandra Mașaleru [1], Larisa Anghel [1], Cristian Stătescu [1], Radu Andy Sascău [1] and Florin Mitu [1,3]

[1] Department of Medical Specialties I, Faculty of Medicine, Grigore T. Popa University of Medicine and Pharmacy, 700111 Iași, Romania; ioana-madalina.chiorescu@umfiasi.ro (I.M.Z.); cozma.dima@umfiasi.ro (C.L.D.-C.); maria.leon@umfiasi.ro (M.M.L.); sebastian.gavril@umfiasi.ro (R.S.G.); mihai.c.roca@umfiasi.ro (M.R.); dan-alexandru.costache@umfiasi.ro (A.D.C.); alexandra.mastaleru@umfiasi.ro (A.M.); larisa.anghel@umfiasi.ro (L.A.); cristian.statescu@umfiasi.ro (C.S.); radu.sascau@umfiasi.ro (R.A.S.); florin.mitu@umfiasi.ro (F.M.)

[2] Pharmacology, Clinical Pharmacology and Algeziology, Department of Morpho-Functional Sciences II, Faculty of Medicine, Grigore T. Popa University of Medicine and Pharmacy, 700111 Iași, Romania

[3] Academy of Medical Sciences of Romania, Ion C. Brătianu Boulevard No 1, 030167 Bucharest, Romania

* Correspondence: cristina.ghiciuc@umfiasi.ro (C.M.G.); doina.cojocaru@umfiasi.ro (D.C.C.)

Abstract: Arterial stiffness naturally increases with age and is a known predictor of cardiovascular morbimortality. Blood flow restriction (BFR) training involves decreasing muscle blood flow by applying a strap or a pneumatic cuff during exercise. BFR induces muscle hypertrophy even at low intensities, making it an appealing option for older, untrained individuals. However, BFR use in patients with cardiovascular comorbidities is limited by the increased pressor and chronotropic response observed in hypertensive elderly patients. Furthermore, the impact of BFR on vascular function remains unclear. We conducted a comprehensive literature review according to PRISMA guidelines, summarizing available data on the acute and long-term consequences of BFR training on vascular function. Although evidence is still scarce, it seems that BFR has a mild or neutral long-term impact on arterial stiffness. However, current research shows that BFR can cause an abrupt, albeit transient, increase in PWV and central blood pressure. BFR and, preferably, lower-body BFR, should be prescribed with caution in older populations, especially in hypertensive patients who have an exacerbated muscle metaboreflex pressor response. Longer follow-up studies are required to assess the chronic effect of BFR training on arterial stiffness, especially in elderly patients who are usually unable to tolerate high-intensity resistance exercises.

Keywords: blood flow restriction training; vascular stiffness; pulse wave velocity; vascular aging; resistance training

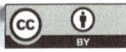

1. Introduction

Resistance training in addition to aerobic exercise is associated with lower cardiovascular risk and all-cause mortality [1]. Current cardiovascular prevention guidelines recommend a resistance training protocol consisting of 1–3 sets of 8–12 repetitions at 60–80% of the patient's repetition maximum (1RM), with 8–10 various exercises involving different major muscle groups performed at least 2 days per week [1,2]. However, elderly patients with associated osteoarthritis and cardiovascular disease are unable to withstand high mechanical stress. Such patients are usually prescribed lower-resistance training regiments, 40–50% of 1RM, along with a greater number of repetitions per set (10–15) [3]. However, exercise intensities below 70% of 1RM usually fail to produce significant muscle hypertrophy or strength gain, and several studies have approached the use of low-intensity BFR (blood flow restriction) training as an alternative strength training modality in patients with stable coronary artery disease [4,5].

Resistance training with BFR involves decreasing muscle blood flow by applying a strap or a blood pressure cuff during exercise. BFR allows effective training of skeletal muscles at lower intensities, making it suitable for untrained subjects and patients with orthopedic comorbidities [6], with muscle hypertrophy occurring even at low-intensity training (20% of 1RM) [7]. However, this technique is rarely used in patients with cardiovascular comorbidities due to safety concerns [2].

Arterial stiffness is a pivotal element in the pathogenesis of cardiovascular disease, considered an independent predictor of cardiovascular mortality and event risk [8]. Arterial stiffening is naturally associated with aging, but is accelerated in the presence of respiratory, metabolic, and cardiovascular comorbidities. Vascular stiffness is usually assessed as the aortic pulse wave travel velocity (PWV), but AIx is also accepted as a surrogate arterial stiffness parameter [9].

In healthy populations, regular exercise has a beneficial impact on vascular function. However, the acute and chronic effects of training seem to vary with different types of exercise modalities, especially in patients with coexisting health issues. Aerobic training reduces central arterial stiffness, but more recently, HIIT (high-intensity interval training) seems to have a more pronounced beneficial impact on endothelial function and arterial stiffness, mediated by the upregulation of the arterial endothelial nitric oxide synthase [10]. On the other hand, previous studies have shown conflicting impacts of resistance training on arterial stiffness [11,12]. Current evidence suggests that while high-intensity resistance training increases PWV [11], lower training intensities have a beneficial impact on vascular stiffness [12]. However, low-intensity resistance training does not correct sarcopenia, an issue which can easily be addressed with the use of BFR. Several systematic reviews and meta-analyses have analyzed the impact of low-intensity BFR training on vascular stiffness. However, they did not include all available studies (due to insufficient reported data and significant variations in protocol [13]) and provided divergent results [14–17]. For instance, Maga et al. [13] did not report significant differences in changes between BFR and non-BFR training, but included both aerobic and resistance BFR training protocols in their meta-analysis. While Pereira et al. [17] found no significant difference between low-intensity BFRE and high-intensity non-BFRE, regarding PWV, the meta-analysis conducted by Liu et al. [14] reported that BFR resistance training is more effective for regulating arterial compliance compared to traditional RT. Contrary to the results of Amorim et al. [16], another recent meta-analysis [15] showed that low-resistance BFR training in older adults will improve not only CAVI and ABI, but also flow-mediated dilation.

As previous studies have been inconsistent, the scope of this review is to summarize all current evidence regarding the impact of BFR resistance training on arterial stiffness parameters.

2. Materials and Methods

The population targeted in the current review are patients of all ages, with and without cardiovascular comorbidities, undergoing arterial stiffness assessment. The primary intervention was BFR resistance training, either isolated or compared to high-load resistance training or controls (no training).

2.1. Electronic Search Strategy

We conducted a comprehensive literature review of the articles currently available in the EMBASE, MEDLINE and PubMed databases, according to PRISMA guidelines. We used the following keywords: "blood flow restriction", "blood flow occlusion", "KAATSU training", "arterial stiffness", "PWV" and "pulse wave velocity". This review was carried out according to the Preferred Reporting Items for Systematic Review and Meta-Analysis (PRISMA) checklist [18]. We applied the following selection criteria:

- Study type: retrospective, cross-sectional or prospective analysis, case reports and case series;
- Language: English;

- Types of participants: patients of all ages with and without cardiovascular comorbidities, undergoing arterial stiffness assessment;
- Follow-up duration: without restrictions;
- Outcome: acute and chronic arterial stiffness changes with BFR training.

Reviews, case reports, studies available only as abstracts (including conference abstracts) and dissertations were excluded from this analysis.

2.2. Arterial Stiffness Assessment

We selected studies evaluating arterial stiffness as well as other parameters of vascular function.

Primary indicator: arterial stiffness assessment (pulse wave velocity: PWV; augmentation index: AIx; cardio-ankle vascular index: CAVI; ankle-brachial ratio: ABI).

Secondary indicators: endothelial dysfunction assessment (flow-mediated dilation: FMD).

3. Results

We identified a total of 11 literature reports compatible with the beforementioned selection criteria: four studies that assessed the acute influence of BFR training on arterial stiffness (Table 1) and seven studies that examined the medium-to-long-term impact on BFR on vascular function (Table 2).

The acute impact of BFR training on arterial stiffness was studied in small populations of young, healthy individuals. AIx was analyzed before, during and post- 10–55 min of exercise. Rossow et al. [19] reported that AIx decreases during BFR training (more substantially when using a wide cuff) but returns to baseline 15 min after exercise. Figueroa et al. [20] reported a decrease in AIx which persisted 30 min after lower-body resistance training (with and without BFR). Contrary to these results, in two separate studies [21,22], Tai et al. documented increases in AIx after upper- and lower-body resistance training, with or without BFR, which persisted 10 and 25 min post-exercise. At 10 min post-exercise, AIx increased more with upper- versus lower-body training (with or without BFR) and at 25 min post-exercise AIx increased more with upper-body training without BFR versus upper-body training with BFR [21].

We identified seven studies that assessed the long-term influence of BFR on arterial stiffness. Two of them included young, healthy individuals: Although 4 weeks of low-load lower-body BFR (but not high-load resistance training without BFR) improved PWV by 5% in a small group of healthy young men [6], Clark et al. [23] did not document a significant change in PWV or ABI after 4 weeks of low-load lower-body BFR in a smaller mixed-gender group (14 m, 2 f). A single study included middle-aged adults, in which lower-body low-resistance BFR training increased PWV only in the BFR randomized limb (no significant change in the free flow limb) [24]. Two studies focused on healthy, elderly adults and found no change in CAVI, FMD, or ABI after 12 weeks upper- [7] or lower-body [25] low-load BFR training. And finally, two other studies assessed the impact of low-intensity BFR in healthy, older women and showed no impact on CAVI and ABI after 12 weeks of upper- [26] or lower-body [27] BFR training.

Table 1. Acute influence of BFR training on arterial stiffness.

Authors	Population	Study Design	Arterial Stiffness Parameter	Results
Tai et al. [21]	Young individuals performing regular resistance training (≥3 days/week for at least 1 year) N = 23 (14 m, 9 f)	Non-randomized Pulse wave reflections assessed at rest, 10, 25, 40 and 55 min after upper- and lower-body resistance training with and without BFR Upper-body training—latissimus dorsi pulldown and chest press Lower-body training—leg extensions and leg curls Regular training (no BFR) protocol—four sets of eight repetitions at 70% of 1RM with 60 s and 2 min rests between sets and exercises BFR protocol—30-15-15-15 repetitions at 30% of 1RM, with 30 s and 2 min of rest between sets and exercises Cuff pressure—40% AOP, maintained during rest intervals Arterial stiffness assessed before training and post-training (after 10, 25, 40, and 55 min of rest in supine position)	AIx, AIx75 (SphygmoCor XCEL, AtCor Medical, Sydney, Australia)	Upper-body resistance training with or without BFR significantly increase AIx and AIx75 At 10 min post exercise—AIx and AIx75 increased more with upper-body RE +/− BFR versus lower-body RE +/− BFR At 25 min post-exercise—AIx75 increased more with upper-body RE without BFR versus upper-body RE with BFR. Upper-body RE without BFR also induced higher AIx75 at 25 min post-exercise compared to upper-body RE with BFR. No absolute values provided in the manuscript
Tai et al. (b) [22]	Young men performing regular resistance training (≥3 days/week for at least 1 year) N = 16	AIx and AIx75 assessed in controls and 10 min after low-load BFR and high-load resistance training Low-load BFR training consisted of four sets of 30, 15, 15, and 15 bench press repetitions at 30% of 1RM (30 s rest between sets) The high-load training consisted of four sets of eight Bench press repetitions at 70% of 1RM (1 min rest between sets) For the control measurements, the participants rested in the supine position for 10 min, in order to match the body position of the resistance exercises The tension of the wrap was determined using a visual analog scale of perceived pressure (7 out of 10).	AIx, AIx75 (SphygmoCor XCEL, AtCor Medical, Sydney, Australia)	AIx, AIx75 increased after low-load BFR and after high-load training compared to rest and control Low-load BFR and high-load resistance training resulted in similar increases in AIx and AIx75 No absolute values provided in the manuscript

Table 1. *Cont.*

Authors	Population	Study Design	Arterial Stiffness Parameter	Results
Rossow et al. [19]	Young healthy individuals N = 27 (13 m, 14 f)	Randomized cross-over study AIx and AIx75 measured at rest, upon inflation, mid-exercise, immediately post-, 5 min and 15 min post-exercise. Participants performed two separate BFR training sessions at 20% of 1RM with two different cuffs (narrow-elastic and wide-non-elastic) The exercise protocol consisted of four sets of knee extension at 20% of 1RM and: 30 repetitions, 30 s rest, 15 repetitions, 60 s rest, 15 repetitions, 30 s rest, 15 repetitions. Cuff pressure was 130% of resting SBP. Cuffs remained inflated throughout the exercise session (including rest periods).	AIx (SphygmoCor, AtCor Medical, Sydney, Australia)	AIx decreased during BFR but returned to baseline 15 min after exercise. Wide cuff use was associated with a more substantial decrease in AIx: Wide cuff—AIx decreased from 9% to −4% mid-exercise and to −9% immediately post-exercise Narrow cuff—AIx decreased from 6%, to 1% mid-exercise and to 0% immediately post-exercise
Figueroa et al. [20]	Young, physically active, healthy subjects N = 23 (12 f, 11 m)	Prospective, randomized cross-over AIx measured at baseline, 2 and 30 min post-exercise Participants performed three separate sessions—control session (no training), low-intensity resistance exercise (40% of 1RM) and low-intensity resistance training with BFR During control, subjects rested on the seated leg extension machine. Training protocol consisted of seated bilateral leg flexion and extension at 40% of 1RM, performed until fatigue, with a 1 min inter-set rest, with and without BFR. Cuff pressure was set at 100 mmHg. Cuffs were deflated during rest periods.	AIx (SphygmoCor, AtCor Medical, Sydney, Australia)	No significant change in AIx during the control session In the low-intensity resistance training group without BFR AIx decreased from 7% (baseline) to −6% (30 min post exercise) In the BFR training group, AIx decreased from 4% (baseline) to −4% (30 min post exercise)

BFR: resistance training with blood flow restriction; 1RM: one-repetition maximum; SBP: systolic blood pressure; N: number; m: male; f: female; HLRT: high-load resistance training; AOP: arterial occlusion pressure; RE: resistance exercise; AIx: augmentation index; AIx75: augmentation index at 75 beats per minute.

Table 2. Long-term influence of BFR training on arterial stiffness.

Authors	Population	Study Design	Arterial Stiffness Parameter	Results
Horiuchi et al. [6]	Healthy young men (18–30 years) N = 24 (12—low-load BFR, 12—high load resistance training no BFR)	Prospective randomized control trial haPWV measured before training, at 2 weeks and after 4 weeks of training In the HLRT group, participants performed bilateral knee extensions and leg presses (75% of 1RM)—3 × 10 repetitions with 2 min rest intervals, 4 days/week, for 4 weeks In the BFR group, participants performed low-intensity (30% of 1RM) bilateral knee extensions and leg presses, 4 × 20 repetitions with 30 s rest intervals, 4 days/week, for 4 weeks haPWV assessed before training and after 2 and 4 weeks of training. Occlusive pressure was set at 1.3 × SBP. The cuff was inflated during the entire training session	haPWV Vasera-1000 (Fukuda-Denshi Co., Ltd., Tokyo, Japan)	haPWV improved by 5% after BFR (Δ − 0.32 m/s), 95% CI (−0.51–−11.8) haPWV did not significantly vary after HLRT (+1% (Δ + 0.03 m/s), 95% CI (−0.17–0.23)
Yasuda et al. [7]	Healthy elderly adults aged 61–85 years (low load-BFR N = 7, low load resistance training without BFR N = 7)	Prospective trial FMD and CAVI assessed before the start of the study and 3–7 days after the 12 weeks training period Participants performed two training sessions/week. Each session consisted of low-load (30% of 1RM) elastic band bilateral arm curls and triceps press-downs—75 repetitions (30, 15, 15, and 15 repetitions, 30 s rests between each set) for both exercises (90 s rests between different exercises). For the BFR group (seven patients) cuff pressure was gradually inflated from 30 to 120 mm Hg on the first day of training. Cuff pressure was increased by 10–20 mm Hg at each subsequent training session until 270 mm Hg, if tolerated The mean cuff pressure throughout training was 196 +/− 18 mm Hg. Cuff pressure removed after completion of the two exercises	FMD—UNEX EF (Unex Co. Ltd., Nagoya, Japan) CAVI and ABI—VS-1500 system (Fukuda Denshi Co., Ltd., Tokyo, Japan).	No significant change in CAVI ($p = 0.150$), FMD ($p = 0.116$) and ABI ($p = 0.485$) after 12 weeks in either group

Table 2. Cont.

Authors	Population	Study Design	Arterial Stiffness Parameter	Results
Yasuda et al. (b) [26]	Healthy older women (61–85 years old) (low load BFR N = 7, low load training without BFR N = 7)	Prospective randomized trial Arterial stiffness assessed before, after 12 weeks of training, and after 12 weeks of detraining Both groups performed two training sessions/week for 12 weeks. Each session consisted of low-load (30% of 1RM) elastic band bilateral arm curls and triceps press-downs—75 repetitions (30, 15, 15, and 15 repetitions, 30 s rests between each set) for both exercises (90 s rests between different exercises), with or without BFR (according to randomized group allocation) For the BFR group (seven patients) cuff pressure was gradually inflated from 30 to 120 mm Hg on the first day of training. Cuff pressure was increased by 10–20 mm Hg at each subsequent training session until 270 mm Hg, if tolerated The mean cuff pressure throughout training was 202 +/− 8 mm Hg. Cuff pressure removed after completion of the two exercises During the detraining period (12 weeks), participants stopped resistance training, and returned to their normal daily activities as prior to the resistance training period	FMD—UNEX EF (Unex Co. Ltd., Nagoya, Japan) CAVI and ABI—VS-1500 system (Fukuda Denshi Co., Ltd., Tokyo, Japan).	No significant changes in arterial FMD, CAVI and ABI over the duration of the study.
Yasuda et al. (c) [25]	Healthy elderly subjects, 61–84 years old (BFR training N = 9, control (no training) N = 10)	During the 12 weeks detraining period, participants returned to their normal daily activities Prospective randomized Vascular function assessed before and 3–7 days after the final training session. The BFR training group performed two training sessions/week for 12 weeks. Each session consisted of low-load knee extensions (20% of 1RM) and leg press exercises (30% of 1RM)—75 repetitions (30, 15, 15, and 15 repetitions), 30 s rests between each set, for both exercises (90 s rests between different exercises) Cuff pressure was set at 120 mm Hg for the first day of training and then gradually increased by 10–20 mm Hg at each subsequent training session until 270 mm Hg, if tolerated Cuffs remained inflated during both exercises and rest periods	FMD—UNEX EF (Unex Co. Ltd., Nagoya, Japan) CAVI and ABI—VS-1500 system (Fukuda Denshi Co., Ltd., Tokyo, Japan).	No significant change in CAVI and ABI in either group. FMD tended to improve in BFR group (2.8 +/− 2.0%, 4.4 +/− 2.5%, $p = 0.09$).

Table 2. *Cont.*

Authors	Population	Study Design	Arterial Stiffness Parameter	Results
Yasuda et al. (d) [27]	Healthy, physically active elderly women, 61–86 years old (low-intensity BFR N = 10, middle to high-intensity training N = 10, no training N = 10)	Prospective, randomized Vascular function assessed before and 3–7 days after the final training session Participants randomized to low-intensity BFR or middle to high-intensity resistance training performed squat and elastic bands knee extension exercises, 2 days/week for 12 weeks Training protocol in he low-intensity BFR (35–45% of 1RM) group consisted of 75 repetitions (30, 15, 15, and 15). A 30 s resting period between sets was allocated for both exercises and a 90 s rest interval was allocated between the two exercises In the middle- to high-intensity group (70–90% of 1RM) the training protocol consisted of 37–38 repetitions (13, 13 (from the 1st to the 12th training session) or 12 (from the 13th to the 24th training session), and 12). A 30 s rest period between sets was allocated for both exercises and a 90 s rest interval was allocated between the two exercises For the BFR group cuff pressure was gradually inflated from 50 to 120 mm Hg on the first day of training. Cuff pressure was increased by 10–20 mm Hg at each subsequent training session until 200 mm Hg, if tolerated The mean cuff pressure throughout training was 161 +/− 12 mm Hg. Cuffs remained inflated during both exercises and rest periods.	CAVI and ABI-VS-1500 system (Fukuda Denshi Co., Ltd., Tokyo, Japan). Central AIx (HEM-9000AI, Omron Healthcare Co., Ltd., Kyoto, Japan)	No significant change in central AIx, ABI and CAVI in either group.
Fahs et al. [24]	16 middle-aged adults 40–64 years old (11 m, 5 f) performing lower body low-load resistance training (one limb BFR training, one limb free flow training)	Prospective randomized PWV measured 3 weeks and 1 week before training and 48–96 h after the last training session Participants performed three sessions of training per week for 6 weeks. The training protocol consisted of low-load 30% of 1RM knee extensions, performed in sets of 20 repetitions/minute, to volitional fatigue. For each patient, one limb was randomized to BFR training and one limb to free flow training. For the first 2 weeks, participants completed two sets of exercise per limb per session. During weeks 3–4 participants completed three sets of exercise per limb per session. During weeks 5–6 participants completed four sets of exercise per limb per session. One min rest intervals were allocated between all sets. The order of training (BFR first versus free flow first) alternated with each session During the first week of training, the cuff pressure was set at 150 mmHg or 50% of AOP. During the following weeks cuff pressure was set at 80% AOP (no higher than 240 mmHg). The cuff remained inflated during the entire training session	Femoral PWV (Sphygmocor, Atcor Medical, Sydney, Australia)	BFR limb (PWV increased from 8.9 (0.8) to 9.5 (0.9) m/s), $p < 0.05$ Free flow limb—no significant change in PWV

Table 2. *Cont.*

Authors	Population	Study Design	Arterial Stiffness Parameter	Results
Clark et al. [23]	Young, healthy adults N = 16 (14 m, 2 f) randomized to high load resistance training (N = 5) and low load BFR training (N = 9)	Prospective, randomized PWV measured before training and 2–3 days after training completion Participants performed three sessions of training per week for 4 weeks Participants randomized to high-load resistance training (N = 5) performed 8–12 bilateral knee extensions at 80% of 1RM to volitional failure, with 90 s rest between each set Participants randomized to low-load BFR training (N = 9) performed 8–12 bilateral knee extensions at 30% of 1RM to volitional failure, with a 90 s rest between each set. The cuff pressure was set at 130% resting brachial SBP. The cuff pressure was maintained throughout the entire exercise session	Femoral-tibial PWV (Biopac MP150 Systems, Goleta, CA, USA) ABI (MD6 System, D.E. Hokanson Inc., Bellevue, WA, USA)	No significant changes in PWV or ABI following training for either group ($p > 0.05$).

BFR: resistance training with blood flow restriction; N: number; m: male; f: female; 1RM: one-repetition maximum; HLRT: high-load resistance training; haPWV: heart-ankle pulse wave velocity; ABI: ankle-brachial pressure index; FMD: flow mediated dilation; CAVI: cardio-ankle vascular index; AIx: augmentation index; PWV: pulse wave velocity; SBP: systolic blood pressure; AOP: arterial occlusion pressure.

4. Discussion

Ageing is naturally associated with a certain degree of arterial stiffening, explained by degenerative changes in the arterial wall which accelerate with age (elastin degradation, increase in collagen fibers, and calcification of the aortic media). PWV (inversely related to arterial distensibility) and AIx (a composite parameter that varies with the site and degree of wave reflection) exhibit a non-linear, age-related increase that becomes more prominent after the fifth decade [28]. AIx and PWV are considered more sensitive arterial stiffening markers for young and old adults, respectively [28].

Exercise training improves vascular structure and function [29] and current guidelines recommend both endurance and resistance training for cardiovascular prevention. Long-term high-load resistance training (60–70% of 1RM) promotes muscular fitness, improves lipid profile, and cardiovascular morbi-mortality with a less consistent effect on brachial blood pressure values [30]. However, elderly patients are generally unable to withstand high mechanical stress and are usually prescribed a lower-intensity training protocol [3], which is less effective in correcting sarcopenia, a common finding in heart failure and geriatric populations. Although aerobic training improves arterial stiffness and is an essential instrument in cardiovascular prevention, it does not correct sarcopenia [31]. Muscle loss is addressed by prescribing resistance (strength) training at moderate to high intensities. These are not easily tolerated by elderly patients and transiently reduce central artery compliance even in young, healthy men [32] and are usually avoided in geriatric patients with associated cardiovascular disease. However, low-intensity BFR with moderate vascular restriction (100 mmHg) results in similar muscle adaptations at low intensities (20% of 1RM) [7], explaining the emerging interest in BFR as a critical rehabilitation tool in cardiovascular patients.

For this reason, BFR exercises have emerged as a promising alternative to standard strength training especially for elderly, untrained subjects and those with orthopedic and musculoskeletal impairments. BFR training is performed using a pneumatic cuff inflated in the proximal segment of the exercising limb. The occlusive pressure usually set at 1.3 times of individual SBP [6]. The inflated cuff restricts arterial flow and venous return, inducing local metabolic stress and central hemodynamic changes. Low-intensity BFR (20–30% of 1RM) is similar to standard high-intensity resistance training in increasing muscle mass and strength, independent of age [33]. Research regarding BFR resistance training is sparce, but promising in respect to safety outcomes, with an emerging number of studies focusing on the acute and long-term effects on BFR on arterial stiffness parameters.

4.1. Potential Risks with BFR Resistance Training

Sedentarism has been associated with increased all-cause and cardiovascular mortality, and increased risk of oncologic, cardio-metabolic (dyslipidemia, hypertension, diabetes) and neuropsychiatric complications [34]. However, exercise protocols are prescribed with caution in frail patients in order to avoid adverse outcomes. While regular physical activity favors fibrinolysis, high-intensity exercise may induce a prothrombotic state. This risk could be augmented with BFR, as blood lactate correlated with thrombin-antithrombin III complex concentrations and tissue plasminogen activity peak after BFR [2]. Furthermore, BFR training could cause fine microvascular damage (supported by the slight elevations in IL-6 observed after vascular occlusion) which may trigger local thrombosis [35]. However, D-dimer and fibrin/fibrinogen degradation products do not increase in older adults performing BFR [7,36]. Another concern is the potential tissue damage associated with prolonged hypoxia. Indeed, BFR leads to venous congestion and distention, and potential damage to venous valves. However, Takarada et al. [35] showed that light resistance training (20% of 1RM) combined with occlusion (214 mmHg) does not induce considerable tissue damage (assessed via creatine phosphokinase activity and lipid peroxide levels). Muscle damage can occur after unaccustomed exercise involving a large amount of eccentric contractions, but low-intensity BFR has not been associated with increased creatine phosphokinase or myoglobin concentrations [2], even in older adults [7].

Although thrombotic complications are rarely associated with BFR (a rate of 0.06%, which is lower than thrombosis incidence in the general population) [37] candidates should undergo regular coagulation and blood pressure monitoring, with special attention regarding deep venous thrombosis risk [38]. Diabetes, arterial hypertension, chronic kidney disease, rheumatoid arthritis, cancers, thrombophilia, pregnancy, postpartum, and post-surgery status are associated with higher thrombotic risk. In such cases it is useful to use Caprini or IMPROVE scales and exclude high-risk patients from BFR resistance training [38].

As with all other forms of exercise training, individuals with type 1 diabetes performing BFR training should apply routine screening precautions in order to avoid post-exercise hypoglycemia. These include pre- and post-exercise glycemia checks, assessing ketone levels and adjusting carbohydrate intake before and after exercise [38].

Impaired exercise capacity is a both risk factor and a result of chronic kidney disease. Individuals with end-stage chronic kidney disease are more prone to cardiovascular complications, fragility fractures and musculoskeletal pain and should be gradually and cautiously exposed to BFR. Furthermore, electrolyte imbalances, pulmonary congestion, peripheral edema and excess inter-dialytic weight gain are formal contraindications for exercise training in this population [38].

Compared to free flow exercises, BFR training significantly increases plasma adrenaline concentration and should not be prescribed to patients with recent cerebrovascular events. Skeletal muscle contraction activates the exercise pressor reflex (EPR), which enhances sympathetic nervous response with subsequent hemodynamic implications [39]. High-intensity resistance training at 70–100% of 1RM leads to a significant increase in thoracic pressure and a quasi-complete occlusion of skeletal muscular blood flow due to peripheral mechanical compression. As such, high-intensity resistance training leads to an acute increase in HR, systolic, diastolic, and mean arterial pressure, causing significant hemodynamic strain, proportional with the number of repetitions per set [40].

Despite similar individual perceptual responses, HR and BP (especially diastolic blood pressure) increase to a greater extent during BFR training compared to low- and moderate-intensity strength training [41]. In BFR training the exercise pressor reflex is exacerbated by the mechanical vasculature compression, which is higher than the endogenous muscular compression obtained with high-resistance training [39]. BFR training reduces venous return, causing a decrease in systolic volume. However, cardiac output increases due to a marked increase in HR and cardiac workload. The reduced venous return (cardiac preload) observed with BFR can prove useful in patients with associated cardiac disease [37]. The hemodynamic changes observed after BFR are transient, as HR and BP both naturally decrease 30–60 min after training, a similar pattern to that observed with high-load resistance training [15].

Acute cardiovascular changes in low-load BFR training are similar for young and healthy older adults [42]. However, preexistent hypertension is associated with endothelial dysfunction, elevated sympathetic activity, and altered muscle metabo- and mechano-reflexes, explaining the heightened hemodynamic response observed with BFR training [43]. For instance, although BFR without exercise does not significantly impact BP values in healthy young subjects [44], hypertensive elderly women present a mild to moderate pressor response to resting BFR [40]. Abrupt increases in BP increase the risk of cerebrovascular events, raising concerns regarding the safety of this technique in patients with cardiovascular disease. However, a previous analysis of 18 elderly hypertensive females reported similar pressor response after high-load RT and low-resistance BFR [40], recommending equalization of volumes and recovery times in order to minimize BP elevations during exercise [40]. Although two studies have applied BFR training in patients with stable cardiovascular disease with no reported adverse outcomes [4,5], the safety of BFR training in patients with hypertension or associated cardiovascular disease is yet to be determined in larger studies with a longer follow-up.

Nascimento et al. recently published a set of criteria requiring immediate BFR training termination, including (but not limited to) neurological symptoms (confusion, dizziness, impaired balance), nausea or vomiting, significant arrythmia, decrease in SBP or an acute pressor response, chest pain or discomfort suggesting myocardial ischemia, discoloration or significant pain or temperature change in the affected limb [38].

Increased and prolonged activation of the muscle metaboreflex secondary to BFR training may increase BP and illicit abnormal cardiovascular responses (increased retrograde shear stress, intermittent sympathetic overactivation), which raises concerns in prescribing the exercise program to patients with established cardiovascular disease [43]. Indeed, several adverse outcomes, ranging from mild (dizziness, nausea, subcutaneous hemorrhage) [45] to worrisome rhabdomyolysis and central retinal vein occlusion [46] have been reported with BFR training. However, BFR training rarely leads to serious adverse outcomes when performed according to guidelines, in a controlled clinical environment [47].

4.2. Peripheral Blood Flow Changes in BFR Resistance Training

From a physiological and cellular perspective, exercise upregulates the activity of arterial endothelial nitric oxide synthase, improving endothelial function and reducing arterial stiffness. In healthy individuals, acute aerobic training reduces central arterial stiffness, wave reflections, and it is postulated that regular aerobic exercise may delay vascular aging. On the other hand, acute bouts of resistance exercise may cause a transient increase in central arterial stiffness [10]. Indeed, even in healthy young adults, traditional strength training ($\geq$60% of 1RM) increases sympathetic activity and endothelin 1 levels, inducing an acute transient increase in arterial stiffness (PWV) [37]. Although chronic high-intensity resistance training increases arterial stiffness by 11.6% [11], low training intensities can reduce brachial-ankle PWV [12]. However, the effect of RT on arterial stiffness is more pronounced in young patients, which inherently have low arterial stiffness parameters, which could yield these results clinically insignificant [11]. Furthermore, the increase in arterial stiffness with high-intensity RT is attenuated with simultaneous aerobic training, supporting current guidelines that recommend a combination of both exercise modalities.

With BFR training, the increased shear stress obtained with cuff deflation and reperfusion mechanically stimulates endothelial nitric oxide synthase increasing NO production [48]. As low-intensity resistance training has a beneficial impact on arterial stiffness [12], it was postulated that chronic low-intensity BFR could have a beneficial effect on peripheral vascular function [48].

As shown by Tai et al. [21], upper- and lower-body resistance training exercised have different consequences on vascular stiffness, which can be explained by the variation in transit time of the returning pulse waveform. Upper-body resistance training, with or without BFR is associated with an acute increase in AIx and AIx75, which persists up to 25 min post-exercise [21,22]. On the other hand, with lower-body training (with or without BFR), a significant increase in AIx75 can be observed 10 min after exercise, but not at 25, 40, and 55 min after exercise. As such, current evidence suggests that lower-body resistance training with or without BFR has a lesser impact on pulse wave reflections [21]. Indeed, two other studies documented decreases in AIx after low-resistance lower-body BFR training [19,20] reported similar decreases in AIx 30 min after low-resistance lower-body RE with or without BFR. As arterial stiffness parameters return to baseline shortly after training, the effect could be explained by post-exercise vasodilation [19].

The study of the short- and medium-term impact of BFR resistance training on vascular stiffness has yielded divergent results. Horiuchi et al. [6] showed that 4 weeks of BFR reduces arterial stiffness in healthy young men, as opposed to high-intensity resistance training, which produced the opposite effect. Clark et al. [23] reported no significant change in PWV following 4 weeks of either low-intensity (30% of 1RM) BFR or high-intensity (80% of 1RM) lower-body training in young, healthy adults. On the other hand, Fahs et al. [24] reported a small but statistically significant increase in PWV after 6 weeks of low-load BFR in healthy, middle-aged adults. And lastly, several studies performed in older adults showed that 12 weeks of low-load resistance training (with and without BFR) did not significantly alter vascular function (assessed via CAVI, FMD, and ABI) [7,25–27].

Fahs et al. [24] showed that 6 weeks of progressive low-load resistance exercises increased arterial stiffness in middle-aged adults with associated cardiovascular comorbidities. The effect could be explained by increased oxidative stress and a subsequent reduction in nitric oxide bioavailability. The increase in peripheral arterial stiffness was more prominent with BFR compared to free flow training. The same study observed an inverse relationship between pre-training PWV and the change in PWV, which could suggest that the increase in arterial stiffness could be an adaptive response to external compression (cuff pressure and muscle contractions). Although the average increase in arterial stiffness was mild (0.6 m/s, 6.7%), this could have significant long-term implications, as each 1 m/s increase in PWV leads to a 13–15% increase in mortality [49].

4.3. The Importance of BFR Protocol

The lack of consistency regarding study methodologies and protocols, especially regarding BFR pressures, poses a significant limitation in comparing the results of previous stud=ies.

As shown by Rossow et al. [19], cuff type impacts training outcome, since cardiovascular responses, ratings of perceived exertion and pain are higher with the use of wider, non-elastic cuffs. The authors reported a higher decrease in AIx during BFR with wide cuff use, although arterial stiffness parameters returned to baseline 15 min after exercise [19].

Previous studies have used different protocols regarding applied cuff pressure. Limb occlusion pressure (LOP) and a more personalized approach, is the current guideline-recommended approach in BFR training [47]. LOP provides a more objective way to implement BFR training and understand its long-term effects on vascular function. LOP is also considered to have a lesser risk of acute exercise-related adverse events, especially in high-risk patients.

Another important protocol variation is the implementation of continuous versus intermittent pressure during exercise. When using LOP, both continuous and intermittent BFR provide similar grades of muscle hypertrophy [50,51]. Maintaining cuff pressure during rest intervals increases post-exercise release of noradrenaline and is associated with a heightened brachial blood pressure increase [37]. Intermittent BFR requires cuff deflation during rest periods and is the preferred method for patients with associated risk factors, as it reduces the acute hemodynamic stress to BFR [52], including arterial stiffness measures [20]. With continuous pressure, Rossow et al. [19] noted a decrease in AIx after cuff inflation and that persisted during exercise, but returned to baseline values 5 min post-exercise. However, in another study which used intermittent BFR [20], AIx dropped below baseline 30 min post-exercise, emphasizing the importance of protocols.

5. Conclusions

Despite the increasing number of reports that study the effects of BFR training on vascular function, evidence regarding the long-term effects of BFR remains scarce and no firm recommendation can be made at this point. Furthermore, interpretation of the current literature data is limited by the wide variation in sample sizes, population characteristics, but also BFR protocols (cuff pressure, number of repetitions, training duration, etc.).

Overall, it seems that BFR has a mild or neutral long-term impact on arterial stiffness. However, current research shows that BFR can cause an abrupt, albeit transient, increase in PWV and central blood pressure, even in healthy young people. This effect seems to be more prominent in elderly and hypertensive individuals with an exacerbated muscle metaboreflex pressor response. BFR and, preferably, lower-body BFR, should be prescribed with caution in older populations with preexisting cardiovascular comorbidities.

Further research should focus on developing safe BFR protocols regarding potential moderator variables (age, sex, cuff pressure, training frequency, and intensity) and on the long-term follow-up of vascular stiffness variations with BFR training.

Author Contributions: Conceptualization, I.M.Z., C.M.G. and F.M.; methodology, I.M.Z., C.M.G. and F.M.; validation, M.M.L.; investigation, I.M.Z., M.M.L. and A.M.; resources, M.R. and D.C.C.; writing—original draft preparation, C.S., R.A.S., A.D.C. and L.A.; writing—review and editing, A.M., M.M.L., C.L.D.-C. and R.S.G.; visualization, R.S.G.; supervision, F.M. All authors have read and agreed to the published version of the manuscript.

Funding: This research received no external funding.

Institutional Review Board Statement: Not applicable.

Conflicts of Interest: The authors declare no conflict of interest.

References

1. Visseren, F.L.J.; Mach, F.; Smulders, Y.M.; Carballo, D.; Koskinas, K.C.; Bäck, M.; Benetos, A.; Biffi, A.; Boavida, J.-M.; Capodanno, D.; et al. 2021 ESC Guidelines on Cardiovascular Disease Prevention in Clinical Practice. *Eur. Heart J.* **2021**, *42*, 3227–3337. [CrossRef]
2. Loenneke, J.P.; Wilson, J.M.; Wilson, G.J.; Pujol, T.J.; Bemben, M.G. Potential Safety Issues with Blood Flow Restriction Training: Safety of Blood Flow-Restricted Exercise. *Scand. J. Med. Sci. Sports* **2011**, *21*, 510–518. [CrossRef]
3. Garber, C.E.; Blissmer, B.; Deschenes, M.R.; Franklin, B.A.; Lamonte, M.J.; Lee, I.-M.; Nieman, D.C.; Swain, D.P. Quantity and Quality of Exercise for Developing and Maintaining Cardiorespiratory, Musculoskeletal, and Neuromotor Fitness in Apparently Healthy Adults: Guidance for Prescribing Exercise. *Med. Sci. Sports Exerc.* **2011**, *43*, 1334–1359. [CrossRef]
4. Madarame, H.; Kurano, M.; Fukumura, K.; Fukuda, T.; Nakajima, T. Haemostatic and Inflammatory Responses to Blood Flow-Restricted Exercise in Patients with Ischaemic Heart Disease: A Pilot Study. *Clin. Physiol. Funct. Imaging* **2013**, *33*, 11–17. [CrossRef]
5. Kambič, T.; Novaković, M.; Tomažin, K.; Strojnik, V.; Jug, B. Blood Flow Restriction Resistance Exercise Improves Muscle Strength and Hemodynamics, but Not Vascular Function in Coronary Artery Disease Patients: A Pilot Randomized Controlled Trial. *Front. Physiol.* **2019**, *10*, 656. [CrossRef]
6. Horiuchi, M.; Stoner, L.; Poles, J. The Effect of Four Weeks Blood Flow Restricted Resistance Training on Macro- and Micro-Vascular Function in Healthy, Young Men. *Eur. J. Appl. Physiol.* **2023**, *123*, 2179–2189. [CrossRef]
7. Yasuda, T.; Fukumura, K.; Uchida, Y.; Koshi, H.; Iida, H.; Masamune, K.; Yamasoba, T.; Sato, Y.; Nakajima, T. Effects of Low-Load, Elastic Band Resistance Training Combined with Blood Flow Restriction on Muscle Size and Arterial Stiffness in Older Adults. *J. Gerontol. A Biol. Sci. Med. Sci.* **2015**, *70*, 950–958. [CrossRef]
8. Laurent, S.; Boutouyrie, P.; Asmar, R.; Gautier, I.; Laloux, B.; Guize, L.; Ducimetiere, P.; Benetos, A. Aortic Stiffness Is an Independent Predictor of All-Cause and Cardiovascular Mortality in Hypertensive Patients. *Hypertension* **2001**, *37*, 1236–1241. [CrossRef]
9. Townsend, R.R. Arterial Stiffness: Recommendations and Standardization. *Pulse* **2016**, *4*, 3–7. [CrossRef] [PubMed]
10. Kresnajati, S.; Lin, Y.-Y.; Mündel, T.; Bernard, J.R.; Lin, H.-F.; Liao, Y.-H. Changes in Arterial Stiffness in Response to Various Types of Exercise Modalities: A Narrative Review on Physiological and Endothelial Senescence Perspectives. *Cells* **2022**, *11*, 3544. [CrossRef] [PubMed]
11. Miyachi, M. Effects of Resistance Training on Arterial Stiffness: A Meta-Analysis. *Br. J. Sports Med.* **2013**, *47*, 393–396. [CrossRef] [PubMed]
12. Okamoto, T.; Masuhara, M.; Ikuta, K. Effect of Low-Intensity Resistance Training on Arterial Function. *Eur. J. Appl. Physiol.* **2011**, *111*, 743–748. [CrossRef]
13. Maga, M.; Wachsmann-Maga, A.; Batko, K.; Włodarczyk, A.; Kłapacz, P.; Krężel, J.; Szopa, N.; Sliwka, A. Impact of Blood-Flow-Restricted Training on Arterial Functions and Angiogenesis—A Systematic Review with Meta-Analysis. *Biomedicines* **2023**, *11*, 1601. [CrossRef]
14. Liu, Y.; Jiang, N.; Pang, F.; Chen, T. Resistance Training with Blood Flow Restriction on Vascular Function: A Meta-Analysis. *Int. J. Sports Med.* **2021**, *42*, 577–587. [CrossRef]
15. Zhang, T.; Tian, G.; Wang, X. Effects of Low-Load Blood Flow Restriction Training on Hemodynamic Responses and Vascular Function in Older Adults: A Meta-Analysis. *Int. J. Environ. Res. Public. Health* **2022**, *19*, 6750. [CrossRef]
16. Amorim, S.; Rolnick, N.; Schoenfeld, B.J.; Aagaard, P. Low-intensity Resistance Exercise with Blood Flow Restriction and Arterial Stiffness in Humans: A Systematic Review. *Scand. J. Med. Sci. Sports* **2021**, *31*, 498–509. [CrossRef]
17. Pereira-Neto, E.A.; Lewthwaite, H.; Boyle, T.; Johnston, K.; Bennett, H.; Williams, M.T. Effects of Exercise Training with Blood Flow Restriction on Vascular Function in Adults: A Systematic Review and Meta-Analysis. *PeerJ* **2021**, *9*, e11554. [CrossRef]
18. Liberati, A.; Altman, D.G.; Tetzlaff, J.; Mulrow, C.; Gøtzsche, P.C.; Ioannidis, J.P.A.; Clarke, M.; Devereaux, P.J.; Kleijnen, J.; Moher, D. The PRISMA Statement for Reporting Systematic Reviews and Meta-Analyses of Studies That Evaluate Healthcare Interventions: Explanation and Elaboration. *BMJ* **2009**, *339*, b2700. [CrossRef]
19. Rossow, L.M.; Fahs, C.A.; Loenneke, J.P.; Thiebaud, R.S.; Sherk, V.D.; Abe, T.; Bemben, M.G. Cardiovascular and Perceptual Responses to Blood-Flow-Restricted Resistance Exercise with Differing Restrictive Cuffs. *Clin. Physiol. Funct. Imaging* **2012**, *32*, 331–337. [CrossRef] [PubMed]

20. Figueroa, A.; Vicil, F. Post-Exercise Aortic Hemodynamic Responses to Low-Intensity Resistance Exercise with and without Vascular Occlusion. *Scand. J. Med. Sci. Sports* **2011**, *21*, 431–436. [CrossRef] [PubMed]
21. Tai, Y.L.; Marshall, E.M.; Parks, J.C.; Kingsley, J.D. Hemodynamic Response and Pulse Wave Analysis after Upper- and Lower-Body Resistance Exercise with and without Blood Flow Restriction. *Eur. J. Sport Sci.* **2022**, *22*, 1695–1704. [CrossRef]
22. Tai, Y.L.; Marshall, E.M.; Glasgow, A.; Parks, J.C.; Sensibello, L.; Kingsley, J.D. Pulse Wave Reflection Responses to Bench Press with and without Practical Blood Flow Restriction. *Appl. Physiol. Nutr. Metab.* **2019**, *44*, 341–347. [CrossRef]
23. Clark, B.C.; Manini, T.M.; Hoffman, R.L.; Williams, P.S.; Guiler, M.K.; Knutson, M.J.; McGlynn, M.L.; Kushnick, M.R. Relative Safety of 4 Weeks of Blood Flow-Restricted Resistance Exercise in Young, Healthy Adults. *Scand. J. Med. Sci. Sports* **2011**, *21*, 653–662. [CrossRef]
24. Fahs, C.A.; Rossow, L.M.; Thiebaud, R.S.; Loenneke, J.P.; Kim, D.; Abe, T.; Beck, T.W.; Feeback, D.L.; Bemben, D.A.; Bemben, M.G. Vascular Adaptations to Low-Load Resistance Training with and without Blood Flow Restriction. *Eur. J. Appl. Physiol.* **2014**, *114*, 715–724. [CrossRef]
25. Yasuda, T.; Fukumura, K.; Fukuda, T.; Uchida, Y.; Iida, H.; Meguro, M.; Sato, Y.; Yamasoba, T.; Nakajima, T. Muscle Size and Arterial Stiffness after Blood Flow-Restricted Low-Intensity Resistance Training in Older Adults. *Scand. J. Med. Sci. Sports* **2014**, *24*, 799–806. [CrossRef]
26. Yasuda, T.; Fukumura, K.; Iida, H.; Nakajima, T. Effects of Detraining after Blood Flow-Restricted Low-Load Elastic Band Training on Muscle Size and Arterial Stiffness in Older Women. *SpringerPlus* **2015**, *4*, 348. [CrossRef]
27. Yasuda, T.; Fukumura, K.; Tomaru, T.; Nakajima, T. Thigh Muscle Size and Vascular Function after Blood Flow-Restricted Elastic Band Training in Older Women. *Oncotarget* **2016**, *7*, 33595–33607. [CrossRef]
28. McEniery, C.M.; Yasmin; Hall, I.R.; Qasem, A.; Wilkinson, I.B.; Cockcroft, J.R.; ACCT Investigators. Normal Vascular Aging: Differential Effects on Wave Reflection and Aortic Pulse Wave Velocity: The Anglo-Cardiff Collaborative Trial (ACCT). *J. Am. Coll. Cardiol.* **2005**, *46*, 1753–1760. [CrossRef] [PubMed]
29. Baumgartner, L.; Weberruß, H.; Oberhoffer-Fritz, R.; Schulz, T. Vascular Structure and Function in Children and Adolescents: What Impact Do Physical Activity, Health-Related Physical Fitness, and Exercise Have? *Front. Pediatr.* **2020**, *8*, 103. [CrossRef] [PubMed]
30. Cornelissen, V.A.; Fagard, R.H.; Coeckelberghs, E.; Vanhees, L. Impact of Resistance Training on Blood Pressure and Other Cardiovascular Risk Factors: A Meta-Analysis of Randomized, Controlled Trials. *Hypertension* **2011**, *58*, 950–958. [CrossRef]
31. Horiuchi, M.; Okita, K. Blood Flow Restricted Exercise and Vascular Function. *Int. J. Vasc. Med.* **2012**, *2012*, 543218. [CrossRef] [PubMed]
32. Miyachi, M.; Kawano, H.; Sugawara, J.; Takahashi, K.; Hayashi, K.; Yamazaki, K.; Tabata, I.; Tanaka, H. Unfavorable Effects of Resistance Training on Central Arterial Compliance: A Randomized Intervention Study. *Circulation* **2004**, *110*, 2858–2863. [CrossRef] [PubMed]
33. Karabulut, M.; Abe, T.; Sato, Y.; Bemben, M.G. The Effects of Low-Intensity Resistance Training with Vascular Restriction on Leg Muscle Strength in Older Men. *Eur. J. Appl. Physiol.* **2010**, *108*, 147–155. [CrossRef] [PubMed]
34. Park, J.H.; Moon, J.H.; Kim, H.J.; Kong, M.H.; Oh, Y.H. Sedentary Lifestyle: Overview of Updated Evidence of Potential Health Risks. *Korean J. Fam. Med.* **2020**, *41*, 365–373. [CrossRef]
35. Takarada, Y.; Nakamura, Y.; Aruga, S.; Onda, T.; Miyazaki, S.; Ishii, N. Rapid Increase in Plasma Growth Hormone after Low-Intensity Resistance Exercise with Vascular Occlusion. *J. Appl. Physiol.* **2000**, *88*, 61–65. [CrossRef]
36. Fry, C.S.; Glynn, E.L.; Drummond, M.J.; Timmerman, K.L.; Fujita, S.; Abe, T.; Dhanani, S.; Volpi, E.; Rasmussen, B.B. Blood Flow Restriction Exercise Stimulates mTORC1 Signaling and Muscle Protein Synthesis in Older Men. *J. Appl. Physiol.* **2010**, *108*, 1199–1209. [CrossRef] [PubMed]
37. Takano, H.; Morita, T.; Iida, H.; Asada, K.; Kato, M.; Uno, K.; Hirose, K.; Matsumoto, A.; Takenaka, K.; Hirata, Y.; et al. Hemodynamic and Hormonal Responses to a Short-Term Low-Intensity Resistance Exercise with the Reduction of Muscle Blood Flow. *Eur. J. Appl. Physiol.* **2005**, *95*, 65–73. [CrossRef]
38. Nascimento, D.D.C.; Rolnick, N.; Neto, I.V.D.S.; Severin, R.; Beal, F.L.R. A Useful Blood Flow Restriction Training Risk Stratification for Exercise and Rehabilitation. *Front. Physiol.* **2022**, *13*, 808622. [CrossRef]
39. Karabulut, M.; Esparza, B.; Dowllah, I.M.; Karabulut, U. The Impact of Low-Intensity Blood Flow Restriction Endurance Training on Aerobic Capacity, Hemodynamics, and Arterial Stiffness. *J. Sports Med. Phys. Fitness* **2021**, *61*, S0022–S4707. [CrossRef]
40. Pinto, R.R.; Karabulut, M.; Poton, R.; Polito, M.D. Acute Resistance Exercise with Blood Flow Restriction in Elderly Hypertensive Women: Haemodynamic, Rating of Perceived Exertion and Blood Lactate. *Clin. Physiol. Funct. Imaging* **2018**, *38*, 17–24. [CrossRef]
41. Hollander, D.B.; Reeves, G.V.; Clavier, J.D.; Francois, M.R.; Thomas, C.; Kraemer, R.R. Partial Occlusion during Resistance Exercise Alters Effort Sense and Pain. *J. Strength Cond. Res.* **2010**, *24*, 235–243. [CrossRef] [PubMed]
42. Staunton, C.A.; May, A.K.; Brandner, C.R.; Warmington, S.A. Haemodynamics of Aerobic and Resistance Blood Flow Restriction Exercise in Young and Older Adults. *Eur. J. Appl. Physiol.* **2015**, *115*, 2293–2302. [CrossRef] [PubMed]
43. Cristina-Oliveira, M.; Meireles, K.; Spranger, M.D.; O'Leary, D.S.; Roschel, H.; Peçanha, T. Clinical Safety of Blood Flow-Restricted Training? A Comprehensive Review of Altered Muscle Metaboreflex in Cardiovascular Disease during Ischemic Exercise. *Am. J. Physiol. Heart Circ. Physiol.* **2020**, *318*, H90–H109. [CrossRef] [PubMed]
44. Loenneke, J.P.; Fahs, C.A.; Thiebaud, R.S.; Rossow, L.M.; Abe, T.; Ye, X.; Kim, D.; Bemben, M.G. The Acute Hemodynamic Effects of Blood Flow Restriction in the Absence of Exercise. *Clin. Physiol. Funct. Imaging* **2013**, *33*, 79–82. [CrossRef] [PubMed]

45. Yasuda, T.; Meguro, M.; Sato, Y.; Nakajima, T. Use and Safety of KAATSU Training: Results of a National Survey in 2016. *Int. J. KAATSU Train. Res.* **2017**, *13*, 1–9. [CrossRef]
46. Ozawa, Y.; Koto, T.; Shinoda, H.; Tsubota, K. Vision Loss by Central Retinal Vein Occlusion After Kaatsu Training: A Case Report. *Medicine* **2015**, *94*, e1515. [CrossRef]
47. Patterson, S.D.; Hughes, L.; Warmington, S.; Burr, J.; Scott, B.R.; Owens, J.; Abe, T.; Nielsen, J.L.; Libardi, C.A.; Laurentino, G.; et al. Blood Flow Restriction Exercise: Considerations of Methodology, Application, and Safety. *Front. Physiol.* **2019**, *10*, 533. [CrossRef]
48. Paula, S.M.; Fernandes, T.; Couto, G.K.; Jordão, M.T.; Oliveira, E.M.; Michelini, L.C.; Rossoni, L.V. Molecular Pathways Involved in Aerobic Exercise Training Enhance Vascular Relaxation. *Med. Sci. Sports Exerc.* **2020**, *52*, 2117–2126. [CrossRef]
49. Vlachopoulos, C.; Aznaouridis, K.; Stefanadis, C. Prediction of Cardiovascular Events and All-Cause Mortality with Arterial Stiffness: A Systematic Review and Meta-Analysis. *J. Am. Coll. Cardiol.* **2010**, *55*, 1318–1327. [CrossRef]
50. Rodrigues Neto, G.; Silva, J.C.G.D.; Freitas, L.; Silva, H.G.D.; Caldas, D.; Novaes, J.D.S.; Cirilo-Sousa, M.S. Effects of Strength Training with Continuous or Intermittent Blood Flow Restriction on the Hypertrophy, Muscular Strength and Endurance of Men. *Acta Sci. Health Sci.* **2019**, *41*, 42273. [CrossRef]
51. Freitas, E.D.S.; Miller, R.M.; Heishman, A.D.; Ferreira-Júnior, J.B.; Araújo, J.P.; Bemben, M.G. Acute Physiological Responses to Resistance Exercise with Continuous Versus Intermittent Blood Flow Restriction: A Randomized Controlled Trial. *Front. Physiol.* **2020**, *11*, 132. [CrossRef]
52. Neto, G.R.; Sousa, M.S.C.; Costa, P.B.; Salles, B.F.; Novaes, G.S.; Novaes, J.S. Hypotensive Effects of Resistance Exercises with Blood Flow Restriction. *J. Strength Cond. Res.* **2015**, *29*, 1064–1070. [CrossRef]

Disclaimer/Publisher's Note: The statements, opinions and data contained in all publications are solely those of the individual author(s) and contributor(s) and not of MDPI and/or the editor(s). MDPI and/or the editor(s) disclaim responsibility for any injury to people or property resulting from any ideas, methods, instructions or products referred to in the content.

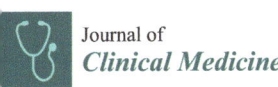 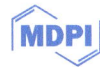

Article

Differences between SCORE, Framingham Risk Score, and Estimated Pulse Wave Velocity-Based Vascular Age Calculation Methods Based on Data from the Three Generations Health Program in Hungary

Helga Gyöngyösi [1,†], Gergő József Szőllősi [2,3,†], Orsolya Csenteri [2], Zoltán Jancsó [2], Csaba Móczár [1], Péter Torzsa [1], Péter Andréka [2], Péter Vajer [2,‡] and János Nemcsik [1,*,‡]

1 Department of Family Medicine, Semmelweis University, 1085 Budapest, Hungary; helgagyongyosi@gmail.com (H.G.); moczar.csaba@semmelweis.hu (C.M.); torzsa.peter@semmelweis.hu (P.T.)
2 Gottsegen National Cardiovascular Center, 1096 Budapest, Hungary; szolgerjozs@gmail.com (G.J.S.); csenteri.orsolya@gmail.com (O.C.); jancso.zoltan.g3@gmail.com (Z.J.); peter.andreka@gokvi.hu (P.A.)
3 Coordination Center for Research in Social Sciences, Faculty of Economics and Business, University of Debrecen, 4032 Debrecen, Hungary
* Correspondence: nemcsik.janos@semmelweis.hu
† These authors contributed equally to this work.
‡ These authors contributed equally to this work.

Abstract: Early vascular ageing contributes to cardiovascular (CV) morbidity and mortality. There are different possibilities to calculate vascular age including methods based on CV risk scores, but different methods might identify different subjects with early vascular ageing. We aimed to compare SCORE and Framingham Risk Score (FRS)-based vascular age calculation methods on subjects that were involved in a national screening program in Hungary. We also aimed to compare the distribution of subjects identified with early vascular ageing based on estimated pulse wave velocity (ePWV). The Three Generations for Health program focuses on the development of primary health care in Hungary. One of the key elements of the program is the identification of risk factors of CV diseases. Vascular ages based on the SCORE and FRS were calculated based on previous publications and were compared with chronological age and with each other in the total population and in patients with hypertension or diabetes. ePWV was calculated based on a method published previously. Supernormal, normal, and early vascular ageing were defined as <10%, 10–90%, and >90% ePWV values for the participants. In total, 99,231 subjects were involved in the study, and among them, 49,191 patients had hypertension (HT) and 15,921 patients had diabetes (DM). The chronological age of the total population was 54.0 (48.0–60.0) years, while the SCORE and FRS vascular ages were 59.0 (51.0–66.0) and 64.0 (51–80) years, respectively. In the HT patients, the chronological, SCORE, and FRS vascular ages were 57.0 (51.0–62.0), 63.0 (56.0–68.0), and 79.0 (64.0–80.0) years, respectively. In the DM patients, the chronological, SCORE, and FRS vascular ages were 58.0 (52.0–62.0), 63.0 (56.0–68.0), and 80.0 (76.0–80.0) years, respectively. Based on ePWV, the FRS identified patients with an elevated vascular age with high sensitivity (97.3%), while in the case of the SCORE, the sensitivity was much lower (13.3%). In conclusion, different vascular age calculation methods can provide different vascular age results in a population-based cohort. The importance of this finding for the implementation in CV preventive strategies requires further studies.

Keywords: vascular age; risk scores; estimated pulse wave velocity

Citation: Gyöngyösi, H.; Szőllősi, G.J.; Csenteri, O.; Jancsó, Z.; Móczár, C.; Torzsa, P.; Andréka, P.; Vajer, P.; Nemcsik, J. Differences between SCORE, Framingham Risk Score, and Estimated Pulse Wave Velocity-Based Vascular Age Calculation Methods Based on Data from the Three Generations Health Program in Hungary. *J. Clin. Med.* **2024**, *13*, 205. https://doi.org/10.3390/jcm13010205

Academic Editors: Paolo Salvi and Andrea Grillo

Received: 17 November 2023
Revised: 28 December 2023
Accepted: 28 December 2023
Published: 29 December 2023

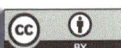

Copyright: © 2023 by the authors. Licensee MDPI, Basel, Switzerland. This article is an open access article distributed under the terms and conditions of the Creative Commons Attribution (CC BY) license (https://creativecommons.org/licenses/by/4.0/).

1. Introduction

Cardiovascular (CV) diseases are still the leading cause of global morbidity and mortality. Proper medication and lifestyle changes can lead to a reduction in their adverse impacts, in particular in the case of hypertension [1]. The cornerstone of primary prevention is to identify high-risk patients. The calculation of CV risk and its communication by the physician may make patients aware of the possible consequences, and they can become more motivated about healthy lifestyles and the long-term use of proper medication. Demonstration of the absolute CV risk is not always convincing as the numeric value that represents this risk in percentage can be relatively low with the risk of misinterpretation. The concept of vascular age was created to demonstrate if the patient's vasculature is older than their chronological age, which might be more convincing for long-term adherence [2].

The Framingham Risk Score (FRS), which is a widely used method for stratifying CV risk, was introduced in 2008. It was derived from the data of 8491 participants in the Framingham study [2]. Over a 12-year follow-up period, 1174 participants experienced their first CV event. FRS offers sex-specific estimates of an individual's 10-year risk of developing a fatal or non-fatal CV event. The paper that introduced FRS also presented the concept of vascular age calculation. This approximation is based on first the calculation of the FRS for an individual and then determining the age of a person with the same predicted risk but with all other risk factors falling within the normal ranges [2].

The Systematic Coronary Risk Evaluation (SCORE) is also a commonly used tool for estimating the 10-year risk of fatal CV events. This estimation is based on a combined database from 12 European cohort studies, primarily conducted in the general population. The database includes 205,178 subjects, corresponding to 2.7 million person–years of follow-up, during which 7934 CV deaths occurred, including 5652 from coronary heart disease [3]. Additionally, a method for calculating vascular age based on the SCORE was also published [4]. The definition of vascular age in the SCORE shows similarities with the vascular age concept in the FRS. In both cases, it represents the age of a person with the same CV risk but with all risk factors falling within the normal ranges. Essentially, this represents a CV risk solely attributed to age and gender [4].

Aortic stiffness, as measured by carotid–femoral pulse wave velocity, is a standalone predictor of future events in individuals with hypertension In the Systolic Blood Pressure Intervention Trial (SPRINT) population, estimated pulse wave velocity (ePWV) was a reliable predictor of the primary outcome and all-cause death, independently of the FRS [5].

There are previous studies which have investigated the differences between the calculated vascular ages evaluated with CV risk-based methods. In one of our previous papers published in the topic and evaluating 172 participants, significant differences were observed in the vascular age values calculated with the FRS or SCORE, as well as in the proportion of individuals with impaired vascular age when assessed with the measured PWV, FRS, or SCORE [6].

The aim of our study was to compare SCORE and FRS-based vascular age calculation methods and their relation to early vascular ageing based on ePWV on a huge population-based sample in Hungary.

2. Materials and Methods

2.1. Three Generations for Health Program

The Three Generations for Health program is organized by the National Directorate General for Hospitals in partnership with the Gottsegen György National Cardiovascular Center of Hungary. The main objectives of the program focus on reducing mortality rates related to coronary heart disease and CV ailments, exhibiting a seamless alignment with Health Sector Strategy of Hungary's goals [7]. The main goals of the Three Generations for Health program are the evolution of primary health care and collaboration between the participants involved in general practitioners' services through cooperation with the health promotion offices and also local governments [7]. Alongside evaluating the population's CV risk, another goal of this program is to introduce healthy lifestyle practices and tools of primary prevention. The program involves 806 general practitioner practices across the country; the initiative targets three generations of participants (0–18 years, 40–65 years, and 65+ years) and aims to reduce mortality from coronary heart disease and CV diseases in alignment with Hungary's Health Sector Strategy. Therefore, this initiative embodies a comprehensive strategy for assessing cardiovascular risk, combining medical methodologies, technological advancements, and strategic alignment with national health goals.

The study was performed in respect of the guidelines of the Declaration of Helsinki with the respect of the Regulation 2016/679—Protection of natural persons regarding the processing of human data. All participants enrolled in the Three Generations for Health program provided their informed consent. According to the Medical Research Council, no approval from an ethics committee was needed as all procedures were performed in compliance with the applicable standards and regulations, paying full regard to the decision made by the government.

2.2. Calculation of Vascular Age Using the Framingham Risk Score

The calculation of vascular age using the FRS was carried out following the methods of D'Agostino et al., which details the process of FRS calculation [2]. The calculation provides sex-specific results and considers age, total cholesterol, high density lipoprotein cholesterol (HDL), brachial systolic blood pressure, ongoing smoking, and the presence of diabetes or treated hypertension. The original publication also provides an estimation of vascular age, first with FRS calculation and next with the calculation as the age of a subject with the same risk but with all risk factor levels in the normal ranges [2]. In the FRS vascular age calculation, the highest value is designated as '80+' but in our calculations, we considered the age of 80 years for these participants.

2.3. Calculation of Vascular Age Using the Systematic Coronary Risk Evaluation (SCORE) Risk Score

The SCORE risk score calculation considers age, sex, smoking status, brachial systolic blood pressure, and total cholesterol, and it is different in low and high CV risk European countries [3]. The procedure for estimating vascular age using the SCORE framework shows similarities with the FRS-based method, as the vascular age of the subject is equal to the age of somebody with the same CV risk but without any risk factors, meaning a risk only due to gender and age. The calculated vascular ages with the two SCORE charts (designed for high- and low-risk countries) were in high agreement, suggesting the widespread applicability of this concept [4].

2.4. Calculation of ePWV

The equation of the ePWV was described in the study of Greve et al. [8] and was derived by the Reference Values for Arterial Stiffness' Collaboration [9]. Age and MBP were used to evaluate ePWV following the formula:

$$ePWV = 9.587 - 0.402 \times age + 4.560 \times 10^{-3} \times age^2 - 2.621 \times 10^{-5} \times age^2 \times MBP + 3.176 \times 10^{-3} \times age \times MBP - 1.832 \times 10^{-2} \times MBP.$$

The mean BP was calculated as diastolic BP (DBP) + 0.4 (SBP − DBP).

2.5. Supernormal, Normal, and Early Vascular Ageing

Supernormal, normal, and early vascular ageing were defined as <10%, 10–90%, and >90% ePWV values for the participants, following the study of Bruno RM et al. [10].

2.6. Statistical Analysis

Categorical data are presented as frequencies and as medians and interquartile ranges for data measured on a continuous scale. Data analysis was performed using chi-squared tests for categorical variables. Data measured on a continuous scale were analyzed using Kruskal–Wallis tests due to the non-symmetric distribution of the data in all cases. The p-values from statistical analyses were considered significant if the p-values from the procedure were less than 0.05. Stata Statistical Software (version 13.0, Stata Corp, College Station, TX, USA) was used for the statistical analysis, and $p < 0.05$ was considered significant.

3. Results

During the data collection period between January 2019 and January 2022, 99,231 subjects were involved in the study, and among them, 49,191 patients had hypertension (HT) and 15,921 patients had diabetes (DM). Table 1 provides the demographic data and baseline laboratory parameters.

Table 1. Demographic data and baseline laboratory parameters. Data are presented as the median (interquartile ranges). BP, blood pressure, ePWV, estimated pulse wave velocity, and HDL-cholesterol, high-density lipoprotein cholesterol.

n	99,231
Age (years)	54.0 (48.0–60.0)
Men (%)	40,443 (40.8)
Women (%)	58,788 (59.2)
Hypertension (%)	49,191 (49.6)
Diabetes (%)	15,921 (16.0)
Smoking (%)	28,956 (29.2)
Systolic BP (mmHg)	130.0 (122.0–130.0)
Diastolic BP (mmHg)	80.0 (76.0–86.0)
ePWV (m/s)	9.0 (8.1–10.0)
Cholesterol (mmol/L)	5.4 (4.7–6.2)
HDL-cholesterol (mmol/L)	1.4 (1.2–1.7)

The median chronological age in the whole cohort was 54.0 (48.0–60.0) years, the median vascular ages calculated with the SCORE and FRS were 59.0 (51.0–66.0) and 64.0 (51.0–80.0) years, respectively. In the HT patients, the chronological, SCORE, and FRS vascular ages were 57.0 (51.0–62.0), 63.0 (56.0–68.0), and 79.0 (64.0–80.0) years, respectively ($p < 0.05$). In the DM patients, the chronological, SCORE, and FRS vascular ages were 58.0 (52.0–62.0), 63.0 (56.0–68.0), and 80.0 (76.0–80.0) years, respectively ($p < 0.05$). In participants without HT or DM, the chronological, SCORE, and FRS vascular ages did not differ in clinically significant manner (51.0 (45.0–57.0), 54.0 (47.0–62.0), and 51.0 (45.0–64.0), respectively). Figure 1 demonstrates the chronological and vascular ages calculated with the SCORE and FRS in the whole group, in HT patients, in DM patients, and in participants without HT or DM.

Based on our previous publication [6], groups of subjects were created based on the arbitrary threshold of a 2-year difference between SCORE vascular age or FRS vascular age, compared with chronological age defining the following groups:

- Age difference < −2 years: SCORE−, FRS−: supernormal vascular ageing;
- Age difference between −2 and 2 years: SCORE normal, FRS normal: normal vascular ageing;
- Age difference > 2 years: SCORE+, FRS+: early vascular ageing.

Based on this definition, 17,210 (17.3%) and 10,608 (10.7%) of the patients fell into the normal vascular ageing category according to the SCORE and FRS, respectively. A total of 57,433 (57.9%) subjects were SCORE− and 24,588 (24.5%) subjects were SCORE+. Based on FRS vascular age calculation, 18,659 (18.8%) patients were FRS− and 69,964 (70.5%) patients were FRS+.

The ePWV in the total population, HT patients, and DM patients was 9.0 (8.1–10.0) m/s, 9.6 (8.7–10.3) m/s, and 9.7 (8.8–10.4) m/s, respectively. Table 2. describes the characteristic of the supernormal, normal, and early vascular ageing patients based on ePWV. In all ePWV-based vascular ageing categories, FRS vascular age was higher compared with SCORE vascular age ($p < 0.05$). Among the patients with early vascular aging, 2718 (27.7%) had neither HT nor DM.

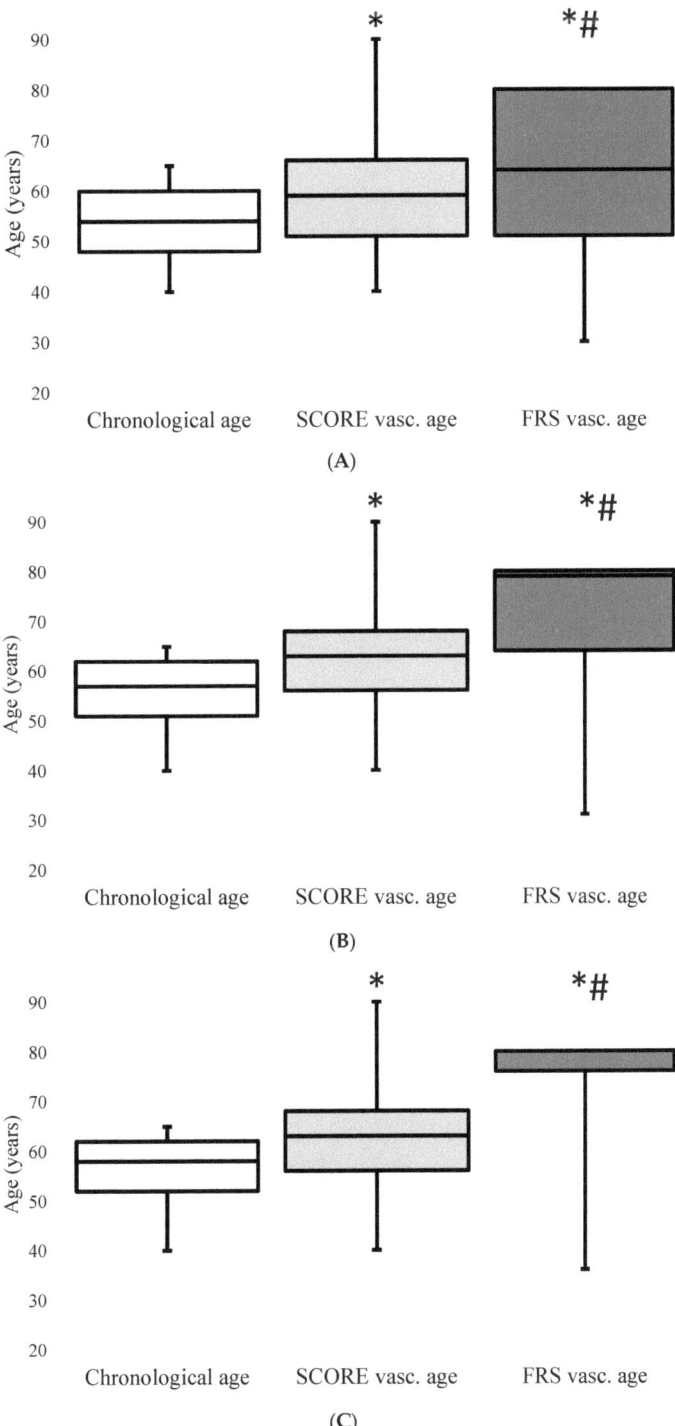

Figure 1. Cont.

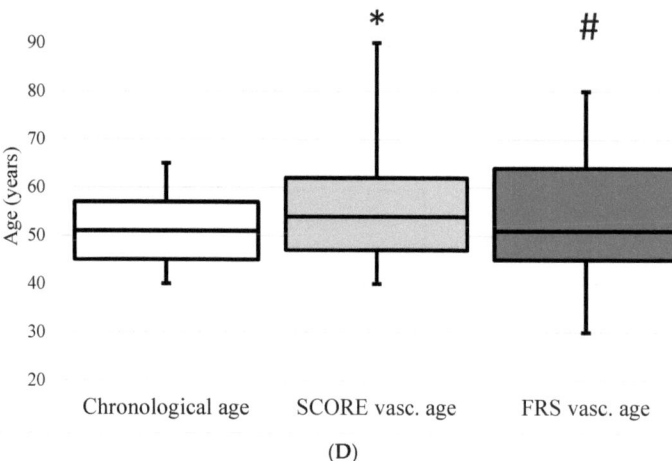

(D)

Figure 1. The chronological age and the vascular age calculated based on the Systematic Coronary Risk Evaluation (SCORE vasc. age) and the vascular age calculated based on the Framingham Risk Score (FRS vasc. age) in the total population (**A**), patients with hypertension (**B**), patients with diabetes (**C**), and patients without diabetes or hypertension (**D**). Data are presented as the median (interquartile ranges in error bars). * $p < 0.05$ compared with chronological age; # $p < 0.05$ compared with SCORE vasc. Age.

Table 2. Characteristics of the study participants in relation to their ePWV-based vascular ageing status. Data are presented as the median (interquartile ranges) SCORE vascular age and vascular age based on the Systematic Coronary Risk Evaluation method and FRS vascular ag based on the Framingham Risk Score method. ePWV, estimated pulse wave velocity, and HDL-cholesterol, high-density lipoprotein cholesterol.

	Supernormal Vascular Aging	Normal Vascular Aging	Early Vascular Aging
N (%)	10,557 (10.6)	78,855 (79.5)	9819 (9.9)
Men (%)	2671 (25.3)	32,703 (41.5)	5069 (51.6)
Women (%)	7886 (74.7)	46,152 (58.5)	4750 (48.4)
Chronological age (years)	51.0 (45.0–60.0)	54.0 (48.0–61.0)	57.0 (48.0–62.0)
SCORE vascular age (years)	52.0 (46.0–60.0)	59.0 (51.0–66.0)	67.00 (58.0–74.0)
FRS vascular age (years)	59.0 (48.0–80.0)	64.0 (51.0–80.0)	80.0 (68.0–80.0)
ePWV (m/s)	7.80 (6.9–8.7)	9.0 (8.2–9.9)	10.6 (9.80–11.5)
Hypertension (%)	2892 (27.4)	39,436 (50.0)	6863 (69.9)
Diabetes (%)	935 (8.9)	12,936 (16.4)	2050 (20.9)
No hypertension or diabetes (%)	7375 (69.8)	36,757 (46.6)	2718 (27.7)
Smoking (%)	2844 (26.9)	22,851 (29.0)	3261 (33.2)
Systolic BP (mmHg)	115.0 (110.0–120.0)	130.0 (125.0–140.0)	157.0 (150.0–167.0)
Diastolic BP (mmHg)	70.0 (67.0–72.0)	80.0 (78.0–85.0)	95.00 (90.0–100.0)
Cholesterol (mmol/L)	5.3 (4.6–6.1)	5.4 (4.7–6.2)	5.60 (4.81–6.40)
HDL-cholesterol (mmol/L)	1.5 (1.2–1.8)	1.40 (1.2–1.7)	1.4 (1.2–1.7)

Table 3 demonstrates the overlap between participants identified as having supernormal, normal, and early vascular ages with the three different methods. The FRS identified patients with EVA based on ePWV with higher sensitivity (97.3%) compared to the SCORE (13.3%); however, the ratio of the FRS+ patients was high in all vascular ageing categories. Differences between the SCORE and FRS-based vascular ageing categories were significant in all settings ($p < 0.05$).

Table 3. Overlap between participants identified as having supernormal, normal, or early vascular ageing with the different methods. Data are presented as the median (interquartile ranges); categorical parameters are presented as n (%). SCORE- and FRS- were defined as >2 years younger compared with chronological age. Those between −2−+2 years were defined as normal and those >2 years older were defined as SCORE+ and FRS+.

	Supernormal Vascular Aging	Normal Vascular Aging	Early Vascular Aging
FRS− (n %)	5521 (52.3)	13,077 (16.6)	61 (0.1)
FRS normal (n %)	1554 (14.7)	8854 (11.2)	200 (0.6)
FRS+ (n %)	3482 (33)	56,924 (72.2)	9558 (97.3)
SCORE− (n %)	2776 (26.3)	47,742 (60.5)	6915 (70.4)
SCORE normal (n %)	1868 (17.7)	13,742 (17.4)	1600 (16.3)
SCORE+ (n %)	5913 (56.0)	17,371 (22.1)	1304 (13.3)

Elevated vascular age was determined based on the SCORE and FRS in 24.8%, and 70.5%, respectively. However, only 3.9% of the FRS+ patients were SCORE+ as well, and in SCORE+ patients, the overlap with FRS+ was 11%. Approximately 13.7% of the FRS+ patients were found to have early vascular ageing based on ePWV, and only 5.3% of the SCORE+ patients were confirmed by ePWV. Approximately 97.3% of the ePWV+ patients were FRS+; on the other hand, only 13.3% of the ePWV+ subjects were SCORE+. With all three methods, only 1.1% of the subjects were found to be older than their chronological age. Figure 2 demonstrates the overlap between subjects identified with early vascular ageing through the use of different methods.

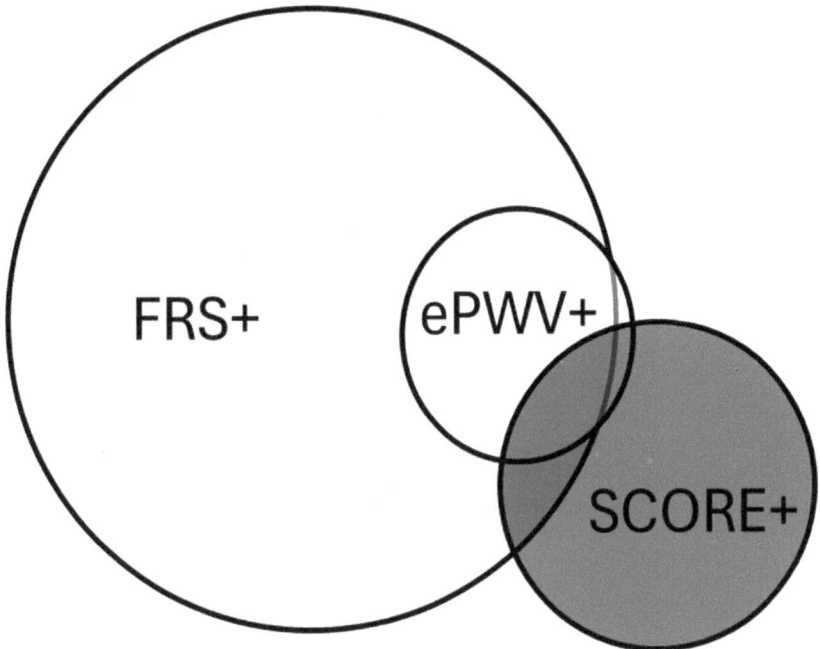

Figure 2. Overlap between subjects identified with early vascular ageing as having more than 2 years of difference compared to their chronological age with the Framingham Score-based method (FRS+), the SCORE-based method (SCORE+), or above 90% with estimated pulse wave velocity (ePWV+).

4. Discussion

This is the first study, which confirmed our previous findings in a population-based cohort using SCORE and FRS-based vascular age calculation methods, to identify different patients with early vascular ageing. Marked differences were found between the vascular age values calculated with the FRS or SCORE in patients with diabetes and hypertension, suggesting that in these conditions, the FRS-based method could be more convincing in risk communication. Based on ePWV, subjects with early vascular ageing were identified with high sensitivity using the FRS-based method, while only a small proportion of the participants were identified by the SCORE.

Our findings about the differences between FRS-based and SCORE-based vascular age calculation methods in patients with treated hypertension or diabetes are in line with previous findings. The FRS-based method resulted in a markedly higher vascular age in those treated for hypertension and diabetes in two of our previous studies, with 172 and 241 subjects involved [6,11], and in the study of Kozakova et al. including 528 participants [12]. In that study, the FRS vascular age was higher compared to the SCORE vascular age in the early vascular ageing group which was based on the common carotid artery distensibility coefficient [12]. The present, population-based study also confirms these findings, suggesting that in these conditions, the FRS-based method might be more convincing in CV risk communication than the SCORE-based method. In subjects free of hypertension or diabetes, however, there were significant differences between the groups, but the clinical significance is moderate, so the two methods might be used interchangeably.

In our present, population-based study, only minor overlap was found between patients with early vascular ageing evaluated with the different methods. This finding is in line with two of our previous studies. Vecsey-Nagy et al. found that 83.4% and 93.8% of the population had an elevated vascular age based on the FRS and SCORE, respectively, while only 42.3% had an elevated vascular age based on CACS. Approximately 38.2% of the patients were found to be older than their chronological age with all three methods [11]. In the other previous study of our lab, 78.5% and 32% of the population were found to be FRS+ and SCORE+ and 40.1% were PWV+. Approximately 9.3% of the subjects' vascular ages were found to be higher than their chronological age with all three methods [6]. These findings confirm marked differences between the identified patients with early vascular ageing and warrants further studies and consensus to overcome these methodological differences.

Vascular age calculation methods can also be divided into functional and morphological measurement-based categories, besides risk score-based ones. In line with our findings, recent publications have discovered marked differences between functional and morphological methods as well. Both in the study of Yurdadogan T et al. and Sigl M et al., in a high proportion of subjects, significant differences were found between the PWV-based (functional) and carotid artery intima–media thickness-based (morphological) methods in the identification of early vascular ageing [13,14]. Besides these emerging problems, the hypothesis that vascular ageing communication is superior to communication of the absolute CV risk in percentage has not been proven yet. Moreover, in low-risk patients, an internet-based survey with a short-term follow-up (2 weeks) failed to prove the superior effectiveness of vascular age communication on the intention to change one's lifestyle [15]. However, a recent review paper nicely summarizes the clinical potential of the vascular ageing concept and the added value of vascular ageing biomarkers to established biomarkers in the prediction of CV outcomes [16].

In contrast with the clinical use of risk scores, namely SCORE2 and SCORE2-OP, which are strongly recommended (class of recommendation: I, level of evidence: B) both in the recent CV prevention and hypertension guidelines [17,18], the use of vascular age as an alternative risk communication strategy is not involved in guidelines. Maybe by fulfilling the gaps in evidence and confirming the effectiveness of the clinical utility of different methods, the vascular age concept could have a place in future guidelines.

The marked differences between the calculated vascular ages can rely on the methodological characteristics. The SCORE risk calculator includes a lower number of risk factors compared with the FRS and considers the risk of 10-year CV mortality, which might underestimate the absolute risk of a young patient with several CV risk factors [4]. Otherwise, the FRS integrates treated risk factors as well, like hypertension and diabetes, and, in contrast with SCORE populations, patients with diabetes were also involved in the Framingham study and the factor of treated hypertension was also registered. Additionally, FRS predicts non-lethal CV events besides CV mortality [2,3]. The differences between the SCORE- and FRS-derived vascular ages in hypertensive and diabetic patients could be explained by these facts. In the case of ePWV, in contrast with risk score-based methods, its calculation is more dependent on the measured blood pressure, so it is more measurement-based, similar to PWV and CACS.

It is also worth mentioning that ePWV is only an estimation, which means that it cannot totally substitute the measurement. Moreover, there are different methods for ePWV calculation as well, with their own limitations. In the Mobil-O-Graph device, the ARCSolver method is used for PWV estimation [19], which is a predictor of CV outcome in patients with suspected coronary artery disease (in line with the ePWV method applied in our present study) [20], but it did not work well in patients with Marfan syndrome [21]. Additionally, in the MORGAM Project which included 107,599 subjects in 38 cohorts from 11 countries, ePWV (the same method like in our present paper) was only associated with all-cause mortality and not CV mortality after adjustment for traditional CV risk factors [22]. These results suggest that in the case of ePWV, similar to vascular age calculation methods, more work is needed to describe its strengths and limitations before its routine use in clinical practice.

This study has limitations that should be considered. This was a cross-sectional study which does not allow us to draw conclusions about the outcome of patients with different vascular age results. Prospective data and head-to-head comparison of different preventive strategies based on different vascular age calculation methods are necessary to clarify which method is the most effective. Additionally, when we determined the vascular age categories, we chose an arbitrary threshold of 2 years' difference, which is not based on consensus but was previously used in one of our studies [6].

5. Conclusions

We confirmed our previous results [6], in a population-based cohort, that different vascular age calculation methods can provide different vascular age results and identify different subjects with early vascular ageing. The importance of this finding for implementation in CV preventive strategies requires further studies.

Author Contributions: H.G. helped with the data analysis and wrote the manuscript draft. G.J.S. analyzed the data and critically reviewed the manuscript. O.C., Z.J., C.M., P.T., P.A. and P.V. helped with the data collection and critically reviewed the manuscript. J.N. planned the present study and wrote the draft and the final version of the manuscript. All authors have read and agreed to the published version of the manuscript.

Funding: This research was funded by the Ministry of Human Resources (Government Decision No. 1234/2017 (IV. 28.)) on the first phase of the health sector policy program related to the National Public Health Strategy.

Informed Consent Statement: Informed consent was obtained from all subjects involved in the study.

Data Availability Statement: The data presented in this study are available on request from the corresponding author. The data are not publicly available due to privacy.

Acknowledgments: We would like to thank all of the GPs who participated in the project and helped us by providing accurate data.

Conflicts of Interest: The authors declare no conflicts of interest.

References

1. Ettehad, D.; Emdin, C.A.; Kiran, A.; Anderson, S.G.; Callender, T.; Emberson, J.; Chalmers, J.; Rodgers, A.; Rahimi, K. Blood pressure lowering for prevention of cardiovascular disease and death: A systematic review and meta-analysis. *Lancet* **2016**, *387*, 957–967. [CrossRef] [PubMed]
2. D'Agostino, R.B., Sr.; Vasan, R.S.; Pencina, M.J.; Wolf, P.A.; Cobain, M.; Massaro, J.M.; Kannel, W.B. General cardiovascular risk profile for use in primary care: The Framingham Heart Study. *Circulation* **2008**, *117*, 743–753. [CrossRef] [PubMed]
3. Conroy, R.M.; Pyörälä, K.; Fitzgerald, A.P.; Sans, S.; Menotti, A.; De Backer, G.; De Bacquer, D.; Ducimetière, P.; Jousilahti, P.; Keil, U.; et al. Estimation of ten-year risk of fatal cardiovascular disease in Europe: The SCORE project. *Eur. Heart J.* **2003**, *24*, 987–1003. [CrossRef] [PubMed]
4. Cuende, J.I.; Cuende, N.; Calaveras-Lagartos, J. How to calculate vascular age with the SCORE project scales: A new method of cardiovascular risk evaluation. *Eur. Heart J.* **2010**, *31*, 2351–2358. [CrossRef] [PubMed]
5. Vlachopoulos, C.; Terentes-Printzios, D.; Laurent, S.; Nilsson, P.M.; Protogerou, A.D.; Aznaouridis, K.; Xaplanteris, P.; Koutagiar, I.; Tomiyama, H.; Yamashina, A.; et al. Association of Estimated Pulse Wave Velocity with Survival: A Secondary Analysis of SPRINT. *JAMA Netw. Open* **2019**, *2*, e1912831. [CrossRef]
6. Gyöngyösi, H.; Kőrösi, B.; Batta, D.; Nemcsik-Bencze, Z.; László, A.; Tislér, A.; Cseprekál, O.; Torzsa, P.; Eörsi, D.; Nemcsik, J. Comparison of Different Cardiovascular Risk Score and Pulse Wave Velocity-Based Methods for Vascular Age Calculation. *Hear. Lung Circ.* **2021**, *30*, 1744–1751. [CrossRef]
7. Available online: https://gokvi.hu/harom-generacioval-az-egeszsegert-program-kardiovaszkularis-prevencio-az-alapellatasban (accessed on 1 February 2022).
8. Greve, S.V.; Blicher, M.K.; Kruger, R.; Sehestedt, T.; Gram-Kampmann, E.; Rasmussen, S.; Vishram, J.K.; Boutouyrie, P.; Laurent, S.; Olsen, M.H. Estimated carotid-femoral pulse wave velocity has similar predictive value as measured carotid-femoral pulse wave velocity. *J. Hypertens.* **2016**, *34*, 1279–1289. [CrossRef]
9. Reference Values for Arterial Stiffness' Collaboration. Determinants of pulse wave velocity in healthy people and in the presence of cardiovascular risk factors: 'Establishing normal and reference values'. *Eur. Heart J.* **2010**, *31*, 2338–2350. [CrossRef]
10. Bruno, R.M.; Nilsson, P.M.; Engström, G.; Wadström, B.N.; Empana, J.P.; Boutouyrie, P.; Laurent, S. Early and Supernormal Vascular Aging: Clinical Characteristics and Association with Incident Cardiovascular Events. *Hypertension* **2020**, *76*, 1616–1624. [CrossRef]
11. Vecsey-Nagy, M.; Szilveszter, B.; Kolossváry, M.; Boussoussou, M.; Vattay, B.; Merkely, B.; Maurovich-Horvat, P.; Radovits, T.; Nemcsik, J. Correlation between Coronary Artery Calcium- and Different Cardiovascular Risk Score-Based Methods for the Estimation of Vascular Age in Caucasian Patients. *J. Clin. Med.* **2022**, *11*, 1111. [CrossRef]
12. Kozakova, M.; Morizzo, C.; Jamagidze, G.; Chiappino, D.; Palombo, C. Comparison between Carotid Distensibility-Based Vascular Age and Risk-Based Vascular Age in Middle-Aged Population Free of Cardiovascular Disease. *J. Clin. Med.* **2022**, *11*, 4931. [CrossRef] [PubMed]
13. Yurdadogan, T.; Malsch, C.; Kotseva, K.; Wood, D.; Leyh, R.; Ertl, G.; Karmann, W.; Müller-Scholden, L.; Morbach, C.; Breunig, M.; et al. Functional versus morphological assessment of vascular age in patients with coronary heart disease. *Sci. Rep.* **2021**, *11*, 18164. [CrossRef] [PubMed]
14. Sigl, M.; Winter, L.; Schumacher, G.; Helmke, S.C.; Shchetynska-Marinova, T.; Amendt, K.; Duerschmied, D.; Hohneck, A.L. Comparison of Functional and Morphological Estimates of Vascular Age. *Vivo* **2023**, *37*, 2178–2187. [CrossRef] [PubMed]
15. Bonner, C.; Jansen, J.; Newell, B.R.; Irwig, L.; Teixeira-Pinto, A.; Glasziou, P.; Doust, J.; McKinn, S.; McCaffery, K. Is the "Heart Age" Concept Helpful or Harmful Compared to Absolute Cardiovascular Disease Risk? An Experimental Study. *Med. Decis. Mak.* **2015**, *35*, 967–978. [CrossRef] [PubMed]
16. Climie, R.E.; Alastruey, J.; Mayer, C.C.; Schwarz, A.; Laucyte-Cibulskiene, A.; Voicehovska, J.; Bianchini, E.; Bruno, R.M.; Charlton, P.H.; Grillo, A.; et al. Vascular ageing: Moving from bench towards bedside. *Eur. J. Prev. Cardiol.* **2023**, *30*, 1101–1117. [CrossRef] [PubMed]
17. Visseren, F.L.J.; Mach, F.; Smulders, Y.M.; Carballo, D.; Koskinas, K.C.; Bäck, M.; Benetos, A.; Biffi, A.; Boavida, J.M.; Capodanno, D.; et al. 2021 ESC Guidelines on cardiovascular disease prevention in clinical practice: Developed by the Task Force for cardiovascular disease prevention in clinical practice with representatives of the European Society of Cardiology and 12 medical societies With the special contribution of the European Association of Preventive Cardiology (EAPC). *Rev. Esp. Cardiol.* **2022**, *75*, 429. [CrossRef] [PubMed]
18. Mancia, G.; Kreutz, R.; Brunström, M.; Burnier, M.; Grassi, G.; Januszewicz, A.; Muiesan, M.L.; Tsioufis, K.; Agabiti-Rosei, E.; Algharably, E.A.E.; et al. 2023 ESH Guidelines for the management of arterial hypertension The Task Force for the management of arterial hypertension of the European Society of Hypertension: Endorsed by the International Society of Hypertension (ISH) and the European Renal Association (ERA). *J. Hypertens.* **2023**, *41*, 1874–2071. [CrossRef]
19. Weber, T.; Wassertheurer, S.; Hametner, B.; Parragh, S.; Eber, B. Noninvasive methods to assess pulse wave velocity: Comparison with the invasive gold standard and relationship with organ damage. *J. Hypertens.* **2015**, *33*, 1023–1031. [CrossRef]
20. Hametner, B.; Wassertheurer, S.; Mayer, C.C.; Danninger, K.; Binder, R.K.; Weber, T. Aortic Pulse Wave Velocity Predicts Cardiovascular Events and Mortality in Patients Undergoing Coronary Angiography: A Comparison of Invasive Measurements and Noninvasive Estimates. *Hypertension* **2021**, *77*, 571–581. [CrossRef]

21. Salvi, P.; Furlanis, G.; Grillo, A.; Pini, A.; Salvi, L.; Marelli, S.; Rovina, M.; Moretti, F.; Gaetano, R.; Pintassilgo, I.; et al. Unreliable Estimation of Aortic Pulse Wave Velocity Provided by the Mobil-O-Graph Algorithm-Based System in Marfan Syndrome. *J. Am. Heart Assoc.* **2019**, *8*, e04028. [CrossRef]
22. Vishram-Nielsen, J.K.K.; Laurent, S.; Nilsson, P.M.; Linneberg, A.; Sehested, T.S.G.; Greve, S.V.; Pareek, M.; Palmieri, L.; Giampaoli, S.; Donfrancesco, C.; et al. Does Estimated Pulse Wave Velocity Add Prognostic Information?: MORGAM Prospective Cohort Project. *Hypertension* **2020**, *75*, 1420–1428. [CrossRef] [PubMed]

Disclaimer/Publisher's Note: The statements, opinions and data contained in all publications are solely those of the individual author(s) and contributor(s) and not of MDPI and/or the editor(s). MDPI and/or the editor(s) disclaim responsibility for any injury to people or property resulting from any ideas, methods, instructions or products referred to in the content.

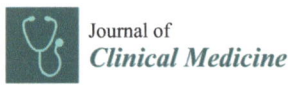 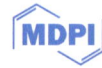

Review

Atrial Fibrillation and Early Vascular Aging: Clinical Implications, Methodology Issues and Open Questions—A Review from the VascAgeNet COST Action

Giacomo Pucci [1,2], Andrea Grillo [3,*], Kalliopi V. Dalakleidi [4], Emil Fraenkel [5], Eugenia Gkaliagkousi [6], Spyretta Golemati [7], Andrea Guala [8,9], Bernhard Hametner [10], Antonios Lazaridis [6], Christopher C. Mayer [10], Ioana Mozos [11], Telmo Pereira [12,13], Dave Veerasingam [14], Dimitrios Terentes-Printzios [15] and Davide Agnoletti [16,17]

1. Unit of Internal Medicine, Santa Maria University Hospital, 05100 Terni, Italy
2. Department of Medicine and Surgery, University of Perugia, 06125 Perugia, Italy
3. Department of Medicine, Surgery and Health Sciences, University of Trieste, 34149 Trieste, Italy
4. Biomedical Simulations and Imaging (BIOSIM) Laboratory, School of Electrical and Computer Engineering, National Technical University of Athens, 15780 Athens, Greece
5. 1st Department of Internal Medicine, Faculty of General Medicine, Pavol Jozef Šafárik University, 04011 Košice, Slovakia
6. 3rd Department of Internal Medicine, Aristotle University of Thessaloniki, Papageorgiou General Hospital, 54124 Thessaloniki, Greece
7. Medical School, National and Kapodistrian University of Athens, 10675 Athens, Greece; sgolemati@med.uoa.gr
8. Vall d'Hebrón Research Institute (VHIR), 08035 Barcelona, Spain
9. CIBER CV, Instituto de Salud Carlos III, 28029 Madrid, Spain
10. AIT Austrian Institute of Technology, Center for Health & Bioresources, Medical Signal Analysis, 1210 Vienna, Austria
11. Department of Functional Sciences—Pathophysiology, Center for Translational Research and Systems Medicine, "Victor Babes" University of Medicine and Pharmacy, 300173 Timisoara, Romania
12. H&TRC—Health & Technology Research Center, Coimbra Health School, Polytechnic University of Coimbra, 3000-331 Coimbra, Portugal
13. Laboratory for Applied Research in Health (Labinsaúde), Polytechnic University of Coimbra, 3000-331 Coimbra, Portugal
14. Department of Cardiothoracic Surgery, Galway University Hospitals, H91 YR71 Galway, Ireland
15. First Department of Cardiology, Hippokration Hospital, Medical School, National and Kapodistrian University of Athens, 11527 Athens, Greece
16. Cardiovascular Internal Medicine, IRCCS Azienda Ospedaliero—Universitaria di Bologna, 40138 Bologna, Italy; davide_agnoletti@hotmail.com
17. Cardiovascular Internal Medicine, Medical and Surgical Sciences Department, University of Bologna, 40138 Bologna, Italy
* Correspondence: andr.grillo@gmail.com

Citation: Pucci, G.; Grillo, A.; Dalakleidi, K.V.; Fraenkel, E.; Gkaliagkousi, E.; Golemati, S.; Guala, A.; Hametner, B.; Lazaridis, A.; Mayer, C.C.; et al. Atrial Fibrillation and Early Vascular Aging: Clinical Implications, Methodology Issues and Open Questions—A Review from the VascAgeNet COST Action. *J. Clin. Med.* **2024**, *13*, 1207. https://doi.org/10.3390/jcm13051207

Academic Editor: Christian-Hendrik Heeger

Received: 8 January 2024
Revised: 2 February 2024
Accepted: 18 February 2024
Published: 20 February 2024

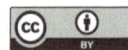

Copyright: © 2024 by the authors. Licensee MDPI, Basel, Switzerland. This article is an open access article distributed under the terms and conditions of the Creative Commons Attribution (CC BY) license (https://creativecommons.org/licenses/by/4.0/).

Abstract: Atrial fibrillation (AF), the most common cardiac arrhythmia, is associated with adverse CV outcomes. Vascular aging (VA), which is defined as the progressive deterioration of arterial function and structure over a lifetime, is an independent predictor of both AF development and CV events. A timing identification and treatment of early VA has therefore the potential to reduce the risk of AF incidence and related CV events. A network of scientists and clinicians from the COST Action VascAgeNet identified five clinically and methodologically relevant questions regarding the relationship between AF and VA and conducted a narrative review of the literature to find potential answers. These are: (1) Are VA biomarkers associated with AF? (2) Does early VA predict AF occurrence better than chronological aging? (3) Is early VA a risk enhancer for the occurrence of CV events in AF patients? (4) Are devices measuring VA suitable to perform subclinical AF detection? (5) Does atrial-fibrillation-related rhythm irregularity have a negative impact on the measurement of vascular age? Results showed that VA is a powerful and independent predictor of AF incidence, however, its role as risk modifier for the occurrence of CV events in patients with AF is debatable. Limited and inconclusive data exist regarding the reliability of VA measurement in the presence of rhythm irregularities associated with AF. To date, no device is equipped with tools capable of detecting AF during VA measurements. This represents a missed opportunity to effectively perform CV prevention in people at high risk. Further advances are needed to fill knowledge gaps in this field.

Keywords: vascular aging; atrial fibrillation; arteriosclerosis; cardiovascular disease; endothelial dysfunction; arterial stiffness; pulse wave velocity; flow mediated dilation

1. Introduction

Atrial fibrillation (AF), the most common sustained cardiac arrhythmia, is associated with a high burden of cardiovascular (CV) morbidity and mortality, mainly related to an increased risk of cardioembolic stroke and heart failure [1]. The global cumulative mortality attributed to AF was 0.51% in 2017, reflecting an 81% relative increase over the past two decades [1]. The prevalence of AF is currently increasing and is expected to rise in the coming years across all age groups and regions [2]. This is primarily attributed to the growing burden of comorbidities, socioeconomic deprivation and AF risk factors such as hypertension, obesity, diabetes and ischemic heart disease [3].

From a pathophysiological point of view, AF is defined as a supraventricular tachyarrhythmia marked by uncoordinated atrial electrical activation, leading to ineffective atrial contraction and causing an irregular heart rhythm. From a clinical perspective, AF is classified as paroxysmal (PAF, episodes lasting less than one week), persistent (continuously sustained beyond 7 days, including episodes terminated by cardioversion) or permanent (stable AF rhythm with no further attempts to restore/maintain sinus rhythm) [4]; long-standing persistent AF (continuously sustained for an extended period, typically lasting beyond 12 months); valvular/non-valvular AF (valvular AF indicates the presence of moderate/severe mitral stenosis or a mechanical prosthetic heart valve(s)). The classification of lone AF, referring to AF without any other cardiorespiratory diseases or risk factors, is now dismissed.

Notably, asymptomatic AF poses a challenge to clinicians, potentially causing delays in establishing preventive strategies [5]. It is estimated that one out of ten ischemic strokes is related to a previously unknown history of AF [6]. This could be prevented by implementing digital systems and mobile health technologies for AF screening and detection, especially in individuals at risk [7].

The term vascular aging (VA) is commonly used to describe the deterioration of both structural and functional components of the arterial tree, although a universally acknowledged definition is still lacking [8].

1.1. Structural Arterial Properties: The Arterial Stiffness

At a structural level, the process of VA is identified with the progressive stiffening of the arterial tree, namely arterial stiffness (AS). This process mainly occurs at the level of large elastic arteries such as the aorta and the carotid arteries, where a mechanical remodeling of the arterial wall is observed [9]. The most commonly used method for the non-invasive estimation of arterial stiffness is the measure of the pulse wave velocity (PWV), which represents the velocity of the pressure waves generated from the systolic contraction along a defined arterial segment. Most commonly, the carotid–femoral PWV (cfPWV) is used as a marker of aortic stiffness. CfPWV has been associated with adverse clinical outcomes in several population settings [10], and predicts CV outcome better than chronological aging [11,12]. Several other methods used for arterial stiffness estimation are summarized in Table 1.

Table 1. Description of vascular aging biomarkers.

Vascular Aging Biomarker	Method of Measurement
Carotid–femoral pulse wave velocity (cfPWV)	Ratio of traveled distance between the carotid and femoral pulse site and transit time between common carotid and common femoral artery; based on tonometers, piezoelectronic sensors, cuffs or Doppler ultrasound, either simultaneously or sequentially, using ECG for gating.
Heart–femoral pulse wave velocity (hfPWV)	Ratio of traveled distance between the heart and femoral pulse sites and transit time starting from second heart sound; based on tonometers, ECG and microphones.
Brachial–ankle pulse wave velocity (baPWV)	Ratio between traveled distance and transit time calculated with occlusive cuffs placed at brachial artery and ankle; cardio-ankle vascular index is a variation using a phonocardiogram and occlusive cuffs.
Arterial stiffness index (ASI)	Marker of arterial stiffness calculated by dividing height by the timing of reflected waves from finger photoplethysmography
Cardio-ankle vascular index (CAVI)	Marker of arterial stiffness based on the stiffness parameter β, reflecting arterial properties from origin of the ascending aorta to the ankle.
Brachial pulse pressure (PP)	Measured using validated sphygmomanometers; brachial pulse pressure defined as systolic minus diastolic BP.
Central pulse pressure (cPP)	Central pulse pressure based on waveforms recorded at the radial, brachial or carotid artery, mainly using tonometers or cuffs; waveforms are calibrated with measured brachial BP leading to central systolic BP and pulse pressure.
Augmentation index (AIx)	The ratio between central augmented pressure and pulse pressure, as a surrogate indicator of wave reflections and left ventricular loading.
Pulse pressure amplification (PPA)	Central to peripheral pulse pressure amplification (peripheral PP/central PP) is due to both cardiac and arterial factors: ventricular ejection, arterial stiffness, amplitude and timing of wave reflection. VA reduces PPA values.
Brachial artery flow-mediated dilation (FMD)	Flow-mediated dilation induces the release of nitric oxide, resulting in vasodilation that can be measured by ultrasound imaging of the diameter of the brachial artery after an ischemia induced by arterial occlusion using a cuff, which is released after 5 min, leading to reactive hyperemia.
Aortic distensibility	Measure of aortic elasticity estimated by the relative change in diameter, area or volume divided by the pulse pressure generating this change; may be measured by echocardiography or by MRI.
Carotid artery distensibility	Measure of carotid artery elasticity estimated by the ratio between relative change in diameter or volume and the pulse pressure generating this change; usually measured by carotid ultrasound.

1.2. Functional Arterial Properties: The Endothelial Dysfunction

At a functional level, the hallmark of VA is the impairment of endothelial function, which is the result of a decrease in nitric oxide synthase (eNOS) expression in endothelial cells and that, in turn, promotes the development of a prothrombotic state [13] and atherosclerosis [9]. This process, namely the endothelial dysfunction (ED), is hastened by oxidative stress and occurs in response to both physiological aging and systemic inflammation [14,15]. Flow-mediated dilation (FMD), usually assessed at the brachial artery, has been established as a reliable and reproducible technique for assessment of ED [16,17], and has been independently associated with vascular disease and adverse CV events [18].

The exposure to CV risk factors, including smoking, obesity, hypertension, diabetes and hypercholesterolemia, promotes the development of both early VA and AF. Therefore, measurement of VA biomarkers such as PWV and brachial FMD in people with AF, or at risk for it, has a strong rationale and large expected impact on clinical practice to better characterize the individual CV risk and to provide targeted interventions.

However, there are some issues undermining the measurement of VA biomarkers, especially in patients with AF. First, the changing of heart period and stroke volume brings questions regarding the accuracy of measurement of VA biomarkers. The measure of PWV by sequential tonometry in a given arterial segment is exposed to an increased variability in the time it takes for the pressure wave to travel between two points. Additionally, changes in stroke volume can also affect measurements based on pulse volume and flow detection, such as FMD. For this reason, measurement of VA in patients with AF is underused and little is known about the prognostic value of VA biomarkers in patients with AF.

With all these premises, a network of scientists and clinicians from the COST Action VascAgeNet (CA18216) [19] identified a list of five clinical and practical key questions regarding the relationship between VA biomarkers and AF and critically reviewed the literature, with a special focus on studies using PWV and ED measures as reference methods for the evaluation of structural and functional arterial properties, in order to find potential answers. The list of question is the following:

1. Are VA biomarkers associated with AF?
2. Does early VA predict AF occurrence better than chronological aging?
3. Is early VA a risk enhancer for the occurrence of CV events in AF patients?
4. Are devices measuring VA suitable to perform subclinical AF detection?
5. Is the measurement of VA negatively influenced by AF-related rhythm irregularities?

2. Materials and Methods

The search was performed using PubMed/MEDLINE databases with relevant keywords on the topics. We selected peer-reviewed articles published from inception to 31 December 2023. Papers written in languages other than English, not pertinent to the present review or whose full text was not available were excluded. The complete search string incorporated inclusive keywords on VA (e.g., "vascular ageing", "vascular aging", "vascular senescence"), arterial stiffness (e.g., "arterial stiffness", "arterial compliance", "pulse wave velocity", "PWV", "augmentation index", "AIx", "central blood pressure", "pulse pressure"), subclinical atherosclerosis ("carotid intima-media thickness"), ED ("flow mediated dilation") and inclusive keywords on AF ("atrial fibrillation", "paroxysmal atrial fibrillation", "persistent atrial fibrillation"). The pertinent papers were evaluated and eventually included in the final manuscript. We considered all papers in open-access and non-open-access journals. A flow chart of the review process, the search strategy summary and the checklist for the narrative review are provided in Figure 1 and Table S1 (Supplementary Materials).

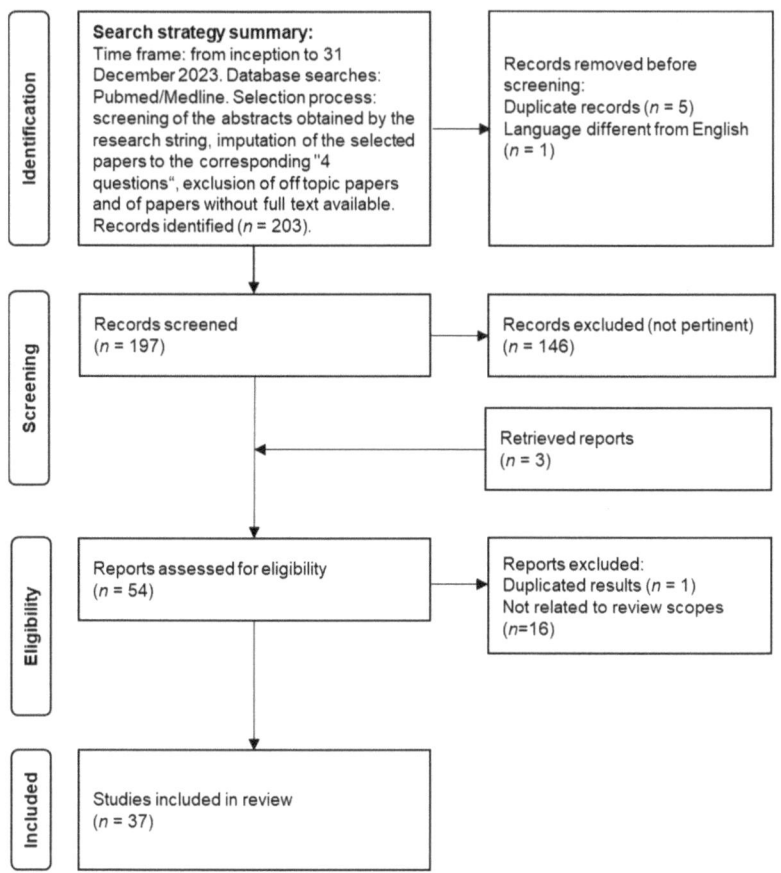

Figure 1. Flow chart of the review process.

3. Results

From the 203 papers identified, we included 37 papers, offering an overview of the current literature. Practical recommendations for the use of VA measures in the context of AF were formulated in agreement between the authors and are presented in italics at the beginning of each paragraph.

The included studies are organized in Table 2, and their results according to method are summarized in Figure 2. For more clarity, a detailed description of each VA biomarker included in the present study is provided in Table 2.

Table 2. Summary of results from clinical studies in adult humans organized according to methodology questions.

Year, Author, Country	Method (Biomarker)	Population	Study Design	Main Results	Q1	Q2	Q3	Q4	Q5
2018, Caluwé R et al., Belgium [20]	SphygmoCor (cfPWV, AIx, central pulse pressure)	34 patients with AF	Experimental study: before and after cardioversion for AF	Good agreement before and after cardioversion for cfPWV and cPP, moderate agreement for AIx.				light green	yellow
2007, Skalidis EI et al., Greece [21]	Brachial artery FMD and NMD (FMD, NMD)	46 patients with AF and 25 controls	Experimental study, before and after electrical cardioversion	FMD improved after successful cardioversion, while NMD was not significantly altered. High agreement in Bland–Altman analysis.		light green			
2016, Chen SC et al., Taiwan [22]	Omron VP-1000 (baPWV)	167 patients with AF	Longitudinal observational study	In patients with AF, a high baPWV was independently associated with increased CV events.		green	green	green	
2021, Shchetynska-Marinova T et al., Germany [23]	Echocardiography (aortic distensibility)	151 patients with AF and 54 controls	Longitudinal observational study	AF was associated with reduced aortic distensibility, left atrial size and pulse pressure. The incidence of AF recurrences increased with loss of aortic distensibility.	light green	green	green	green	
2011, Chen LY et al., USA [24]	SphygmoCor (cfPWV)	118 patients with AF, 274 controls	Observational, case-control study	CfPWV was associated with NT-proBNP level in AF.		green	green	green	
2015, Perri L et al., Italy [25]	Brachial artery FMD (FMD)	514 non-valvular AF patients	Experimental prospective study	In patients with AF, low FMD (<4.6%) independently predicted CV events.		green	green	green	
2022, Zhang J et al., China [26]	Brachial artery FMD (FMD)	291 with paroxysmal AF	Longitudinal observational study	FMD was a predictor of CV events in patients with PAF.		green	green	light green	
2016, Chen LY et al., USA [27]	IMT, carotid distensibility (Echodoppler), aortic PWV (Complior)	13,907 ARIC, 6640 MESA, 5220 Rotterdam Study	Longitudinal observational study	Higher IMT and greater arterial stiffness were associated with higher AF incidence, with modest improvement in AF risk prediction.		green	green		
2021, Almuwaqqat Z et al., USA [28]	Omron VP-1000 (cfPWV)	3882 elderly participants of ARIC	Longitudinal observational study	Low (first quartile) and high (third and fourth quartiles) cfPWV were associated with higher AF risk.		green			
2016, Shaikh AY et al., USA [29]	Arterial tonometry (cfPWV, CPP, AIx). Doppler ultrasound (FMD)	5797 Framingham tonometry sample; 3921 ED sample	Retrospective observational study	Higher AIx and central pressure, lower FMD were associated with increased risk of incident AF.		green			

Table 2. Cont.

Year, Author, Country	Method (Biomarker)	Population	Study Design	Main Results	Questions 1	2	3	4	5
2022, Nagayama D et al., Japan [30]	VaSera cardio-ankle vascular index (CAVI)	47,687 cross-sectional study; 5418 cohort study	Cross-sectional and longitudinal study	CAVI was independently associated with AF. CAVI ≥8.0 was an independent predictor for AF incidence.					
2014, Roetker NS et al., USA [31]	Brachial oscillometry, MRI (pulse pressure, aortic distensibility)	6630 participants from the MESA	Longitudinal observational study	Higher levels of systolic and pulse pressure were associated with increased risk of AF. Aortic distensibility was not consistently associated with the risk of AF.					
2012, Valbusa F et al., Italy [32]	Brachial oscillometry (pulse pressure)	350 patients with type 2 diabetes mellitus	Longitudinal observational study	Increased pulse pressure independently predicted incident AF in 10-year follow-up.					
2012, Larstorp AC et al., Norway [33]	Oscillometry (pulse pressure)	8810 hypertensive patients	Longitudinal observational study	Pulse pressure was the strongest single BP predictor of new-onset AF.					
2007, Mitchell G et al., USA [34]	Brachial oscillometry (pulse pressure)	5331 Framingham Heart Study participants initially free from AF	Longitudinal observational study	Pulse pressure was associated with increased risk for AF (adjusted hazard ratio, 1.26 per 20 mm Hg increment; $p = 0.001$).					
2021, Matsumoto K et al., USA [35]	ABPM, SphygmoCor (central BP, ambulatory BP)	769 participants in sinus rhythm	Longitudinal observational study	ABPM was a better independent predictor of incident AF than central BP.					
2022, Shchetynska-Marinova T et al., Germany [36]	Echocardiography (aortic distensibility)	151 patients with AF who underwent pulmonary vein isolation	Longitudinal observational study	Reduced aortic distensibility and increased atrial size were associated with AF recurrence.					
2013, Lau DH et al., Australia [37]	SphygmoCor (Central BP, AIx)	68 patients with lone AF undergoing successful catheter ablation	Longitudinal observational study	Central pulse pressure ≥ 45 mmHg and augmentation pressure ≥ 12 mmHg were both associated with lower survival free from AF.					
2016, Fumagalli S et al., Italy [38]	VaSera Cardio-ankle vascular index (CAVI)	31 patients with AF	Longitudinal observational study	After cardioversion, AF persistence at follow-up was associated with higher CAVI.					
2015, Kizilirmak F et al., Turkey [39]	Mobil-O-Graph (central pulse pressure, PWV, AIx)	103 patients with PAF, 103 controls	Longitudinal observational study	Increased arterial stiffness markers were associated with AF occurrence but not predicted recurrence after catheter ablation.					

Table 2. Cont.

Year, Author, Country	Method (Biomarker)	Population	Study Design	Main Results	Questions 1	2	3	4	5
2019, Zekavat SM et al., USA [40]	Finger photoplethysmography (ASI)	225,636 UK Biobank participants	Genome-wide association study, Mendelian randomization	Genetic predisposition to higher ASI was significantly associated with increased risk of incident and prevalent AF					
2010, Drager LF et al., Portugal [41]	SphygmoCor, echocardiography (cf-PWV, left atrial diameter)	73 middle-aged patients	Observational study	Left atrial diameter is associated with pulse wave velocity independently of common determinants.					
2008, Lantelme P et al., France [42]	Complior, ABPM, echocardiography (cfPWV, 24 h PP, left atrial diameter)	310 hypertensive patients	Observational study	Left atrial diameter is associated with cfPWV and 24 h PP independently from classical determinants (e.g., age, BMI, LV dimensions and geometry).					
2021, Garg PK et al., USA [43]	Brachial artery FMD (FMD)	2027 elderly patients	Longitudinal observational study	The risk of incident AF was not dependent on baseline FMD when analysis was adjusted for confounders.					
2021, Pauklin P et al., Estonia [44]	Oscillometry, SphygmoCor (cfPWV, central BP, pressure amplification)	76 patients with AF	Observational study	Patients with AF had significantly higher cSBP, cPP, PWV compared to healthy controls. Positive correlation of left atrial diameter and volume with PWV.					
2017, Cui R et al., Japan [45]	Omron HEM9000AI (AIx)	4264 participants	Longitudinal observational study	AIx values, but not brachial or central pulse pressures, were positively and independently associated with the prevalence of AF.					
2009, Doi M et al., Japan [46]	Omron HEM9000AI (radial Aix)	122 patients with PAF (in sinus rhythm), 122 controls	Observational Case-control study	AIx was significantly higher in patients with PAF than in subjects without PAF.					
2005, Shi D et al., China [47]	Omron VP-1000 (brachial-ankle PWV)	132 patients with hypertension and AF (78 paroxysmal, 84 persistent) and 136 with only hypertension	Observational study	Patients with AF and hypertension presented higher baPWV values than hypertension alone. Persistent AF was associated with higher baPWV than PAF.					
2008, Lee SH et al., Republic of Korea [48]	VP-2000 (heart-femoral PWV)	35 subjects with sinus rhythm, 33 subjects with AF	Observational case-control study	Patients with AF had higher hfPWV than those in sinus rhythm. AF was an independent predictor of increased hfPWV together with age and systolic BP.					

Table 2. Cont.

Year, Author, Country	Method (Biomarker)	Population	Study Design	Main Results	Questions 1	2	3	4	5
2014, Miyoshi T et al., Japan [49]	VaSera cardio-ankle vascular index (CAVI)	91 patients with PAF compared with 90 matched controls	Case-control study	CAVI was significantly higher in patients with PAF than in controls.	light green				
2014, Fumagalli S et al., Italy [50]	VaSera cardio-ankle vascular index (CAVI)	33 patients with AF	Observational study	CAVI obtained immediately after cardioversion was associated with short AF duration and left atrial diameter.	light green				
2021, Chung GE et al., Korea [51]	VaSera cardio-ankle vascular index (CAVI)	8048 subjects	Longitudinal observational study	High CAVI was associated with AF in those with intermediate or high CV risk.	light green				
2020, Heshmat-Ghahdarijani K et al., Iran [52]	Brachial artery FMD (FMD)	43 patients with AF and 51 controls	Case-control study	FMD of patients with AF was significantly lower than controls.	light green				
2004, Guazzi M et al., Italy [53]	Brachial artery FMD	35 patients with lone AF undergoing external cardioversion	Longitudinal observational study	Brachial FMD improved after cardioversion and returned to basal values in subjects with AF recurrency.	yellow				
2019, Börschel CS et al., Germany [54]	Brachial artery FMD and peripheral arterial tonometry (PAT ratio)	15,010 subjects (466 AF)	Observational study	FMD and PAT were compromised in individuals with AF, but associations were mediated by age and classical risk factors.	light green				
2021, Khan AA et al., United Kingdom [55]	Brachial artery FMD	30 patients with permanent AF vs. 31 patients with PAF	Case-control study	Duration and frequency of AF lead to worsening endothelial function.	light green				
2013, Polovina M et al., Serbia [56]	Brachial artery FMD and NMD	38 patients with persistent AF and 28 controls	Observational case-control study	FMD of AF patients was significantly lower than FMD of healthy controls. No differences in median NMD values.	light green				

Questions: 1. Correlation of AF and VA. 2. Prediction of AF. 3. Prognostic value of VA in AF. 4. Detection of AF with devices. 5. Accuracy of measurement of VA in AF. Colors legend: Dark green: Significant association in a prospective study. Light green: Significant association. Yellow: Neutral or absent association. Abbreviations: ABPM: ambulatory blood pressure monitoring. ARIC: Atherosclerosis Risk in Communities. MESA: Multi-Ethnic Study of Atherosclerosis. Complete list of abbreviations at the end. Instruments: SphygmoCor (ATCOR, Sidney, Australia), Omron VP-1000, VP-2000 and HEM9000AI (Omron, Kyoto, Japan), VaSera (Fukuda Denshi, Tokyo, Japan), Mobil-O-Graph (IEM GmbH, Aachen, Germany).

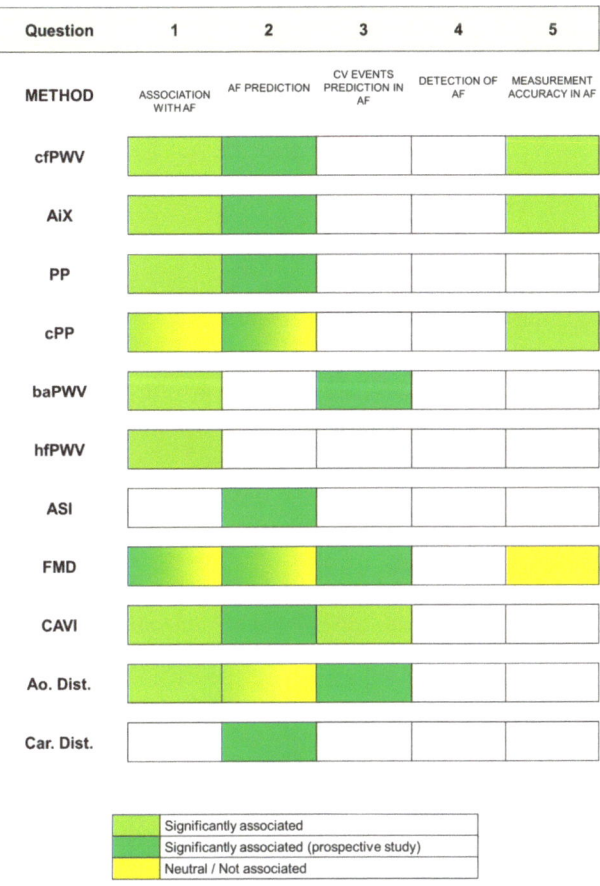

Figure 2. Results of included studies according to methods and the five questions considered in the paper.

3.1. Question 1—Are VA Biomarkers Associated with AF?

Answer: There is substantial evidence, although partly derived from small studies, that subjects with AF have early VA compared to subjects in sinus rhythm. This association is largely explained by concomitant CV risk factors, such as hypertension, dyslipidemia and diabetes mellitus, which are often present in people with AF. However, at least for measures of AS, there is also evidence that this association remains significant after multiple adjustment.

In a case–control study, 76 patients with either permanent or paroxysmal AF were compared to a control group of 75 healthy individuals. Compared to patients in sinus rhythm, patients with AF had higher PWV (8.0 m/s vs. 7.2 m/s, $p < 0.001$), central SBP (118 mm Hg vs. 114 mm Hg, $p = 0.033$), central PP (39 mm Hg vs. 37 mm Hg, $p = 0.035$) and lower PP amplification (PPA), measured as the ratio between peripheral and central PPs (1.24 vs. 1.30, $p = 0.015$). The relationship between cfPWV and AF remained significant after adjustment for age, sex, heart rate, weight, MAP and glomerular filtration rate [44]. In a large cross-sectional study conducted on Japanese men and women ($n = 4264$, age range 40–79 years), the PPA was negatively associated with the prevalence of AF and total arrhythmia, independently of CV risk factors. In a multivariate model adjusted for age, sex, BMI, heart rate, SBP, smoking, alcohol consumption, serum total and HDL cholesterol, triglycerides, diabetes mellitus and use of antihypertensive and lipid-lowering medications, as compared with subjects in the highest tertile of PPA, subjects in the lower tertile of PPA showed higher odds of having AF (OR 3.4, 95%CI 1.4–8.6). No significant associations between either brachial or central PP and AF prevalence were reported [45].

In a study by Doi et al., 122 patients with PAF were compared with 122 age- and sex-matched controls without PAF. All subjects were in sinus rhythm. AIx was calculated from the radial artery waveform using applanation tonometry. After adjustment for age, sex, heart rate and medications, AIx was significantly higher in patients with than without PAF (89 ± 1.0 vs. 82 ± 1.0%, $p < 0.001$). Each 10% increase in AIx was associated with higher odds of PAF (OR 1.6, 95%CI 1.13–2.25) [46]. These data suggest that AF remains associated with increased arterial stiffness even after restoration of sinus rhythm.

Similarly, other measures of AS, such as baPWV and heart–femoral PWV (hfPWV), were found to be higher in subjects with AF than in controls, independently of confounders. The former (baPWV) was evaluated in a population of 132 patients with hypertension and AF (78 with PAF and 84 with persistent AF) compared to 136 patients with hypertension in sinus rhythm. In a multivariate logistic regression model adjusted for multiple CV risk factors, each unit increase in baPWV corresponded to 10.4% increased risk of having AF. Interestingly, this association was no longer significant after further adjustment for uric acid, suggesting that this factor could be implicated in the mechanism of AF development in the presence of early VA [47]. The latter (hfPWV) was found to be higher in 35 subjects with AF compared to 33 subjects in sinus rhythm (1028 ± 222 vs. 923 ± 110 cm/s, $p = 0.03$). Together with age and systolic BP, the presence of AF was an independent predictor of increased hfPWV [48].

AS, measured by CAVI, also showed an association with AF. When 91 patients with PAF, after restoring sinus rhythm, were compared with 90 age- and sex-matched subjects without PAF, CAVI was significantly higher in the former compared to the latter group (9.0 ± 1.0 vs. 8.7 ± 0.8, $p < 0.01$). This difference, even if clinically small, remained significant after adjustment for age, gender, heart rate and use of antihypertensive and antiarrhythmic drugs [49]. In a study conducted in 33 subjects (mean age 73 ± 12 years) with persistent AF undergoing external cardioversion, CAVI was inversely correlated with AF duration, independently of age and cardiac chamber dimensions [50]. CAVI also showed a correlation with AF in large cross-sectional studies, such as the study by Chung et al. that enrolled 8048 subjects screened for CV disease who underwent electrocardiogram and CAVI. The prevalence of AF was significantly higher in the high group (2.2% in subjects with CAVI ≥ 8) compared with the low group (1% in subjects with CAVI < 8, $p < 0.001$). Multivariate analysis further depicted the association of CAVI ≥ 8 with AF prevalence as independent of age, sex and CV risk factors (OR = 2.06, 95%CI 1.40–3.05, $p < 0.001$). The association of CAVI with AF was also evaluated in subgroups stratified according to the Framingham risk score. Higher odds were found in people at intermediate (OR 3.06, 95%CI 1.39–6.74) and high (OR 3.88, 95%CI 1.14–13.17) CV risk [51]. In 164 subjects with AF, compared to 652 controls after propensity score matching, significantly higher odds of AF were found at each 1-unit increase in CAVI (OR 1.37, 95%CI 1.08–1.22, $p = 0.008$) [30].

Several studies focused on the association between ED and AF. Subjects younger than 60 years with AF and without any other CV risk factor (defined as lone AF, $n = 43$), compared to age- and sex-matched controls ($n = 51$), showed significantly lower values of FMD (5.8 ± 3.9% vs. 7.6 ± 4.4%, $p = 0.04$) [52]. In subjects with AF undergoing restoration of regular sinus rhythm, brachial FMD did significantly improve after cardioversion (0.32 ± 0.07 mm during AF, 0.42 ± 0.08 mm after cardioversion, $p < 0.01$). In 10 patients who underwent a further AF relapse, FMD returned to pre-cardioversion values (0.33 ± 0.07 mm, $p < 0.05$ vs. post-cardioversion) [53]. Another study observed a short-term improvement in FMD, which was observed in 32 patients after 24 h of restoration of sinus rhythm (FMD during AF rhythm 8.4 ± 3.8%, FMD after 24 h of sinus rhythm restoration 10.7 ± 3.9%, $p < 0.001$) [21].

Although these findings support the hypothesis of an independent association between ED and AF, they are, however, counterbalanced by results from other studies. Indeed, in a large cohort study conducted in a sample of 15,010 individuals from the general population, the odds of having reduced FMD in patients with AF ($n = 466$, 3.1% of the population) was no longer significant after multiple adjustment to age, sex, heart rate, BMI, diabetes, smoking status, LDL/HDL cholesterol ratio and SBP (OR 1.03, 95%CI 0.88–1.21, $p = 0.59$) [54].

Long duration of arrythmia and the frequency of AF episodes showed, in some studies, some degree of association with worsening endothelial function. In a study by Khan et al. [55], ED measured by brachial FMD was significantly different between 30 subjects with permanent AF vs. 31 subjects with PAF (3.1% vs. 5.9%, $p = 0.02$). Contrary to FMD, nitroglycerine-mediated vasodilation (NMD), a measure of endothelium-independent vasoreactivity, seems not to be affected by AF. In 38 subjects with lone AF compared to 28 healthy controls matched by age, gender and atherosclerotic risk factors, no difference between groups were found in terms of NMD [56]. Similar results were observed in another study where endothelium-independent vasodilation did not change after sinus rhythm restoration by cardioversion in 46 patients with AF [21].

3.2. Question 2—Does VA Predict the Occurrence of AF Better Than Chronological Aging?

Answer: The role of arterial stiffness as an independent predictor of AF incidence is supported by the results of large-scale prospective observational studies and Mendelian randomization studies. A variety of markers of VA, including cfPWV, augmentation pressure and AIx, CAVI, elevated central and peripheral PP and aortic and carotid distensibility, showed (chronological) age-independent associations with the future occurrence of AF. In many cases, however, this association was mediated by increased BP levels which could, at least in part, confound the association between VA and AF. Arterial stiffness was also an independent predictor of AF recurrences after restoration of sinus rhythm. Associations were also found between arterial stiffness and features of cardiac remodeling, such as left atrial enlargement, pathophysiologically linked to a higher risk of AF incidence. The evidence in favor of FMD as a risk factor for AF incidence is weaker and partly counterbalanced by negative findings.

Results from three large-scale, population-based, cohort studies (the Atherosclerosis Risk in Communities, ARIC, Study, $n = 13{,}907$, the Multi-Ethnic Study of Atherosclerosis, MESA, $n = 6640$, and the Rotterdam Study, $n = 5220$) investigated the prognostic ability of measures of VA in predicting the future occurrence of AF [27]. All these studies adopted carotid distensibility as a marker of AS. In the Rotterdam Study and in a subcohort of the ARIC study, measures of cfPWV were also available. Concerning carotid distensibility, in multivariate models adjusted for multiple confounders including age, ethnicity, use of antihypertensive medication, current smoking, diabetes, history of heart failure and history of myocardial infarction, the hazard ratios (HR) associated with a 1 SD increase in carotid distensibility were 0.90 (95%CI 0.83–0.97, $p < 0.001$) in the ARIC Study and 0.83 (95%CI 0.70–0.98, $p < 0.001$) in the MESA. However, the results became not significant when height, weight, systolic and diastolic BP were included in the models (both $p > 0.05$). In the Rotterdam Study, the HR of AF associated with carotid distensibility was no longer significant after multiple adjustment (0.98, 95%CI 0.83–1.15, $p = 0.78$). In both cases, the loss of significance in multivariate models after adjustment for BP could be attributed to the functional influence of BP values on PWV. Indeed, PWV is consistently dependent on the wall stretch caused by the distending pressure and the passive loss of compliance of the arterial wall [57].

Similarly, cfPWV in the Rotterdam Study showed an independent association with AF incidence (HR 1.15, 95%CI 1.03–1.29, $p = 0.016$ per 1 SD increase in cfPWV), which was lost when the model was adjusted for BP [56]. In the ARIC Study, cfPWV demonstrated a U-shaped association with AF risk: in Cox regression models adjusted for age, race, center, sex, education levels and hemodynamic and clinical factors, the HR for incident AF in the first, third and fourth quartiles were 1.49 (95%CI 1.06–2.10), 1.59 (95%CI 1.14–2.10) and 1.56 (95%CI 1.10–2.19), respectively, compared to those in the second quartile, which was taken as a reference [28].

The predictive role of arterial stiffness for AF incidence was also analyzed in the Framingham Heart Study offspring and third-generation cohorts. Among 5797 participants (mean age 61 ± 10 years) followed up for an average period of 7.1 years, cfPWV, AIx and cPP were all univariately associated with increased risk of AF incidence [29]. In fully adjusted models, only AIx remained significantly associated with AF incidence (HR 1.16, 95%CI 1.02–1.32).

In a cohort study conducted in a Japanese population (n = 5418), baseline CAVI values $\geq$ 8.0, along with age $\geq$ 65 years and male sex, were found to independently predict the incidence of AF (n = 22, 0.41%) over 4 years (HR 5.27, 95%CI 1.6–17.3) [30].

In a subcohort of the MESA (3441 participants aged 45–84 years followed up for 7.8 years), high pulse pressure and low aortic distensibility measured by magnetic resonance imaging (MRI) were both univariately associated with the development of AF. In a multivariate analysis, after adjustment for age, sex, ethnicity, education, height, body mass index, smoking status, antihypertensive treatment, diabetes, left ventricular mass, heart rate and MAP, and after excluding aortic distensibility outliers, only PP remained significantly associated with AF risk, whereas aortic distensibility lost its significance. Each 1 SD increase in PP was independently associated with a 45% increased risk of AF (HR 1.45 95%CI: 1.13–1.87, p = 0.004) [31]. Increased PP independently predicted incident AF also in 350 patients with type 2 diabetes who were free from AF at baseline who were followed up for 10 years (adjusted OR: 1.76 for each SD increment, 95%CI 1.1–2.8, p = 0.01) [29]. The Losartan Intervention for Endpoint Reduction in Hypertension Study (LIFE Study) included 9193 patients with essential hypertension and electrocardiographic LV hypertrophy followed up for a period of 5 years. Increased brachial PP, either baseline or in treatment, was independently associated with a higher risk of new-onset AF in multivariate Cox regression analysis (HR per 10 mmHg baseline PP increase: 1.24, 95%CI 1.14–1.35, HR per 10 mmHg in-treatment PP increase 1.21, 95%CI 1.11–1.33 for in-treatment PP, both p < 0.001). PP was equivalent to SBP and DBP in predicting new-onset AF, but when included in the same statistical model, PP was demonstrated to be the strongest predictor [33]. In another study from the Framingham Heart Study cohort, the predictive power of increased PP for AF incidence was evaluated in a large general population including 5331 individuals followed for 12 years. After adjustment for a substantial number of confounders, the hazard ratio of new-onset AF associated with a 20 mmHg PP increase was 1.26 (95%CI 1.12–1.43, p < 0.001) [32]. It is worth noting that: (i) the increase in PP is dependent on both the physiological aging process and the associated increase in arterial stiffness induced by CV risk factors; (ii) an increase of 20 mmHg in PP can be observed over the lifespan only after several decades [58].

The prognostic superiority of central over peripheral BP measurement in incident AF was also observed in a predominantly older population-based cohort including 769 participants in sinus rhythm with no history of AF or stroke (mean age 70.5 years). Over 9.5 years, AF occurred in 83 participants. No peripheral BP value showed a significant association with incident AF. By contrast, after adjustment for age, sex, race and the number of antihypertensive drugs, both central SBP (HR 1.12 for 10 mmHg increment, 95%CI 1.00–1.25, p = 0.047) and central PP (HR 1.16 for 10 mmHg increment, 95%CI 1.00–1.34, p = 0.048) showed predictive value for AF incidence [34]. These results are of importance given that central PP, rather than peripheral PP, is more strongly linked to the age-related stiffening of large arteries [59].

In a cohort of 151 patients (mean age 71.9 years, mean follow-up 21 months) with AF, who restored sinus rhythm after pulmonary vein isolation, AS, evaluated by aortic distensibility (AD) of the descending aorta using transesophageal echocardiography, was found to be an independent predictor of AF recurrence (OR 3.6, 95%CI 2.8–4.1) [36]. In a study including 68 patients with AF who underwent a successful catheter ablation procedure, higher AF recurrence rates during a mean follow-up of 3 years were found in patients with higher values of peripheral PP, central PP and augmented pressure [37]. Among 31 older patients (mean age 78 ± 7 years) undergoing electrical cardioversion,

CAVI was directly related to the risk of AF recurrence: for each one-unit increase in CAVI, the HR for AF recurrence was 2.31 (95%CI 1.01–5.25) [38]. However, in these two latter cases, the regression models were not adjusted for relevant confounders (e.g., age).

In a cohort of 103 patients with PAF, compared to age- and sex-matched controls, left atrial diameter was significantly correlated with augmented pressure and AIx (both $p < 0.001$). Interestingly, left atrial diameter was the only independent predictor of AF recurrences following cardiac ablation over a follow-up period of 6 months [39].

A genome-wide association study, with Mendelian randomization including 225,636 participants from the UK Biobank, demonstrated a significant association between genetically determined increased levels of a photoplethysmography-derived arterial stiffness index (ASI) and the incidence of AF (OR, 1.8 per SD ASI phenotype, 95%CI, 1.4–2.2) [40]. This Mendelian randomization approach provides evidence of the causal inference between arterial stiffness and AF.

Indirect Markers of AF

AS was frequently found to be associated to well-established cardiac markers associated with increased risk of developing AF, such as LV hypertrophy, LV diastolic dysfunction and elevated LV filling pressure that, in turn, can result in an elevated left atrial pressure leading to left atrial dilation. In a study including 43 younger patients (aged 46 ± 8 years), with moderate to severe obstructive sleep apnea, a cfPWV > 10 m/s significantly correlated with left atrial diameter ($r = 0.45$; $p < 0.001$) both in univariate and multivariate analysis [41]. In a study conducted on 310 middle-aged hypertensive patients, cfPWV and elevated PP measured over 24 h were significantly and directly associated with left atrial diameter ($r = 0.27$ and $r = 0.32$, respectively, both $p < 0.001$) even after adjustment for age, sex, body mass index, indexes of LV structure and geometry and filling pressure [42]. However, regarding the limitations of echocardiographic assessment, which is prone to measurement errors, we should consider that the LA overload is reasonably mediated by LV alterations.

The role of ED in predicting AF incidence was evaluated in a subcohort of 3921 (mean age 58 ± 9 years) participants of the Framingham Heart Study. In this study, FMD was negatively associated with the future occurrence of AF in univariate and multivariate analyses (adjusted HR 0.79, 95%CI 0.63–0.99) [27]. Contrasting results were observed in a cohort of 2027 old individuals enrolled in the Cardiovascular Health Study (mean age 78.3 years). Over a median follow-up of 11 years, 754 incident AF cases occurred. After adjustment for age, sex, race, height, weight, CV disease, cigarette smoking, hypertension, diabetes, kidney function, C-reactive protein, physical activity, alcohol consumption and statins, the risk of AF did not differ according to baseline FMD (HR per FMD unit increment 1.01, 95%CI 0.97–1.05) [43]. Therefore, in comparison to positive findings observed in the Framingham Heart Study, results from this study suggested that, at least in older individuals, the utility of brachial FMD as a risk marker for AF was minimal.

3.3. Question 3—Is Early VA a Risk Enhancer for the Occurrence of CV Events in AF Patients?

Answer: The prognostic impact of measures of VA on future CV events in patients with AF has been tested only in small-scale, short-term, longitudinal studies and remains a matter of investigation. Data are also limited concerning the role of ED as a risk enhancer for adverse CV events in AF patients. Data from studies using changes in surrogate markers of CV prognosis as the primary endpoint are also extremely scarce.

Chen et al. assessed arterial stiffness by measuring brachial–ankle PWV (baPWV) in 167 patients with persistent AF. After a median follow-up of 26 months, the authors found that high baPWV was independently associated with an increased risk of a composite outcome including CV death, non-fatal stroke and myocardial infarction and hospitalization for heart failure. This association remained significant after adjusting for multiple CV risk factors (HR = 1.150; 95%CI: 1.034–1.279, $p = 0.01$). Most importantly, they demonstrated that baPWV had an incremental value in CV outcome prediction, pointing towards the usefulness of this marker in the risk stratification of these patients [22]. In another study, arterial stiffness was assessed by aortic distensibility during transesophageal echocardiography in 151 patients with AF before successful restoration of sinus rhythm with pulmonary vein isolation. Fifty-four controls with similar CV risk profile were also enrolled in the study. Results showed that, after a median follow-up of 21 months, decreased aortic distensibility was univariately associated with a composite endpoint that included AF recurrences, stroke, acute decompensated heart failure, cardiovascular and all-cause hospitalizations. Subjects in the lowest quartile of aortic distensibility showed an increased number of composite events as compared to those in the third quartile ($p = 0.03$) and in the fourth quartile ($p = 0.001$) [23].

The association between arterial stiffness and future CV event was also assessed using indirect descriptors of future CV events in AF. In a cohort of 117 patients with paroxysmal or persistent AF compared to 274 controls, cfPWV was independently associated with plasma N-terminal pro-B-type natriuretic peptide (NT-proBNP), which is considered a surrogate marker of CV prognosis ($\beta = 0.234$; 95%CI: 0.100–0.367, $p = 0.001$). Interestingly, only in patients with paroxysmal or persistent AF were increased values of cfPWV related to greater NT-proBNP plasma levels, whereas this was not observed in the control group, suggesting a relationship between AF, increased arterial stiffness and adverse CV outcomes [24].

The prognostic significance of ED, measured by FMD, in AF patients was evaluated in a cohort of 514 individuals with AF followed up for an average period of 24 months. A composite endpoint of CV events, defined as the occurrence of stroke/transient ischemic attack, myocardial infarction, urgent revascularization and CV death, occurred in 44 patients. In a Cox proportional hazards analysis, after multiple adjustment for other CV risk factors such as MI, history of stroke/TIA, heart failure, treatment with statins, smoking habits, gender and age, individuals with an FMD below 4.6% were at increased risk of CV events (HR 2.20 95%CI 1.13–4.28, $p = 0.020$) [25]. In another prospective observational study, FMD was measured by ultrasound in 291 patients with a positive history of PAF lasting no longer than six months. After a mean follow up of 33 months, subjects with FMD lower than 5.9% showed a doubled rate of composite adverse CV events, which included cardiovascular death, non-fatal myocardial infarction, stroke and heart failure hospitalization (37.1% versus 18% in patients with FMD > 5.9%, $p < 0.001$), which remained significant after adjustment for classical CV risk factors (HR: 3.036, 95%CI 1.546–5.963, $p = 0.01$) [26].

3.4. Question 4—Are Devices Measuring VA Suitable to Perform Subclinical AF Detection?

Answer: The implementation of AF screening in the VA diagnostic approach remains an unmet need.

For many patients, measurement of VA biomarkers with automated devices might represent a unique opportunity to effectively diagnose AF. It could be supposed that individuals currently prescribed VA assessment for clinical purposes are individuals with a high burden of CV risk factor and therefore at high risk of developing AF. In these patients, targeted AF screening and early AF detection could potentially prevent the risk of ischemic stroke and AF-related complications [4]. Despite the potential benefits and the relatively simple technological advances needed for implementation, there are no data regarding the performance of devices measuring VA in AF detection.

Photopletysmogram (PPG) signals are proposed as promising tools to assess VA. Indeed, the time taken for the PPG pulse wave to travel the arterial tree is a function of AS. Moreover, pulse wave shapes could reflect changes in VA [60]. Noteworthily, the detection of rhythm irregularities through the analysis of peripheral PPG signals is a promising application for AF detection in patients at risk [61]. However, at present, there is no device that combines these two technologies into a single apparatus.

Devices using oscillometric techniques may also contribute to AF screening. Blood pressure monitors which detect AF from oscillometry-based algorithms have been in the market for a few years, with very high sensitivity and specificity rates, ranging from 90 to

100% [62]. The algorithm for diagnosis, based on pulse irregularity, could be implemented in devices measuring central blood pressure or pulse wave velocity from oscillometric cuffs.

3.5. Question 5—Does Atrial-Fibrillation-Related Rhythm Irregularity Have a Negative Impact on the Measurement of Vascular Age?

Answer: From these limited available data (two studies), measurements of biomarkers of arterial structure during AF appear reliable. Results about reliability of FMD measurement during AF are, to date, inconclusive.

In a clinical study, cfPWV and cPP assessed by applanation tonometry were estimated in 34 patients with AF before and after successful electrical cardioversion [20]. After adjustment for post-procedural changes in mean arterial pressure (MAP) and heart rate, the intra-class correlation coefficient for both cfPWV and cPP was 0.89 (95%CI 0.79–0.95 for cfPWV, 0.72–0.95 for cPP), consistent with good reliability [63]. By contrast, measures of wave reflection such as central augmentation index (AIx) showed only moderate reliability (ICC = 0.59; 95%CI 0.17–0.80).

The reliability of FMD measurement was assessed in 32 patients with AF by comparing measures obtained before and 24 h after successful electrical cardioversion [21]. In this study, reliability was not formally tested using ICC but using a 2-sided t-test for independent samples, with further calculation of 95% confidence intervals from a Bland–Altman plot. As compared with FMD measurement taken during AF rhythm, FMD 24 h after restoration of sinus rhythm was, on average, significantly higher and showed high heterogeneity (FMD during AF rhythm 8.4 ± 3.8%, FMD 24 h after sinus rhythm restoration 10.7 ± 3.9%, $p < 0.001$, 95%CI for mean difference 1.15–3.65). The lack of appropriate statistics to assess reliability and the large time difference do not allow making definite conclusions about reliability of FMD during AF rhythm.

4. Discussion

In this paper, we aimed to review and summarize state-of-the-art data from the literature exploring the potential link between mechanical and functional biomarkers of VA and the presence and severity of AF. We aimed to find answers to five clinically and methodologically relevant questions and identify open and unanswered issues, including the cross-sectional association between VA and AF, the predictive role of VA for AF incidence, the role of VA as a risk enhancer for CV events in AF patients, the accuracy of VA measurement in AF rhythm and the performance of devices measuring VA in detecting AF rhythm.

This review was conceived as part of the work plan of the VascAgeNet COST action (COST Action CA18216) which is to refine, harmonize and promote the VA concept, to bring innovations in CV research from bench to bedside and to establish assessment of VA in clinical practice [19].

Our results showed that VA has a cross-sectional relationship with AF and is also independently associated with increased risk of incident AF. This was found for several biomarkers of arterial structure, such as PWV as a proxy measure of AS, wave reflection, arterial distensibility and VA-related measures of central hemodynamics such as central PP. A visual summary of the degree of the association between each measure of VA according to methodology questions is provided in Figure 2. Although less pronounced, there is substantial evidence of an independent link between VA biomarkers related to arterial function, such as brachial FMD, and AF.

The relationship between VA and AF has a profound rationale and is supported by shared common etiological mechanisms, such as elevated BP values and several other CV risk factors. Since BP is a surrogate marker of cardiac and arterial load, it is important to identify which temporal relationship exists between increased AS, elevated BP and AF and whether or at which level this process could be reverted by therapeutic approaches. There is robust evidence to support the hypothesis that increased arterial stiffness could precede the pathogenesis of elevated BP [64]. Therefore, measurement of arterial stiffness and VA in clinical practice could be the first ideal screening step to tackle the AF burden by identifying and targeting interventions in individuals with elevated AS at risk of developing hypertension and subsequent CV events, including AF. A further factor possibly influencing the link between FA and arterial stiffness is that both contribute to blood pressure variability, which is a potential independent risk factor for cardiovascular complications. Both the fluctuations of blood pressure induced by FA and the aging of vessels may cause an increased blood pressure variability in the short term [65]. In turn, an increased blood pressure variability is associated with an increased incidence of FA [66] and with cardiovascular outcomes among patients with FA [67], making this association a topic of major interest for future research.

The promotion of a healthier lifestyle early in life through increasing physical activity, healthy diet, smoking cessation, weight control, lowering stress and normalization of sleep patterns was found to be associated with lower levels of arterial stiffness [61]. There is also strong evidence that AF has an independent association with ED, measured by FMD of the brachial artery. However, this association seems to be largely explained by concomitant CV risk factors, such as hypertension, dyslipidemia and diabetes, which are known to negatively affect the endothelial function, and it is currently unknown whether ED could be reverted by therapeutic approaches. However, to our knowledge, no study has investigated the role of more stringent therapeutic goals aiming at a better VA control on AF-related outcomes.

Even though increased arterial stiffness has been described as a predictor of AF, available evidence regarding its prognostic value for CV events in patients with AF is far from conclusive. This is due to the lack of relevant data, often originating from underpowered studies with high heterogeneity in terms of arterial stiffness markers, as well as to the methods for assessing AS. To this end, larger, prospective, community-based cohorts with longer follow-up periods are needed. The prognostic value of ED for future CV events is understudied in AF patients and further studies are needed specifically targeting this population.

At the methodological level, there are still few data regarding the performance of devices measuring arterial stiffness in detecting AF. Given that a considerable proportion of patients with AF are undiagnosed, developing technology would help increase the screening and the detection rates of this condition. The potential outcome of combining screening approaches for the evaluation of VA and AF detection into one single device needs therefore to be tested in future dedicated studies. The measurement of VA biomarkers during irregular cardiac rhythm, as observed in AF with irregular response rate, represents a practical challenge that is not fully overcome. As a consequence, AF patients are often excluded from clinical trials with VA assessment. We showed that, despite preliminary promising results provided by a few methodological studies, substantial research should focus on technological solutions addressing this issue.

5. Conclusions

In conclusion, given the close pathophysiological link between VA and AF, it is reasonable that measurements of arterial stiffness should be implemented in clinical practice in all individuals at risk of developing AF and its adverse consequences to better stratify their risk. The predictive role of both arterial stiffness and ED as CV risk factors in AF patients still needs to be proven in dedicated studies. Future studies and upcoming technologies will be helpful to address the gap of knowledge in this field.

Supplementary Materials: The following supporting information can be downloaded at: https://www.mdpi.com/article/10.3390/jcm13051207/s1, Table S1: Narrative review checklist.

Author Contributions: Conceptualization, A.G. (Andrea Grillo) and D.A.; methodology, G.P., A.G. (Andrea Grillo) and D.A.; data curation, all authors; writing—original draft preparation, G.P., A.G. (Andrea Grillo) and D.A.; writing—review and editing, all authors; visualization, all authors; supervision, D.A.; project administration, D.A.; funding acquisition, B.H., A.G. (Andrea Grillo) and C.C.M. All authors have read and agreed to the published version of the manuscript.

Funding: This article is based upon work from COST Action "Network for Research in Vascular Ageing" (VascAgeNet, CA18216), supported by European Cooperation in Science and Technology (COST, cost.eu). Guala A. has received funding from "la Caixa" Foundation (LCF/BQ/PR22/11920008).

Conflicts of Interest: The authors declare no conflicts of interest.

References

1. Lippi, G.; Sanchis-Gomar, F.; Cervellin, G. Global epidemiology of atrial fibrillation: An increasing epidemic and public health challenge. *Int. J. Stroke* **2020**, *16*, 217–221. [CrossRef]
2. Benjamin, E.J.; Muntner, P.; Alonso, A.; Bittencourt, M.S.; Callaway, C.W.; Carson, A.P.; Chamberlain, A.M.; Chang, A.R.; Cheng, S.; Das, S.R.; et al. Heart disease and stroke statistics—2019 update: A report from the American heart association. *Circulation* **2019**, *139*, e56–e528. [CrossRef]
3. Wu, J.; Nadarajah, R.; Nakao, Y.M.; Nakao, K.; Wilkinson, C.; Mamas, M.A.; Camm, A.J.; Gale, C.P. Temporal trends and patterns in atrial fibrillation incidence: A population-based study of 3·4 million individuals. *Lancet Reg. Health Eur.* **2022**, *17*, 100386. [CrossRef]
4. Hindricks, G.; Potpara, T.; Dagres, N.; Arbelo, E.; Bax, J.J.; Blomström-Lundqvist, C.; Boriani, G.; Castella, M.; Dan, J.-A.; Dilaveris, P.E.; et al. The Task Force for the diagnosis and management of atrial fibrillation of the European Society of Cardiology (ESC) Developed with the special contribution of the European Heart Rhythm Association (EHRA) of the ESC. *Eur. Heart J.* **2021**, *42*, 373–498. [CrossRef] [PubMed]
5. Martinez, C.; Katholing, A.; Freedman, S.B.; Martinez, C.; Katholing, A.; Freedman, S.B. Adverse prognosis of incidentally detected ambulatory atrial fibrillation. *Thromb. Haemost.* **2014**, *112*, 276–286. [CrossRef] [PubMed]
6. Freedman, B.; Potpara, T.S.; Lip, G.Y.H. Stroke prevention in atrial fibrillation. *Lancet* **2016**, *388*, 806–817. [CrossRef] [PubMed]
7. Freedman, B. Screening for Atrial Fibrillation Using a Smartphone: Is There an App for That? *J. Am. Heart Assoc.* **2016**, *5*, e004000. [CrossRef] [PubMed]
8. Climie, R.E.; Alastruey, J.; Mayer, C.C.; Schwarz, A.; Laucyte-Cibulskiene, A.; Voicehovska, J.; Bianchini, E.; Bruno, R.-M.; Charlton, P.H.; Grillo, A.; et al. Vascular ageing: Moving from bench towards bedside. *Eur. J. Prev. Cardiol.* **2023**, *30*, 1101–1117. [CrossRef] [PubMed]
9. Gkaliagkousi, E.; Lazaridis, A.; Dogan, S.; Fraenkel, E.; Tuna, B.G.; Mozos, I.; Vukicevic, M.; Yalcin, O.; Gopcevic, K. Theories and Molecular Basis of Vascular Aging: A Review of the Literature from VascAgeNet Group on Pathophysiological Mechanisms of Vascular Aging. *Int. J. Mol. Sci.* **2022**, *23*, 8672. [CrossRef] [PubMed]
10. Ben-Shlomo, Y.; Spears, M.; Boustred, C.; May, M.; Anderson, S.; Benjamin, E.; Boutouyrie, P.; Cameron, J.; Chen, C.-H.; Cruickshank, J.K.; et al. Aortic Pulse Wave Velocity Improves Cardiovascular Event Prediction. *J. Am. Coll. Cardiol.* **2014**, *63*, 636–646. [CrossRef] [PubMed]
11. Bruno, R.M.; Nilsson, P.M.; Engström, G.; Wadström, B.N.; Empana, J.-P.; Boutouyrie, P.; Laurent, S. Early and Supernormal Vascular Aging: Clinical Characteristics and Association with Incident Cardiovascular Events. *Hypertension* **2020**, *76*, 1616–1624. [CrossRef] [PubMed]
12. Cao, Q.; Li, M.; Wang, T.; Chen, Y.; Dai, M.; Zhang, D.; Xu, Y.; Xu, M.; Lu, J.; Wang, W.; et al. Association of Early and Supernormal Vascular Aging categories with cardiovascular disease in the Chinese population. *Front. Cardiovasc. Med.* **2022**, *9*, 895792. [CrossRef] [PubMed]
13. Lip, G. Does atrial fibrillation confer a hypercoagulable state? *Lancet* **1995**, *346*, 1313–1314. [CrossRef]
14. Cai, H.; Li, Z.; Goette, A.; Mera, F.; Honeycutt, C.; Feterik, K.; Wilcox, J.N.; Dudley, S.C.; Harrison, D.G.; Langberg, J.J.; et al. Downregulation of endocardial nitric oxide synthase expression and nitric oxide production in atrial fibrillation: Potential mechanisms for atrial thrombosis and stroke. *Circulation* **2002**, *106*, 2854–2858. [CrossRef]
15. Khan, A.A.; Thomas, G.N.; Lip, G.Y.H.; Shantsila, A. Endothelial function in patients with atrial fibrillation. *Ann. Med.* **2020**, *52*, 1–11. [CrossRef] [PubMed]
16. Corretti, M.C.; Anderson, T.J.; Benjamin, E.J.; Celermajer, D.; Charbonneau, F.; Creager, M.A.; Deanfield, J.; Drexler, H.; Gerhard-Herman, M.; Herrington, D.; et al. Guidelines for the ultrasound assessment of endothelial-dependent flow-mediated vasodilation of the brachial artery: A report of the International Brachial Artery Reactivity Task Force. *J. Am. Coll. Cardiol.* **2002**, *39*, 257–265. [CrossRef]
17. Thijssen, D.H.J.; Bruno, R.M.; Van Mil, A.C.C.M.; Holder, S.M.; Faita, F.; Greyling, A.; Zock, P.L.; Taddei, S.; Deanfield, J.E.; Luscher, T.; et al. Expert consensus and evidence-based recommendations for the assessment of flow-mediated dilation in humans. *Eur. Heart J.* **2019**, *40*, 2534–2547. [CrossRef]
18. Xu, Y.; Arora, R.C.; Hiebert, B.M.; Lerner, B.; Szwajcer, A.; McDonald, K.; Rigatto, C.; Komenda, P.; Sood, M.M.; Tangri, N. Non-invasive endothelial function testing and the risk of adverse outcomes: A systematic review and meta-analysis. *Eur. Heart J. Cardiovasc. Imaging* **2014**, *15*, 736–746. [CrossRef]
19. Climie, R.E.; Mayer, C.C.; Bruno, R.M.; Hametner, B. Addressing the Unmet Needs of Measuring Vascular Ageing in Clinical Practice—European COoperation in Science and Technology Action VascAgeNet. *Artery Res.* **2020**, *26*, 71–75. [CrossRef]

20. Caluwé, R.; De Vriese, A.S.; Van Vlem, B.; Verbeke, F. Measurement of pulse wave velocity, augmentation index, and central pulse pressure in atrial fibrillation: A proof of concept study. *J. Am. Soc. Hypertens.* **2018**, *12*, 627–632. [CrossRef]
21. Skalidis, E.I.; Zacharis, E.A.; Tsetis, D.K.; Pagonidis, K.; Chlouverakis, G.; Yarmenitis, S.; Hamilos, M.; Manios, E.G.; Vardas, P.E. Endothelial cell function during atrial fibrillation and after restoration of sinus rhythm. *Am. J. Cardiol.* **2007**, *99*, 1258–1262. [CrossRef] [PubMed]
22. Chen, S.-C.; Lee, W.-H.; Hsu, P.-C.; Lin, M.-Y.; Lee, C.-S.; Lin, T.-H.; Voon, W.-C.; Lai, W.-T.; Sheu, S.-H.; Su, H.-M. Association of Brachial–Ankle Pulse Wave Velocity with Cardiovascular Events in Atrial Fibrillation. *Am. J. Hypertens.* **2015**, *29*, 348–356. [CrossRef]
23. Shchetynska-Marinova, T.; Liebe, V.; Papavassiliu, T.; Fernandez, A.d.F.; Hetjens, S.; Sieburg, T.; Doesch, C.; Sigl, M.; Akin, I.; Borggrefe, M.; et al. Determinants of arterial stiffness in patients with atrial fibrillation. *Arch. Cardiovasc. Dis.* **2021**, *114*, 550–560. [CrossRef]
24. Chen, L.Y.; Tai, B.C.; Foo, D.C.; Wong, R.C.; Adabag, A.S.; Benditt, D.G.; Ling, L.H. Carotid-femoral pulse wave velocity is associated with N-terminal pro-B-type natriuretic peptide level in patients with atrial fibrillation. *Heart Asia* **2011**, *3*, 55–59. [CrossRef] [PubMed]
25. Perri, L.; Pastori, D.; Pignatelli, P.; Violi, F.; Loffredo, L. Flow-mediated dilation is associated with cardiovascular events in non-valvular atrial fibrillation patients. *Int. J. Cardiol.* **2015**, *179*, 139–143. [CrossRef] [PubMed]
26. Zhang, J.; Tan, Q.; Lina, W.; Zhaoqian, Z. Endothelial dysfunction predicted cardiovascular events in patients with paroxysmal atrial fibrillation. *SciVee* **2022**, *43*, 708–714. [CrossRef]
27. Chen, L.Y.; Leening, M.J.G.; Norby, F.L.; Roetker, N.S.; Hofman, A.; Franco, O.H.; Pan, W.; Polak, J.F.; Witteman, J.C.; Kronmal, R.A.; et al. Carotid Intima-Media Thickness and Arterial Stiffness and the Risk of Atrial Fibrillation: The Atherosclerosis Risk in Communities (ARIC) Study, Multi-Ethnic Study of Atherosclerosis (MESA), and the Rotterdam Study. *J. Am. Heart Assoc.* **2016**, *5*, e002907. [CrossRef]
28. Almuwaqqat, Z.; Claxton, J.S.; Norby, F.L.; Lutsey, P.L.; Wei, J.; Soliman, E.Z.; Chen, L.Y.; Matsushita, K.; Heiss, G.; Alonso, A. Association of arterial stiffness with incident atrial fibrillation: A cohort study. *BMC Cardiovasc. Disord.* **2021**, *21*, 247. [CrossRef]
29. Shaikh, A.Y.; Wang, N.; Yin, X.; Larson, M.G.; Vasan, R.S.; Hamburg, N.M.; Magnani, J.W.; Ellinor, P.T.; Lubitz, S.A.; Mitchell, G.F.; et al. Relations of Arterial Stiffness and Brachial Flow–Mediated Dilation with New-Onset Atrial Fibrillation: The Framingham Heart Study. *Hypertension* **2016**, *68*, 590–596. [CrossRef]
30. Nagayama, D.; Fujishiro, K.; Nakamura, K.; Watanabe, Y.; Yamaguchi, T.; Suzuki, K.; Shimizu, K.; Saiki, A.; Shirai, K. Cardio-Ankle Vascular Index is Associated with Prevalence and New-Appearance of Atrial Fibrillation in Japanese Urban Residents: A Retrospective Cross-Sectional and Cohort Study. *Vasc. Health Risk Manag.* **2022**, *18*, 5–15. [CrossRef]
31. Roetker, N.S.; Chen, L.Y.; Heckbert, S.R.; Nazarian, S.; Soliman, E.Z.; Bluemke, D.A.; Lima, J.A.; Alonso, A. Relation of Systolic, Diastolic, and Pulse Pressures and Aortic Distensibility with Atrial Fibrillation (from the Multi-Ethnic Study of Atherosclerosis). *Am. J. Cardiol.* **2014**, *114*, 587–592. [CrossRef]
32. Valbusa, F.; Bonapace, S.; Bertolini, L.; Zenari, L.; Arcaro, G.; Targher, G. Increased Pulse Pressure Independently Predicts Incident Atrial Fibrillation in Patients with Type 2 Diabetes. *Diabetes Care* **2012**, *35*, 2337–2339. [CrossRef]
33. Larstorp, A.C.K.; Ariansen, I.; Gjesdal, K.; Olsen, M.H.; Ibsen, H.; Devereux, R.B.; Okin, P.M.; Dahlöf, B.; Kjeldsen, S.E.; Wachtell, K. Association of pulse pressure with new-onset atrial fibrillation in patients with hypertension and left ventricular hypertrophy: The Losartan Intervention For Endpoint (LIFE) reduction in hypertension study. *Hypertension* **2012**, *60*, 347–353. [CrossRef] [PubMed]
34. Mitchell, G.F.; Vasan, R.S.; Keyes, M.J.; Parise, H.; Wang, T.J.; Larson, M.G.; D'agostino, R.B.; Kannel, W.B.; Levy, D.; Benjamin, E.J. Pulse pressure and risk of new-onset atrial fibrillation. *JAMA* **2007**, *297*, 709–715. [CrossRef] [PubMed]
35. Matsumoto, K.; Jin, Z.; Homma, S.; Elkind, M.S.; Schwartz, J.E.; Rundek, T.; Mannina, C.; Ito, K.; Sacco, R.L.; Di Tullio, M.R. Office, central and ambulatory blood pressure for predicting incident atrial fibrillation in older adults. *J. Hypertens.* **2020**, *39*, 46–52. [CrossRef]
36. Shchetynska-Marinova, T.; Kranert, M.; Baumann, S.; Liebe, V.; Grafen, A.; Gerhards, S.; Rosenkaimer, S.; Akin, I.; Borggrefe, M.; Hohneck, A.L. Recurrence of atrial fibrillation after pulmonary vein isolation in dependence of arterial stiffness. *Neth. Heart J.* **2021**, *30*, 198–206. [CrossRef] [PubMed]
37. Lau, D.H.; Middeldorp, M.E.; Brooks, A.G.; Ganesan, A.N.; Roberts-Thomson, K.C.; Stiles, M.K.; Leong, D.P.; Abed, H.S.; Lim, H.S.; Wong, C.X.; et al. Aortic Stiffness in Lone Atrial Fibrillation: A Novel Risk Factor for Arrhythmia Recurrence. *PLoS ONE* **2013**, *8*, e76776. [CrossRef]
38. Fumagalli, S.; Giannini, I.; Pupo, S.; Agostini, F.; Boni, S.; Roberts, A.T.; Gabbai, D.; Di Serio, C.; Gabbani, L.; Tarantini, F.; et al. Atrial fibrillation after electrical cardioversion in elderly patients: A role for arterial stiffness? Results from a preliminary study. *Aging Clin. Exp. Res.* **2016**, *28*, 1273–1277. [CrossRef]
39. Kizilirmak, F.; Guler, G.B.; Guler, E.; Gunes, H.M.; Demir, G.G.; Omaygenc, M.O.; Cakal, B.; Olgun, F.E.; Koklu, E.; Kilicaslan, F. Impact of aortic stiffness on the frequency of paroxysmal atrial fibrillation recurrences. *Acta Cardiol.* **2015**, *70*, 414–421. [CrossRef] [PubMed]
40. Zekavat, S.M.; Roselli, C.; Hindy, G.; Lubitz, S.A.; Ellinor, P.T.; Zhao, H.; Natarajan, P. Genetic Link Between Arterial Stiffness and Atrial Fibrillation. *Circ. Genom. Precis. Med.* **2019**, *12*, e002453. [CrossRef]

41. Drager, L.F.; Bortolotto, L.A.; Pedrosa, R.P.; Krieger, E.M.; Lorenzi-Filho, G. Left atrial diameter is independently associated with arterial stiffness in patients with obstructive sleep apnea: Potential implications for atrial fibrillation. *Int. J. Cardiol.* **2010**, *144*, 257–259. [CrossRef] [PubMed]
42. Lantelme, P.; Laurent, S.; Besnard, C.; Bricca, G.; Vincent, M.; Legedz, L.; Milon, H. Arterial stiffness is associated with left atrial size in hypertensive patients. *Arch. Cardiovasc. Dis.* **2008**, *101*, 35–40. [CrossRef]
43. Garg, P.K.; Bartz, T.M.; Burke, G.; Gottdiener, J.S.; Herrington, D.; Heckbert, S.R.; Kizer, J.R.; Sotoodehnia, N.; Mukamal, K.J. Brachial Flow-Mediated Dilation and Risk of Atrial Fibrillation in Older Adults: The Cardiovascular Health Study. *Vasc. Health Risk Manag.* **2021**, *17*, 95–102. [CrossRef] [PubMed]
44. Pauklin, P.; Eha, J.; Tootsi, K.; Kolk, R.; Paju, R.; Kals, M.; Kampus, P. Atrial fibrillation is associated with increased central blood pressure and arterial stiffness. *J. Clin. Hypertens.* **2021**, *23*, 1581–1587. [CrossRef]
45. Cui, R.; Yamagishi, K.; Muraki, I.; Hayama-Terada, M.; Umesawa, M.; Imano, H.; Li, Y.; Eshak, E.S.; Ohira, T.; Kiyama, M.; et al. Association between markers of arterial stiffness and atrial fibrillation in the Circulatory Risk in Communities Study (CIRCS). *Atherosclerosis* **2017**, *263*, 244–248. [CrossRef]
46. Doi, M.; Miyoshi, T.; Hirohata, S.; Iwabu, A.; Tominaga, Y.; Kaji, Y.; Kamikawa, S.; Sakane, K.; Kitawaki, T.; Kusano, K.F.; et al. Increased Augmentation Index of the Radial Pressure Waveform in Patients with Paroxysmal Atrial Fibrillation. *Cardiology* **2009**, *113*, 138–145. [CrossRef]
47. Shi, D.; Meng, Q.; Zhou, X.; Li, L.; Liu, K.; He, S.; Wang, S.; Chen, X. Factors influencing the relationship between atrial fibrillation and artery stiffness in elderly Chinese patients with hypertension. *Aging Clin. Exp. Res.* **2016**, *28*, 653–658. [CrossRef] [PubMed]
48. Lee, S.-H.; Choi, S.; Jung, J.-H.; Lee, N. Effects of Atrial Fibrillation on Arterial Stiffness in Patients with Hypertension. *Angiology* **2008**, *59*, 459–463. [CrossRef]
49. Miyoshi, T.; Doi, M.; Noda, Y.; Ohno, Y.; Sakane, K.; Kamikawa, S.; Noguchi, Y.; Ito, H. Arterial stiffness determined according to the cardio-ankle vascular index is associated with paroxysmal atrial fibrillation: A cross-sectional study. *Heart Asia* **2014**, *6*, 59–63. [CrossRef]
50. Fumagalli, S.; Gabbai, D.; Nreu, B.; Roberts, A.T.; Boni, S.; Ceccofiglio, A.; Fracchia, S.; Baldasseroni, S.; Tarantini, F.; Marchionni, N. Age, left atrial dimension and arterial stiffness after external cardioversion of atrial fibrillation. A vascular component in arrhythmia maintenance? Results from a preliminary study. *Aging Clin. Exp. Res.* **2014**, *26*, 327–330. [CrossRef]
51. Chung, G.E.; Park, H.E.; Lee, H.; Choi, S.-Y. Clinical significance of increased arterial stiffness associated with atrial fibrillation, according to Framingham risk score. *Sci. Rep.* **2021**, *11*, 4955. [CrossRef]
52. Heshmat-Ghahdarijani, K.; Jangjoo, S.; Amirpoor, A.; Najafian, J.; Khosravi, A.; Heidarpour, M.; Hekmat, M.; Shafie, D. Endothelial dysfunction in patients with lone atrial fibrillation. *ARYA Atheroscler.* **2020**, *16*, 278–283. [CrossRef]
53. Guazzi, M.; Belletti, S.; Tumminello, G.; Fiorentini, C.; Guazzi, M.D. Exercise hyperventilation, dyspnea sensation, and ergoreflex activation in lone atrial fibrillation. *Am. J. Physiol. Circ. Physiol.* **2004**, *287*, H2899–H2905. [CrossRef] [PubMed]
54. Börschel, C.S.; Rübsamen, N.; Ojeda, F.M.; Wild, P.S.; Hoffmann, B.A.; Prochaska, J.H.; Gori, T.; Lackner, K.J.; Blankenberg, S.; Zeller, T.; et al. Noninvasive peripheral vascular function and atrial fibrillation in the general population. *J. Hypertens.* **2019**, *37*, 928–934. [CrossRef] [PubMed]
55. Khan, A.A.; Junejo, R.T.; Alsharari, R.; Thomas, G.N.; Fisher, J.P.; Lip, G.Y.H. A greater burden of atrial fibrillation is associated with worse endothelial dysfunction in hypertension. *J. Hum. Hypertens.* **2021**, *35*, 667–677. [CrossRef]
56. Polovina, M.; Potpara, T.; Giga, V.; Stepanovic, J.; Ostojic, M. Impaired endothelial function in lone atrial fibrillation. *Vojnosanit. Pregl.* **2013**, *70*, 908–914. [CrossRef]
57. Spronck, B.; Heusinkveld, M.H.; Vanmolkot, F.H.; Roodt, J.O.; Hermeling, E.; Delhaas, T.; Kroon, A.A.; Reesink, K.D. Pressure-dependence of arterial stiffness: Potential clinical implications. *J. Hypertens.* **2015**, *33*, 330–338. [CrossRef]
58. Franklin, S.S.; Gustin, W.; Wong, N.D.; Larson, M.G.; Weber, M.A.; Kannel, W.B.; Levy, D. Hemodynamic patterns of age-related changes in blood pressure: The Framingham Heart Study. *Circulation* **1997**, *96*, 308–315. [CrossRef]
59. Yu, S.; McEniery, C.M. Central Versus Peripheral Artery Stiffening and Cardiovascular Risk. *Arter. Thromb. Vasc. Biol.* **2020**, *40*, 1028–1033. [CrossRef] [PubMed]
60. Charlton, P.H.; Paliakaitė, B.; Pilt, K.; Bachler, M.; Zanelli, S.; Kulin, D.; Allen, J.; Hallab, M.; Bianchini, E.; Mayer, C.C.; et al. Assessing hemodynamics from the photoplethysmogram to gain insights into vascular age: A review from VascAgeNet. *Am. J. Physiol. Heart Circ. Physiol.* **2022**, *322*, H493–H522. [CrossRef]
61. Chan, P.; Wong, C.; Poh, Y.C.; Pun, L.; Leung, W.W.; Wong, Y.; Wong, M.M.; Poh, M.; Chu, D.W.; Siu, C.; et al. Diagnostic Performance of a Smartphone-Based Photoplethysmographic Application for Atrial Fibrillation Screening in a Primary Care Setting. *J. Am. Heart Assoc.* **2016**, *5*, e003428. [CrossRef]
62. Park, S.-H.; June, K.J.; Choi, Y.-K. Predictive validity of automated oscillometric blood pressure monitors for screening atrial fibrillation: A systematic review and meta-analysis. *Expert Rev. Med. Devices* **2019**, *16*, 503–514. [CrossRef] [PubMed]
63. Koo, T.K.; Li, M.Y. A Guideline of Selecting and Reporting Intraclass Correlation Coefficients for Reliability Research. *J. Chiropr. Med.* **2016**, *15*, 155–163. [CrossRef] [PubMed]
64. Najjar, S.S.; Scuteri, A.; Shetty, V.; Wright, J.G.; Muller, D.C.; Fleg, J.L.; Spurgeon, H.P.; Ferrucci, L.; Lakatta, E.G. Pulse Wave Velocity Is an Independent Predictor of the Longitudinal Increase in Systolic Blood Pressure and of Incident Hypertension in the Baltimore Longitudinal Study of Aging. *J. Am. Coll. Cardiol.* **2008**, *51*, 1377–1383. [CrossRef] [PubMed]

65. Parati, G.; Bilo, G.; Kollias, A.; Pengo, M.; Ochoa, J.E.; Castiglioni, P.; Stergiou, G.S.; Mancia, G.; Asayama, K.; Asmar, R.; et al. Blood pressure variability: Methodological aspects, clinical relevance and practical indications for management-a European Society of Hypertension position paper. *J. Hypertens.* **2023**, *41*, 527–544. [CrossRef] [PubMed]
66. Kaze, A.D.; Yuyun, M.F.; Fonarow, G.C.; Echouffo-Tcheugui, J.B. Blood Pressure Variability and Risk of Atrial Fibrillation in Adults with Type 2 Diabetes. *JACC Adv.* **2023**, *2*, e100382. [CrossRef]
67. Proietti, M.; Romiti, G.F.; Olshansky, B.; Lip, G.Y. Systolic Blood Pressure Visit-to-Visit Variability and Major Adverse Outcomes in Atrial Fibrillation: The AFFIRM Study (Atrial Fibrillation Follow-Up Investigation of Rhythm Management). *Hypertension* **2017**, *70*, 949–958. [CrossRef]

Disclaimer/Publisher's Note: The statements, opinions and data contained in all publications are solely those of the individual author(s) and contributor(s) and not of MDPI and/or the editor(s). MDPI and/or the editor(s) disclaim responsibility for any injury to people or property resulting from any ideas, methods, instructions or products referred to in the content.

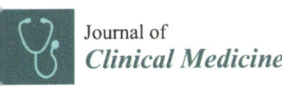 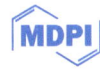

Article

Deterioration of Kidney Function Is Affected by Central Arterial Stiffness in Late Life

Lisanne Tap [1,*], Kim Borsboom [1], Andrea Corsonello [2,3], Fabrizia Lattanzio [2] and Francesco Mattace-Raso [1]

1. Section of Geriatric Medicine, Department of Internal Medicine, Erasmus MC, University Medical Center Rotterdam, 3000 CA Rotterdam, The Netherlands
2. Italian National Research Center on Ageing (IRCCS INRCA), 60124 Ancona, Italy
3. Department of Pharmacy, Health and Nutritional Sciences, University of Calabria, 87100 Cosenza, Italy
* Correspondence: l.tap@erasmusmc.nl; Tel.: +31-107035979

Abstract: Cardiovascular diseases affect kidney function. The aim of this study was to investigate the possible associations between hemodynamic parameters and change in kidney function in individuals aged 75 years and older. Data on hemodynamics and blood and urine samples were collected at baseline and during one-year visits. Hemodynamics were split into two groups based on median values. Changes in the estimated glomerular filtration rate (eGFR) were investigated between low and high groups for each hemodynamic parameter using analysis of variance. Changes in the albumin–creatinine ratio (ACR) were examined as binary outcomes (large increase vs. stable) using logistic regression. The population consisted of 252 participants. Participants in the high central systolic blood pressure (cSBP) group had a greater decline in eGFR than participants in the low cSBP group (−6.3% vs. −2.7%, $p = 0.006$). Participants in the high aortic pulse wave velocity (aPWV) group had a greater decline in eGFR than those in the low aPWV group (−6.8% vs. −2.5%, $p = 0.001$). Other hemodynamic parameters were not associated with eGFR changes. Hemodynamics were not associated with changes in the ACR; aPWV and cSBP appear to be predictors for eGFR decline in older age; monitoring and treatment of elevated stiffness might be helpful in order to prevent kidney function decline.

Keywords: hemodynamics; arterial stiffness; aortic pulse wave velocity; blood pressure; aging; chronic kidney disease; kidney function; cardiovascular disease

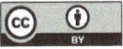

1. Introduction

Chronic kidney disease (CKD) is a common finding in older individuals and is associated with increased risk of morbidity and mortality [1,2]. Individuals in late life, especially those with CKD, are more likely to develop cardiovascular diseases. Several risk factors are known to cause kidney function decline, such as aging, hypertension and diabetes mellitus [1]. In contrast to age, these cardiovascular risk factors are modifiable and therefore important factors in screening and treatment for CKD [2,3].

Relevant cardiovascular age-related changes are decline in cardiac output and stroke volume [4]. Aging also causes changes in vascular walls, which leads to a decrease in the elasticity of the vessels [5]. As a result, vascular resistance and arterial stiffness will increase. These age-related processes can be accelerated by different risk factors like hypertension, hypercholesterolemia and diabetes mellitus [6]. In addition, these age-related changes might also affect the kidney in several ways. Lower cardiac output and stroke volume can alter the renal blood flow, whereas vascular stiffening can expose the microcirculation to hemodynamic stress. Both processes could eventually lead to damage in the kidneys [7,8]. Also, kidney function decline can influence bone mineralization and promotes vascular calcification [9]. This makes cardiovascular diseases both a cause and consequence of kidney function decline.

The association between cardiovascular condition and CKD in older individuals has been investigated. However, the results are conflicting and the possible association, especially in the oldest populations, remains unclear [8,10–14]. The aim of this study was to investigate the effect of hemodynamic parameters on the changes in kidney function within one year in older individuals. We hypothesized that older individuals with poor hemodynamics at baseline would have a greater decline in kidney function during follow up than those with favorable hemodynamics.

2. Materials and Methods

2.1. Study Population

The present study was conducted within the framework of the "Screening for Chronic kidney disease among Older People across Europe" (SCOPE) study, an international, observational and prospective cohort study [15]. A detailed description of the study protocol can be found elsewhere [15]. A comprehensive geriatric assessment (CGA) was performed at baseline and during follow-up visits. Inclusion criteria of the SCOPE study were as follows: participants had to be 75 years or older and had to attend outpatient services or clinics. Patients with end-stage renal disease (ESRD; estimated Glomerular Filtration Rate (eGFR) < 15 mL/min/1.73 m^2) or renal dialysis, end-stage heart failure (New York Heart Association Classification (NYHA) class IV), a history of solid organ or bone marrow transplantation, an active malignancy of metastatic cancer within 24 months prior to the visit, a life expectancy of less than 6 months, a severe cognitive impairment (Mini-Mental State Examination (MMSE) < 10/30) or patients unwilling to provide consent were ineligible for the study.

The subgroup used for the present study consisted of 301 participants enrolled in the Netherlands. In this subset, data from baseline and one-year follow-up visits were used. Participants who could not be followed up and whose hemodynamic or kidney function parameters could not be collected were excluded from the present study. The Medical Ethics Committee of the Erasmus Medical Center in Rotterdam reviewed and approved the SCOPE study. All participants provided written informed consent.

2.2. Hemodynamics and Kidney Function

Blood and urine samples were collected at baseline and after one year of follow up. The BIS 1 (Berlin Initiative study) equation was used to determine kidney function [16]. This creatinine-based formula is accurate for estimating the GFR of older individuals. Calculation of eGFR-BIS1 was performed by using serum creatinine, age and sex of the participants. Also, albuminuria was measured to assess kidney function. Consistent with previous literature, we defined a large increase in the urine Albumin-to-Creatinine Ratio (UACR) as a 2-fold increase in UACR during follow up, the development of a UACR $\geq$ 2.5 g/mol for men who had UACR < 2.5 at baseline or the development of a UACR $\geq$ 3.5 g/mol for women who had UACR < 3.5 at the first visit [11].

Hemodynamic parameters were determined with the Mobil-O-Graph (IEM, Rheinland, Germany) [17]. The Mobil-O-Graph is a non-invasive device for the analysis of peripheral systolic and diastolic blood pressure, mean arterial pressure, pulse pressure and heart rate [18,19]. The software of this device has the ability to analyze these measurements and is able to calculate central blood pressure, aortic pulse wave velocity (aPWV) and the augmentation index. With the software, other hemodynamic parameters were also assessed. These parameters included cardiac output, stroke volume, cardiac index and total peripheral resistance [20].

The parameters used in this study include the following: (central) systolic blood pressure (cSBP), in mmHg; (central) diastolic blood pressure (cDBP) in mmHg; stroke volume, in mL, cardiac output (CO), in L/min; cardiac index [a] (CI) in L/min/m^2); total peripheral resistance (TPR) in s·mmHg/mL); central pulse pressure (cPP) in mmHg; aortic pulse wave velocity (aPWV) in m/s [b].

^a Cardiac index assesses cardiac output values based on body size. It is denoted in liters/minute/body surface area measured in meters squared.
^b Pulse wave velocity is the velocity of the pulse wave to travel between two points in the arterial system, measured in m/s.

2.3. Statistical Analyses

The Shapiro–Wilk normality test was conducted for characteristics and variables to test the normality of the data distribution. Categorical data were expressed in percent prevalence (%). Depending on the normality of the data distribution, continuous data were noted as means ± SD or median [IQR].

The parameters of interest were (c)SBP, (c)DBP, stroke volume, CO, CI, TPR, cPP and aPWV. Each parameter was split into two groups based on the median considering the relatively small group of participants included and the lack of specific reference values for multimorbid older adults. The group with outcomes equal to and below the median were called "low" and the group with outcomes above the median were called "high". The baseline table is also stratified for low and high aPWV. Continuous variables were compared with an independent sample *t*-test or Mann–Whitney U test. Categorical variables were compared with the Chi-square test.

Change in eGFR (in percentage) within one year was investigated in low and high groups for each hemodynamic parameter using analysis of variance (ANOVA). Changes in UACR were examined as binary outcomes (large increase vs. stable) by performing logistic regression. If an association was found between a hemodynamic parameter and change in eGFR or a large increase in UACR, further multivariate analyses were performed using analysis of covariance (ANCOVA) or multivariate logistic regression per parameter. Potential confounders were identified and those with a *p*-value < 0.1 were used in adjusted analysis using different models, where appropriate. Age and sex were not included in the models, since comparable annual eGFR change can be expected for adults above the age of 75 years [21]. *p*-values < 0.05 were considered statistically significant. Statistical analyses were performed using IBM SPSS Statistics version 25 for Windows.

3. Results

In total, 301 participants were enrolled in the SCOPE study in the Netherlands. Eventually, 277 participants were successfully followed up for a period of one year. Patients with missing values were excluded. Therefore, the study population consisted of 252 participants.

3.1. Baseline Characteristics

The health-related baseline characteristics are presented in Table 1. The mean age of the participants was 80.1 ± 4.4 years old and 41.3% of the participants were women. Among all the participants, 71.8% used antihypertensive drugs. Hypertension was found in 176 participants (69.8%) and diabetes mellitus in 65 participants (25.8%). Participants in the high PWV group (aPWV > 12.2 m/s, n = 121) were older than those in the low group (83.0 vs. 76.9 years, *p*-value < 0.001). Participants in the low aPWV group (n = 131) used beta blockers (50.4% vs. 32.2%, *p* = 0.004) and statins more often than participants in the high aPWV group (57.3% vs. 34.7%, *p* < 0.001). Participants in the high aPWV group did not have higher prevalence of cardiovascular events, heart failure, atrial fibrillation or diabetes mellitus compared to the participants in the low aPWV group.

Table 1. Health-related baseline characteristics stratified for aPWV.

	All Participants (n = 252)	aPWV ≤ 12.2 m/s (n = 131)	aPWV > 12.2 m/s (n = 121)	p Value
Age, years	79.1 [76.6–83.0]	76.9 [75.5–78.4]	83.0 [79.6–85.9]	$p < 0.001$
Women, %	41.3	42.7	39.7	$p = ns$
BMI, kg/m^2	26.2 (3.9)	26.4 (3.9)	26.1 (3.9)	$p = ns$
MMSE, score	29 [27–30]	29 [28–30]	28 [28–30]	$p = ns$
ADL independent, %	83.3	86.3	80.2	$p = ns$
iADL independent, %	47.2	58.0	35.5	$p = ns$
Alcohol				$p = ns$
no, (%)	64.3	64.1	64.5	
1–2 units/day, %	26.2	26.7	25.6	
>2 units/day, %	9.5	9.2	9.9	
Smoking				$p = ns$
No, %	29.8	32.1	27.3	
Former, %	65.1	62.6	67.8	
Current, %	9.5	5.3	5.0	
Medication				
Antihypertensives, %	71.8	74.0	69.4	$p = ns$
ACE inhibitor, %	19.8	17.6	22.3	$p = ns$
Beta blocker, %	41.7	50.4	32.2	$p = 0.004$
CA channel blocker, %	23.0	22.1	24.0	$p = ns$
Diuretics, %	19.8	21.4	18.2	$p = ns$
Statins, %	46.4	57.3	34.7	$p < 0.001$
Comorbidities				
Hypertension, %	69.8	64.1	76.0	$p = 0.040$
CVA, %	7.9	6.1	9.9	$p = ns$
TIA, %	14.7	13.0	16.5	$p = ns$
HF, %	12.7	13.0	12.4	$p = ns$
MI, %	17.9	18.3	17.4	$p = ns$
AF, %	17.1	17.6	16.5	$p = ns$
DM, %	25.8	29.8	21.5	$p = ns$
CIRS, severity index	1.8 (0.3)	1.8 (0.3)	1.8 (0.3)	$p = ns$
CIRS, total	12.7 (4.9)	12.8 (4.9)	12.5 (5.0)	$p = ns$

Abbreviations: ADL, activities of daily living; AF; atrial fibrillation; aPWV, aortic pulse wave velocity; BMI, body mass index; CA, calcium; CIRS, Cumulative Illness Rating Scale; CVA, cerebral vascular accident; DM, diabetes mellitus; HF, heart failure; iADL, instrumental activities of daily living; MI, myocardial Infarction; MMSE, Mini-Mental State Examination; TIA, transient ischemic attack. Note: non-normally continuous variables are presented as median [interquartile range] and normally distributed continuous are presented as mean ± SD. Categorical variables are presented as percentages. Continuous variables were compared between the PWV ≤ median and PWV > median with an independent sample t-test or Mann–Whitney U test. Categorical variables were compared with a Chi-square test. p-values < 0.05 were considered statistically significant.

Table 2 describes the hemodynamic and laboratory characteristics at baseline stratified for aPWV. The mean aPWV in the total cohort was 12.4 ± 1.2 m/s. Participants in the high aPWV group in general had higher blood pressure values (both peripheral and central) than participants in the low aPWV group. For instance, the SBP was 158.0 vs. 141.0 mmHg ($p < 0.001$), MAP was 119.4 vs. 107.6 mmHg ($p < 0.001$) and cPP was 49.4 vs. 39.1 mmHg ($p < 0.001$), respectively. The TPR was higher in the high aPWV group than in the low aPWV group (median 1.5 vs. 1.3 s·mmHg/mL, $p = 0.008$). Stroke volume, CO and CI did not differ between groups. At baseline, the mean eGFR in the low aPWV group was 49.0 ± 13.6 mL/min and 46.2 ± 12.7 mL/min in the high aPWV group with no statistically significant difference between the groups. Participants in the high aPWV group had a higher UACR (median 3.4 vs. 1.9 g/mol, $p = 0.008$) than those in the low aPWV group.

Table 2. Hemodynamics and laboratory baseline characteristics stratified for aPWV.

	All Participants (n = 252)	aPWV ≤ 12.2 m/s (n = 131)	aPWV > 12.2 m/s (n =121)	*p* Value
Hemodynamics				
SBP, mmHg	147.0 [135.0–160.0]	141.0 [129.0–151.0]	158.0 [144.0–171.0]	*p* < 0.001
DBP, mmHg	86.2 (11.2)	83.3 (10.1)	89.4 (11.5)	*p* < 0.001
cSBP, mmHg	130.9 (17.5)	123.2 (12.9)	139.3 (18.0)	*p* < 0.001
cDBP, mmHg	86.8 (11.4)	84.0 (10.1)	89.9 (11.9)	*p* < 0.001
MAP, mmHg	113.3 (14.1)	107.6 (11.3)	119.4 (14.3)	*p* < 0.001
HR, beats/min	69.8 (12.1)	67.9 (11.3)	71.8 (12.7)	*p* = 0.014
Stroke volume, mL	75.3 (13.2)	76.5 (14.3)	74.0 (11.9)	*p* = ns
CO, L/min	5.2 (1.0)	5.1 (0.9)	5.3 (1.1)	*p* = ns
CI, L/min/m^2	2.8 [2.3–3.2]	2.7 [2.3–3.2]	2.8 [2.4–3.3]	*p* = ns
TPR, s·mmHg/mL	1.3 [1.1–1.6]	1.3 [1.1–1.5]	1.5 [1.2–1.7]	*P* = 0.008
cPP, mmHg	44.0 (12.8)	39.1 (9.3)	49.4 (13.9)	*p* < 0.001
aPWV, m/s	12.4 (1.2)	11.6 (0.5)	13.4 (0.9)	*p* < 0.001
Kidney function				
eGFR, mL/min	47.6 (13.7)	49.0 (13.6)	46.2 (13.7)	*p* = ns
UACR, g/mol [1]	2.7 [0.9–10.7]	1.9 [0.6–7.5]	3.4 [1.2–12.3]	*p* = 0.008

[1] Missing data of 1 participant for PWV ≤ 12.2 m/s. Abbreviations: aPWV; aortic pulse wave velocity; cDBP, central diastolic blood pressure; CI, cardiac index; CO, cardiac output; cPP, central pulse pressure; cSBP, central systolic blood pressure; DBP, diastolic blood pressure; HR, heart rate; SBP, systolic blood pressure; TPR, total peripheral resistance; UACR; urinary albumin creatinine ratio. Note: non-normally continuous variables are presented as median [interquartile range] and normally distributed continuous are presented as mean ± SD. Categorical variables are presented as n (percentages). Continuous variables were compared between the PWV ≤ median and PWV > median with an independent sample *t*-test or Mann–Whitney U test. Categorical variables were compared with a Chi-square test. *p*-values < 0.05 were considered statistically significant.

3.2. Hemodynamic Parameters and Change in eGFR

Table 3 shows the difference in kidney function expressed in percentage change in eGFR within one year for the different hemodynamic parameters according to median values. Participants in the high cSBP group showed a greater decline in eGFR than the participants in the low cSBP group (−5.9% vs. −3.2%, *p* = 0.042). Likewise, participants in the high aPWV group had a greater decline in eGFR compared to those in the low group (−6.5% vs. −2.8%, *p* = 0.005). The change in eGFR for participants in the high groups of SBP, DBP, cDBP, stroke volume, CO, CI, TPR and cPP did not differ from those in the low groups of those hemodynamic variables.

Table 3. Mean change in eGFR within one year in low group (below median) and high group (above median) of different hemodynamics (n = 252).

Parameter (Median)	Low Group % Change in eGFR (95%CI)	High Group % Change in eGFR (95%CI)	Difference between Groups (95%CI)
SBP (147)	−3.6 (−5.6, −1.6)	−5.6 (−7.1, −3.9)	2.0 (−0.6, 4.5)
DBP (85)	−4.2 (−6.0, −2.4)	−5.0 (−6.8, −3.1)	0.8 (−1.8, 3.4)
cSBP (129)	−3.2 (−5.0, −1.4)	−5.9 (−7.7, −4.1)	**2.7 (0.1, 5.2)**
cDBP (85)	−4.5 (−6.3, −2.7)	−4.6 (−6.4, −2.8)	0.1 (−2.5, 2.7)
Stroke volume (74.6)	−4.0 (−5.8, −2.2)	−5.1 (−6.9, −3.3)	1.1 (−1.5, 3.7)
CO (5.1)	−3.8 (−5.6, −2.0)	−5.3 (−7.1, −3.5)	1.5 (−1.1, 4.1)
CI (2.8)	−4.1 (−6.0, −2.3)	−5.0 (−6.8, −3.2)	0.8 (−1.7, 3.4)
TVR (1.3)	−4.7 (−6.6, −2.7)	−4.5 (−6.2, −2.7)	−0.2 (−2.8, 2.4)
cPP (42)	−3.9 (−5.7, −2.1)	−5.3 (−7.1, −3.4)	1.4 (−1.2, 4.0)
aPWV (12.2)	−2.8 (−4.6, −1.0)	−6.5 (−8.3, −4.6)	**3.7 (1.1, 6.2)**

Abbreviations: aPWV, aortic pulse wave velocity; cDBP, central diastolic blood pressure; CI, cardiac index; CO, cardiac output; cSBP, central systolic blood pressure; cPP, central pulse pressure; DBP, diastolic blood pressure; SBP, systolic blood pressure; TPR, total peripheral resistance; Note: bold is *p* < 0.05.

Figure 1 shows the adjusted mean percentage change in eGFR in participants with low and high cSBP (panels A–C) and in those with low and high aPWV (panels D–F). In the adjusted analyses, participants in the high group of cSBP had a greater decline in eGFR than those in the low group. In the extensive adjusted model (panel C), the mean percentage change in eGFR was −2.7% in the low cSBP group and −6.3% in the high cSBP group ($p = 0.006$). Comparable results were found in the analysis for aPWV, where participants in the high group of aPWV had a greater decline in eGFR than participants in the low group of aPWV. In the extensive adjusted model (panel F), the mean percentage change in eGFR was −2.5% in the low aPWV group and −6.8% in the high aPWV group ($p = 0.001$)

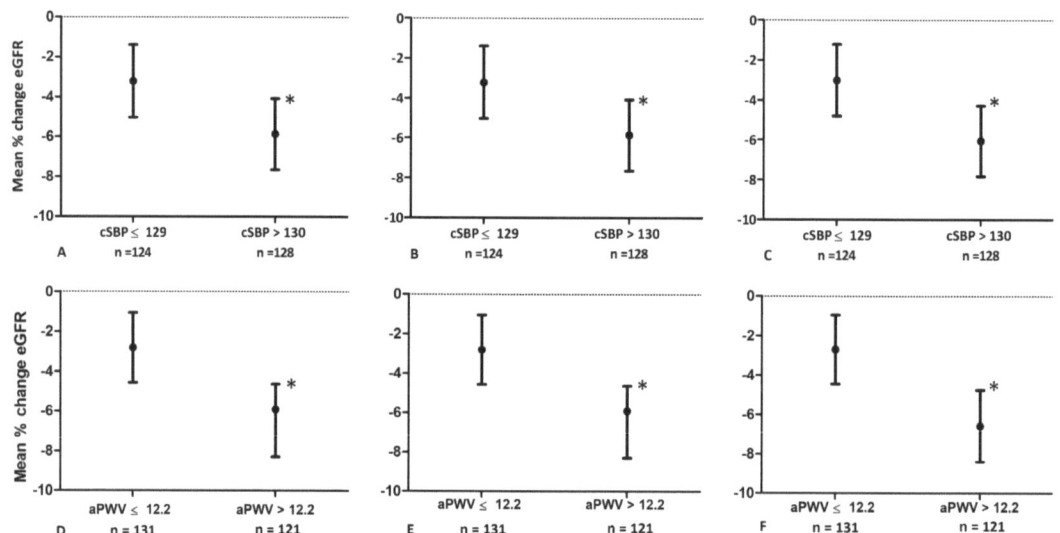

Figure 1. Association between baseline cSBP (panel **A–C**) or baseline aPWV (panel **D–F**) and percentage change in eGFR (n = 252): (**A**) adjusted for baseline eGFR; (**B**) adjusted for baseline eGFR, BMI, and DM; (**C**) adjusted for baseline eGFR, BMI, DM, the use of ACE inhibitors and beta blockers; (**D**) adjusted for baseline eGFR; (**E**) adjusted for baseline eGFR, BMI, DM, and hypertension; (**F**) adjusted for baseline eGFR, BMI, DM, hypertension, the use of ACE inhibitors and beta blockers. Dots represent means and bars represent 95% confidence interval. Significant differences between groups are marked with an asterisk (*). Abbreviations: aPWV, aortic pulse wave velocity; BMI, body mass index; cSBP, central systolic blood pressure; DM, diabetes mellitus; eGFR, estimated glomerular filtration rate.

3.3. Hemodynamic Parameters and Change in UACR

For all hemodynamic parameters, there were no differences between the low and high groups in the association between the baseline parameters and the chance of a large increase in the UACR.

4. Discussion

In the present study in individuals aged 75 years and over, we found that participants in the highest categories of cSBP and aPWV had a greater decline in kidney function within one year than participants in the lowest category of cSBP and aPWV with an additional decline of 2.7% and 3.7% in one year, respectively. These results suggest that increased aortic stiffness has a negative effect on kidney function (even) in older age. All included hemodynamics appeared to have no influence on changes in UACR.

Several mechanisms can explain the found associations. Due to age-related changes in the vascular wall and the presence of additional cardiovascular risk factors, wall elasticity

Table 2. Hemodynamics and laboratory baseline characteristics stratified for aPWV.

	All Participants (n = 252)	aPWV ≤ 12.2 m/s (n = 131)	aPWV > 12.2 m/s (n =121)	p Value
Hemodynamics				
SBP, mmHg	147.0 [135.0–160.0]	141.0 [129.0–151.0]	158.0 [144.0–171.0]	$p < 0.001$
DBP, mmHg	86.2 (11.2)	83.3 (10.1)	89.4 (11.5)	$p < 0.001$
cSBP, mmHg	130.9 (17.5)	123.2 (12.9)	139.3 (18.0)	$p < 0.001$
cDBP, mmHg	86.8 (11.4)	84.0 (10.1)	89.9 (11.9)	$p < 0.001$
MAP, mmHg	113.3 (14.1)	107.6 (11.3)	119.4 (14.3)	$p < 0.001$
HR, beats/min	69.8 (12.1)	67.9 (11.3)	71.8 (12.7)	$p = 0.014$
Stroke volume, mL	75.3 (13.2)	76.5 (14.3)	74.0 (11.9)	p = ns
CO, L/min	5.2 (1.0)	5.1 (0.9)	5.3 (1.1)	p = ns
CI, L/min/m^2	2.8 [2.3–3.2]	2.7 [2.3–3.2]	2.8 [2.4–3.3]	p = ns
TPR, s·mmHg/mL	1.3 [1.1–1.6]	1.3 [1.1–1.5]	1.5 [1.2–1.7]	$P = 0.008$
cPP, mmHg	44.0 (12.8)	39.1 (9.3)	49.4 (13.9)	$p < 0.001$
aPWV, m/s	12.4 (1.2)	11.6 (0.5)	13.4 (0.9)	$p < 0.001$
Kidney function				
eGFR, mL/min	47.6 (13.7)	49.0 (13.6)	46.2 (13.7)	p = ns
UACR, g/mol [1]	2.7 [0.9–10.7]	1.9 [0.6–7.5]	3.4 [1.2–12.3]	$p = 0.008$

[1] Missing data of 1 participant for PWV ≤ 12.2 m/s. Abbreviations: aPWV; aortic pulse wave velocity; cDBP, central diastolic blood pressure; CI, cardiac index; CO, cardiac output; cPP, central pulse pressure; cSBP, central systolic blood pressure; DBP, diastolic blood pressure; HR, heart rate; SBP, systolic blood pressure; TPR, total peripheral resistance; UACR; urinary albumin creatinine ratio. Note: non-normally continuous variables are presented as median [interquartile range] and normally distributed continuous are presented as mean ± SD. Categorical variables are presented as n (percentages). Continuous variables were compared between the PWV ≤ median and PWV > median with an independent sample t-test or Mann–Whitney U test. Categorical variables were compared with a Chi-square test. p-values < 0.05 were considered statistically significant.

3.2. Hemodynamic Parameters and Change in eGFR

Table 3 shows the difference in kidney function expressed in percentage change in eGFR within one year for the different hemodynamic parameters according to median values. Participants in the high cSBP group showed a greater decline in eGFR than the participants in the low cSBP group (-5.9% vs. -3.2%, $p = 0.042$). Likewise, participants in the high aPWV group had a greater decline in eGFR compared to those in the low group (-6.5% vs. -2.8%, $p = 0.005$). The change in eGFR for participants in the high groups of SBP, DBP, cDBP, stroke volume, CO, CI, TPR and cPP did not differ from those in the low groups of those hemodynamic variables.

Table 3. Mean change in eGFR within one year in low group (below median) and high group (above median) of different hemodynamics (n = 252).

Parameter (Median)	Low Group % Change in eGFR (95%CI)	High Group % Change in eGFR (95%CI)	Difference between Groups (95%CI)
SBP (147)	−3.6 (−5.6, −1.6)	−5.6 (−7.1, −3.9)	2.0 (−0.6, 4.5)
DBP (85)	−4.2 (−6.0, −2.4)	−5.0 (−6.8, −3.1)	0.8 (−1.8, 3.4)
cSBP (129)	−3.2 (−5.0, −1.4)	−5.9 (−7.7, −4.1)	**2.7 (0.1, 5.2)**
cDBP (85)	−4.5 (−6.3, −2.7)	−4.6 (−6.4, −2.8)	0.1 (−2.5, 2.7)
Stroke volume (74.6)	−4.0 (−5.8, −2.2)	−5.1 (−6.9, −3.3)	1.1 (−1.5, 3.7)
CO (5.1)	−3.8 (−5.6, −2.0)	−5.3 (−7.1, −3.5)	1.5 (−1.1, 4.1)
CI (2.8)	−4.1 (−6.0, −2.3)	−5.0 (−6.8, −3.2)	0.8 (−1.7, 3.4)
TVR (1.3)	−4.7 (−6.6, −2.7)	−4.5 (−6.2, −2.7)	−0.2 (−2.8, 2.4)
cPP (42)	−3.9 (−5.7, −2.1)	−5.3 (−7.1, −3.4)	1.4 (−1.2, 4.0)
aPWV (12.2)	−2.8 (−4.6, −1.0)	−6.5 (−8.3, −4.6)	**3.7 (1.1, 6.2)**

Abbreviations: aPWV, aortic pulse wave velocity; cDBP, central diastolic blood pressure; CI, cardiac index; CO, cardiac output; cSBP, central systolic blood pressure; cPP, central pulse pressure; DBP, diastolic blood pressure; SBP, systolic blood pressure; TPR, total peripheral resistance; Note: bold is $p < 0.05$.

Figure 1 shows the adjusted mean percentage change in eGFR in participants with low and high cSBP (panels A–C) and in those with low and high aPWV (panels D–F). In the adjusted analyses, participants in the high group of cSBP had a greater decline in eGFR than those in the low group. In the extensive adjusted model (panel C), the mean percentage change in eGFR was −2.7% in the low cSBP group and −6.3% in the high cSBP group ($p = 0.006$). Comparable results were found in the analysis for aPWV, where participants in the high group of aPWV had a greater decline in eGFR than participants in the low group of aPWV. In the extensive adjusted model (panel F), the mean percentage change in eGFR was −2.5% in the low aPWV group and −6.8% in the high aPWV group ($p = 0.001$)

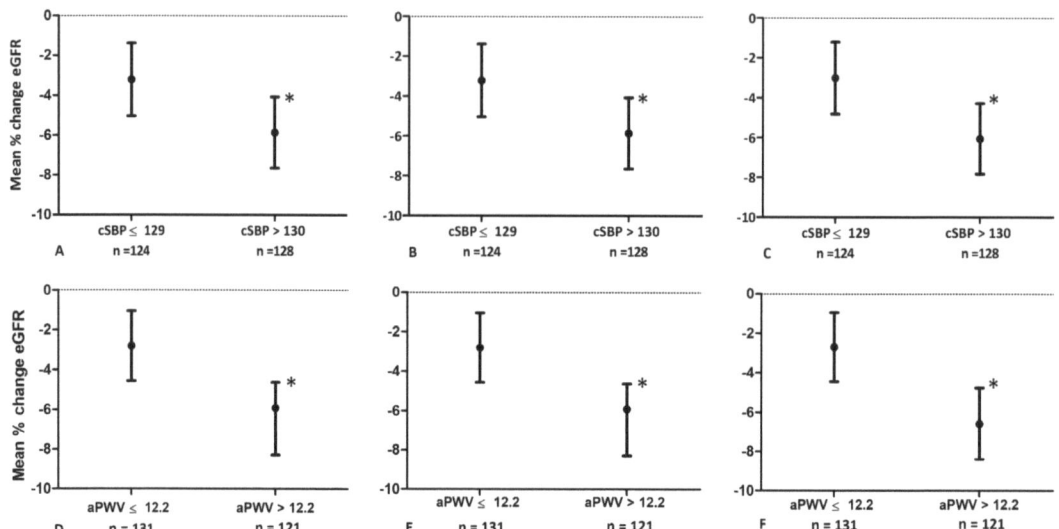

Figure 1. Association between baseline cSBP (panel **A–C**) or baseline aPWV (panel **D–F**) and percentage change in eGFR (n = 252): (**A**) adjusted for baseline eGFR; (**B**) adjusted for baseline eGFR, BMI, and DM; (**C**) adjusted for baseline eGFR, BMI, DM, the use of ACE inhibitors and beta blockers; (**D**) adjusted for baseline eGFR; (**E**) adjusted for baseline eGFR, BMI, DM, and hypertension; (**F**) adjusted for baseline eGFR, BMI, DM, hypertension, the use of ACE inhibitors and beta blockers. Dots represent means and bars represent 95% confidence interval. Significant differences between groups are marked with an asterisk (*). Abbreviations: aPWV, aortic pulse wave velocity; BMI, body mass index; cSBP, central systolic blood pressure; DM, diabetes mellitus; eGFR, estimated glomerular filtration rate.

3.3. Hemodynamic Parameters and Change in UACR

For all hemodynamic parameters, there were no differences between the low and high groups in the association between the baseline parameters and the chance of a large increase in the UACR.

4. Discussion

In the present study in individuals aged 75 years and over, we found that participants in the highest categories of cSBP and aPWV had a greater decline in kidney function within one year than participants in the lowest category of cSBP and aPWV with an additional decline of 2.7% and 3.7% in one year, respectively. These results suggest that increased aortic stiffness has a negative effect on kidney function (even) in older age. All included hemodynamics appeared to have no influence on changes in UACR.

Several mechanisms can explain the found associations. Due to age-related changes in the vascular wall and the presence of additional cardiovascular risk factors, wall elasticity decreases and vascular resistance and arterial stiffness increases [5,6]. Also, elevated arterial stiffness is associated with hypertension [22,23]. Thus, with the stiffening of the arteries, an increase in (central) SBP and increase in aPWV can be observed. Previous studies showed that increased aortic stiffness is associated with changes in the microvascular structure in kidneys [8,11]. Moreover, due to vascular contraction, the arterial flow of the cortex could decrease, both potentially resulting in kidney function decline [8,24]. Increased central blood pressure, as well as increased pulsatility is associated with end-stage organ tissue damage [7], particularly in an autoregulated organ such as the kidney. Since central blood pressure is a direct reflection of the fluctuations in pressure that small arterial vessels face, high cSBP might result in impairment of kidney function [25]. It should be noted that age, blood pressure and aortic stiffness are all intertwined and related. Therefore, the found associations could be the result of the linked age-related microcirculatory changes, including loss of GFR and may not suggest causality.

Our hypothesis suggesting lower cardiac output, cardiac index and stroke volume would be associated with kidney function decline was not confirmed in the present study. As stiffening of the arteries, decline in cardiac output and stroke volume are also age-related changes [26,27], this might not affect kidney perfusion due to sufficient compensation mechanisms. In people with lower cardiac output or stroke volume, redistribution of blood volume in the body could prevent a decrease in blood flow to the kidneys to preserve kidney function [28].

Our finding that aPWV is associated with kidney function decline is in line with previous studies [8,11,12]. Due to different ways of determining kidney function, follow-up time and different age groups, the results could not be completely compared.

In contrast to our results, these previous studies also found an association between cPP as a marker of arterial stiffness and kidney function decline [8,11,12]. A large longitudinal retrospective registry-based cohort found that high-baseline cPP predicted kidney function decline in participants aged 60 to 79 years old, but not in participants above 80 years [29]. This is in line with the present study, with an average age of 80 years, in which we did not find an association between cPP and eGFR decline. Moreover, a community-based study with participants over 85 years old did not find an association between pulse pressure and decline in creatinine clearance [30]. Furthermore, aPWV is a more reliable marker for arterial stiffness than cPP as aPWV is based on arterial properties only, whereas cPP is based on arterial properties and cardiac function [31].

In the present study, pSBP and both cDBP and pDBP were not associated with changes in kidney function. Firstly, fluctuations in the central arteries are a reflection of the pressure that the vessels in kidneys are actually being exposed to [25], which could be an explanation of the found association in central measures but not in peripheral. Secondly, both SBP and DBP increase with age; however, over the age of 60 only SBP increases, whereas DBP remains stable (or even decreases) [32]. This could be another explanation as to why associations between DBP and kidney function were not found.

In the present study, we did not find associations between hemodynamics and changes in UACR. Consistent with our findings, a longitudinal study in participants in the same age group found that higher baseline aPWV and cPP were not associated with UACR increase, which were both analyzed as categorical and continuous variables [11]. Alternatively, in a cohort of the Framingham heart study, higher carotid–femoral PWV at baseline was associated with incident microalbuminuria over a 7- to 10-year period of follow up [33]. This association attenuated after adjustment for different risk factors. The differences in findings could be explained by the use of different cut-off values for albuminuria. Furthermore, differences between study populations, especially age and follow-up time, could account for the differences between previous studies and our results.

Several limitations need to be discussed. First, parameters were split into two groups based on the median considering the relatively small group of participants included and the lack of specific reference values for multimorbid older adults. The high PWV group is older, had higher SBP and PP and lower eGFR at baseline; Despite using multivariate models, intrinsic bias and confounding due to this factor may not be fully eliminated and have an impact on the found results. Second, the study has a relatively short follow-up-time of 1 year. However, despite this small sample size and short follow-up time, we were able to detect significant results. Larger studies with a longer follow-up time might be needed to investigate this topic further. Furthermore, we have focused on older individuals aged 75 years and older and the majority are Caucasian. Therefore, the generalizability could be limited. Survivor bias might also have played a role in attenuating the relationship between hemodynamics and kidney function. In addition, we used the UACR from a random portion of urine, which is a practical method to collect urine in older or frail adults. However, the collection of urine over 24 h is more reliable to investigate albuminuria. Moreover, the Kidney Disease Improving Global Outcomes (KDIGO) suggest that albuminuria could also be transient, suggesting a repeated measurement after three months to confirm this finding [34]. It should also be acknowledged that the Mobil-O-Graph calculates aPWV using an algorithm essentially based on age and blood pressure values, resulting in the interpretation of aPWV as a combined index of vascular aging [18,35]. It should be stated that the Mobil-O-graph is mainly validated for blood pressure and pulse wave analyses; therefore. analyses on other hemodynamics parameters could be less reliable. In addition, there may be evidence of confounding in the reported variables; for instance, the high aPWV group or high cSBP group might have had more nephrosclerosis before the start of the study and thus experience a greater decline in eGFR during the study as a result of this. Unfortunately, we have no information on the trajectories of the patients' kidney function and concomitant pathology before inclusion in the study. Therefore, we adjusted for relevant identified covariates at baseline such as, among others, baseline eGFR, diabetes and hypertension. Finally, there were no restrictions in smoking, drinking coffee or tea or medication use on the day of the measurements, which might have influenced the measurements of arterial stiffness. Nonetheless, circumstances were comparable between the groups. Hence, this should not have affected the results. The present study also has several strengths. One of the strengths is the fact that the BIS 1 equation was used to determine kidney function, which is developed for older populations and gives a more accurate estimation of kidney function [16]. Moreover, a comprehensive geriatric assessment was performed, which is able to capture numerous domains of health status and their complex interactions in older and/or frail adults. To our best knowledge, this is the first study that has investigated various hemodynamics and their effect on kidney function in individuals aged 75 years and over.

5. Conclusions

In conclusion, we found that elevated central aortic stiffness is associated with a greater decline in kidney function in old age. Since aPWV and cSBP both appear to be predictors of eGFR decline, it might be of interest to identify older individuals with elevated aortic stiffness. In this specific population, intensive blood pressure reduction might be justified in order to slow down the process of vascular aging and prevent kidney function decline. It would be of interest to expand the study population to investigate the relationship between hemodynamics and kidney function decline in a large study population and longer follow-up time. Additional functional imaging techniques (sonography, computed tomography, magnetic resonance imaging or positron emission tomography) might also be of additional informative value to better understand the structural changes as a result of vascular and kidney aging.

Author Contributions: Conceptualization, L.T., K.B. and F.M.-R.; methodology, L.T., K.B. and F.M.-R.; software, L.T., K.B., A.C., F.L. and F.M.-R.; validation, L.T., K.B. and F.M.-R.; formal analysis, L.T., K.B. and F.M.-R.; investigation, L.T., K.B. and F.M.-R.; resources, L.T., K.B., A.C., F.L. and F.M.-R.; data curation, L.T., K.B., A.C., F.L. and F.M.-R.; writing—original draft preparation, L.T. and K.B.; writing—review and editing, L.T., K.B., A.C., F.L. and F.M.-R.; visualization, L.T., K.B., A.C., F.L. and F.M.-R.; supervision, F.M.-R.; project administration, A.C. and F.L.; funding acquisition, A.C., F.L. and F.M.-R. All authors have read and agreed to the published version of the manuscript.

Funding: The SCOPE project was granted by the European Union Horizon 2020 program, under the Grant Agreement n°634869.

Institutional Review Board Statement: The study was conducted in accordance with the Declaration of Helsinki, and approved by the Ethics Committees in participating institutions (Erasmus MC University Medical Center Rotterdam, the Netherlands, #MEC-2016-036 #NL56039.078.15, v.4, 7 March 2016).

Informed Consent Statement: Informed consent was obtained from all subjects involved in the study.

Data Availability Statement: Data will be available for SCOPE consortium upon request from the principal investigator, Fabrizia Lattanzio, Italian National Research Center on Aging (IRCCS INRCA), Ancona, Fermo and Cosenza, Italy. f.lattanzio@inrca.it.

Acknowledgments: The authors thank all the investigators of the SCOPE consortium for the collaboration within the SCOPE project. The authors would also like to thank Wave Medical BV Heerenveen, the Netherlands, for their logistic support in performing this study (Mobil-o-graph device).

Conflicts of Interest: The authors declare no conflicts of interest. The funder had no role in the design of the study; in the collection, analyses, or interpretation of data; in the writing of the manuscript; or in the decision to publish the results.

References

1. Kalantar-Zadeh, K.; Jafar, T.H.; Nitsch, D.; Neuen, B.L.; Perkovic, V. Chronic kidney disease. *Lancet* **2021**, *398*, 786–802. [CrossRef] [PubMed]
2. GBD Chronic Kidney Disease Collaboration. Global, regional, and national burden of chronic kidney disease, 1990–2017: A systematic analysis for the Global Burden of Disease Study 2017. *Lancet* **2020**, *395*, 709–733. [CrossRef] [PubMed]
3. Mallappallil, M.; Friedman, E.A.; Delano, B.G.; McFarlane, S.I.; Salifu, M.O. Chronic kidney disease in the elderly: Evaluation and management. *Clin. Pract.* **2014**, *11*, 525–535. [CrossRef] [PubMed]
4. Wu, S.; Jin, C.; Li, S.; Zheng, X.; Zhang, X.; Cui, L.; Gao, X. Aging, Arterial Stiffness, and Blood Pressure Association in Chinese Adults. *Hypertension* **2019**, *73*, 893–899. [CrossRef] [PubMed]
5. Mitchell, G.F. Arterial Stiffness in Aging: Does It Have a Place in Clinical Practice? Recent Advances in Hypertension. *Hypertension* **2021**, *77*, 768–780. [CrossRef] [PubMed]
6. Laurent, S.; Boutouyrie, P.; Cunha, P.G.; Lacolley, P.; Nilsson, P.M. Concept of Extremes in Vascular Aging. *Hypertension* **2019**, *74*, 218–228. [CrossRef] [PubMed]
7. Mitchell, G.F. Effects of central arterial aging on the structure and function of the peripheral vasculature: Implications for end-organ damage. *J. Appl. Physiol. 1985* **2008**, *105*, 1652–1660. [CrossRef]
8. Sedaghat, S.; Mattace-Raso, F.U.; Hoorn, E.J.; Uitterlinden, A.G.; Hofman, A.; Ikram, M.A.; Franco, O.H.; Dehghan, A. Arterial Stiffness and Decline in Kidney Function. *Clin. J. Am. Soc. Nephrol.* **2015**, *10*, 2190–2197. [CrossRef]
9. Lioufas, N.; Hawley, C.M.; Cameron, J.D.; Toussaint, N.D. Chronic Kidney Disease and Pulse Wave Velocity: A Narrative Review. *Int. J. Hypertens.* **2019**, *2019*, 9189362. [CrossRef]
10. Hanberg, J.S.; Sury, K.; Wilson, F.P.; Brisco, M.A.; Ahmad, T.; Ter Maaten, J.M.; Broughton, J.S.; Assefa, M.; Tang, W.H.W.; Parikh, C.R.; et al. Reduced Cardiac Index Is Not the Dominant Driver of Renal Dysfunction in Heart Failure. *J. Am. Coll. Cardiol.* **2016**, *67*, 2199–2208. [CrossRef]
11. Huang, N.; Foster, M.C.; Mitchell, G.F.; Andresdottir, M.B.; Eiriksdottir, G.; Gudmundsdottir, H.; Harris, T.B.; Launer, L.J.; Palsson, R.; Gudnason, V.; et al. Aortic stiffness and change in glomerular filtration rate and albuminuria in older people. *Nephrol. Dial. Transplant.* **2017**, *32*, 677–684. [CrossRef]
12. Madero, M.; Peralta, C.; Katz, R.; Canada, R.; Fried, L.; Najjar, S.; Shlipak, M.; Simonsick, E.; Lakatta, E.; Patel, K.; et al. Association of arterial rigidity with incident kidney disease and kidney function decline: The Health ABC study. *Clin. J. Am. Soc. Nephrol.* **2013**, *8*, 424–433. [CrossRef] [PubMed]
13. Michener, K.H.; Mitchell, G.F.; Noubary, F.; Huang, N.; Harris, T.; Andresdottir, M.B.; Palsson, R.; Gudnason, V.; Levey, A.S. Aortic stiffness and kidney disease in an elderly population. *Am. J. Nephrol.* **2015**, *41*, 320–328. [CrossRef] [PubMed]
14. Temmar, M.; Liabeuf, S.; Renard, C.; Czernichow, S.; Esper, N.E.; Shahapuni, I.; Presne, C.; Makdassi, R.; Andrejak, M.; Tribouilloy, C.; et al. Pulse wave velocity and vascular calcification at different stages of chronic kidney disease. *J. Hypertens.* **2010**, *28*, 163–169. [CrossRef] [PubMed]
15. Corsonello, A.; Tap, L.; Roller-Wirnsberger, R.; Wirnsberger, G.; Zoccali, C.; Kostka, T.; Guligowska, A.; Mattace-Raso, F.; Gil, P.; Fuentes, L.G.; et al. Design and methodology of the screening for CKD among older patients across Europe (SCOPE) study: A multicenter cohort observational study. *BMC Nephrol.* **2018**, *19*, 260. [CrossRef]

16. Schaeffner, E.S.; Ebert, N.; Delanaye, P.; Frei, U.; Gaedeke, J.; Jakob, O.; Kuhlmann, M.K.; Schuchardt, M.; Tölle, M.; Ziebig, R.; et al. Two novel equations to estimate kidney function in persons aged 70 years or older. *Ann. Intern. Med.* **2012**, *157*, 471–481. [CrossRef] [PubMed]
17. Milan, A.; Zocaro, G.; Leone, D.; Tosello, F.; Buraioli, I.; Schiavone, D.; Veglio, F. Current assessment of pulse wave velocity: Comprehensive review of validation studies. *J. Hypertens.* **2019**, *37*, 1547–1557. [CrossRef] [PubMed]
18. Weber, T.; Wassertheurer, S.; Hametner, B.; Parragh, S.; Eber, B. Noninvasive methods to assess pulse wave velocity: Comparison with the invasive gold standard and relationship with organ damage. *J. Hypertens.* **2015**, *33*, 1023–1031. [CrossRef]
19. Weber, T.; Wassertheurer, S.; Rammer, M.; Maurer, E.; Hametner, B.; Mayer, C.C.; Kropf, J.; Eber, B. Validation of a brachial cuff-based method for estimating central systolic blood pressure. *Hypertension* **2011**, *58*, 825–832. [CrossRef]
20. Thomas, W.; Siegfried, W.; Jessica, M.; Carmel Mary, M.; Bernhard, H.; Christopher Clemens, M.; Ronald Karl, B.; Hans-Josef, F.; Gert, K.; Bernhard, M. Validation of a Method to Estimate Stroke Volume from Brachial-cuff Derived Pressure Waveforms. *Artery Res.* **2020**, *26*, 42–47. [CrossRef]
21. Toyama, T.; Kitagawa, K.; Oshima, M.; Kitajima, S.; Hara, A.; Iwata, Y.; Sakai, N.; Shimizu, M.; Hashiba, A.; Furuichi, K.; et al. Age differences in the relationships between risk factors and loss of kidney function: A general population cohort study. *BMC Nephrol.* **2020**, *21*, 477. [CrossRef] [PubMed]
22. Sun, Z. Aging, arterial stiffness, and hypertension. *Hypertension* **2015**, *65*, 252–256. [CrossRef] [PubMed]
23. Zhang, Y.; Lacolley, P.; Protogerou, A.D.; Safar, M.E. Arterial stiffness in hypertension and function of large arteries. *Am. J. Hypertens.* **2020**, *33*, 291–296. [CrossRef] [PubMed]
24. Woodard, T.; Sigurdsson, S.; Gotal, J.D.; Torjesen, A.A.; Inker, L.A.; Aspelund, T.; Eiriksdottir, G.; Gudnason, V.; Harris, T.B.; Launer, L.J.; et al. Mediation analysis of aortic stiffness and renal microvascular function. *J. Am. Soc. Nephrol.* **2015**, *26*, 1181–1187. [CrossRef]
25. Fan, F.; Qi, L.; Jia, J.; Xu, X.; Liu, Y.; Yang, Y.; Qin, X.; Li, J.; Li, H.; Zhang, Y.; et al. Noninvasive Central Systolic Blood Pressure Is More Strongly Related to Kidney Function Decline Than Peripheral Systolic Blood Pressure in a Chinese Community-Based Population. *Hypertension* **2016**, *67*, 1166–1172. [CrossRef] [PubMed]
26. Ogawa, T.; Spina, R.J.; Martin, W.H., 3rd; Kohrt, W.M.; Schechtman, K.B.; Holloszy, J.O.; Ehsani, A.A. Effects of aging, sex, and physical training on cardiovascular responses to exercise. *Circulation* **1992**, *86*, 494–503. [CrossRef]
27. Houghton, D.; Jones, T.W.; Cassidy, S.; Siervo, M.; MacGowan, G.A.; Trenell, M.I.; Jakovljevic, D.G. The effect of age on the relationship between cardiac and vascular function. *Mech. Ageing Dev.* **2016**, *153*, 1–6. [CrossRef]
28. Mullens, W.; Nijst, P. Cardiac Output and Renal Dysfunction: Definitely More Than Impaired Flow. *J. Am. Coll. Cardiol.* **2016**, *67*, 2209–2212. [CrossRef]
29. Vaes, B.; Beke, E.; Truyers, C.; Elli, S.; Buntinx, F.; Verbakel, J.Y.; Goderis, G.; Van Pottelbergh, G. The correlation between blood pressure and kidney function decline in older people: A registry-based cohort study. *BMJ Open* **2015**, *5*, e007571. [CrossRef]
30. van Bemmel, T.; Woittiez, K.; Blauw, G.J.; van der Sman-de Beer, F.; Dekker, F.W.; Westendorp, R.G.; Gussekloo, J. Prospective study of the effect of blood pressure on renal function in old age: The Leiden 85-Plus Study. *J. Am. Soc. Nephrol.* **2006**, *17*, 2561–2566. [CrossRef]
31. Avolio, A.P.; Kuznetsova, T.; Heyndrickx, G.R.; Kerkhof, P.L.M.; Li, J.K. Arterial Flow, Pulse Pressure and Pulse Wave Velocity in Men and Women at Various Ages. *Adv. Exp. Med. Biol.* **2018**, *1065*, 153–168. [CrossRef]
32. Benetos, A.; Petrovic, M.; Strandberg, T. Hypertension Management in Older and Frail Older Patients. *Circ. Res.* **2019**, *124*, 1045–1060. [CrossRef]
33. Upadhyay, A.; Hwang, S.J.; Mitchell, G.F.; Vasan, R.S.; Vita, J.A.; Stantchev, P.I.; Meigs, J.B.; Larson, M.G.; Levy, D.; Benjamin, E.J.; et al. Arterial stiffness in mild-to-moderate CKD. *J. Am. Soc. Nephrol.* **2009**, *20*, 2044–2053. [CrossRef]
34. The Kidney Disease: Improving Global Outcomes (KDIGO) 2012 Clinical Practice Guideline for the Evaluation and Management of Chronic Kidney Disease (CKD). Available online: https://kdigo.org/wp-content/uploads/2017/02/KDIGO_2012_CKD_GL.pdf (accessed on 19 September 2023).
35. Schwartz, J.E.; Feig, P.U.; Izzo, J.L. Pulse Wave Velocities Derived From Cuff Ambulatory Pulse Wave Analysis. *Hypertension* **2019**, *74*, 111–116. [CrossRef]

Disclaimer/Publisher's Note: The statements, opinions and data contained in all publications are solely those of the individual author(s) and contributor(s) and not of MDPI and/or the editor(s). MDPI and/or the editor(s) disclaim responsibility for any injury to people or property resulting from any ideas, methods, instructions or products referred to in the content.

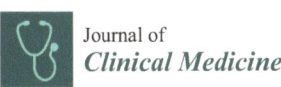

Article

Diabetes-Related Changes in Carotid Wall Properties: Role of Triglycerides

Michaela Kozakova [1,2,†], Carmela Morizzo [3,†], Giuseppe Penno [1,†], Dante Chiappino [4] and Carlo Palombo [3,5,*,†]

[1] Department of Clinical and Experimental Medicine, University of Pisa, 56126 Pisa, Italy; michaela.kozakova@esaote.com (M.K.); giuseppe.penno@unipi.it (G.P.)
[2] Esaote SpA, 16153 Genova, Italy
[3] School of Medicine, Department of Surgical, Medical, Molecular Pathology and Critical Care Medicine, University of Pisa, 56126 Pisa, Italy; carmela.morizzo@unipi.it
[4] Fondazione Toscana G. Monasterio, Massa-Pisa, 56124 Pisa, Italy; dchiappino@gmail.com
[5] Department of Surgical, Medical, Molecular Pathology and Critical Care Medicine, University of Pisa, Via Savi 10, 56126 Pisa, Italy
* Correspondence: carlo.palombo@unipi.it; Tel.: +39-3485840810
† These authors contributed equally to this work.

Abstract: **Background/Objectives:** This study compares the power of the radiofrequency (RF) signal reflected from the media layer (media power) of the common carotid artery (CCA) and the CCA stiffness between individuals with and without type 2 diabetes mellitus (T2DM). It also evaluates the associations of CCA media power with plasma glucose and lipid levels, as well as carotid stiffness. **Methods:** A total of 540 individuals, 115 with and 425 without T2DM (273 males, mean age = 64 ± 8 years) were studied using RF-based tracking of the right CCA. The following parameters were measured: CCA media thickness, luminal diameter, wall tensile stress (WTS), local pulse wave velocity (PWV), and media power. **Results:** Compared to the non-diabetic individuals, the T2DM patients had significantly higher CCA media thickness (652 ± 122 vs. 721 ± 138 microns, $p < 0.005$), luminal diameter (6.12 ± 0.78 vs. 6.86 ± 0.96 mm, $p < 0.0005$), media power (36.1 ± 4.8 vs. 39.3 ± 4.6, $p < 0.0001$), and PWV (7.65 ± 1.32 vs. 8.40 ± 1.89 m/s; $p < 0.01$), but comparable WTS (32.7 ± 10.4 vs. 33.1 ± 10.7 kPa; $p = 0.25$). In the entire population, CCA media power was independently associated with male sex, pulse pressure, current smoking, and T2DM; when T2DM was not included in the model, triglycerides emerged as an independent determinant of media power. The CCA PWV was independently associated with age, pulse pressure, media power, and T2DM. **Conclusions:** Our findings suggest the presence of structural changes in the arterial media of T2DM patients, leading to carotid stiffening and remodeling, aiming to preserve WTS. T2DM-related changes in arterial wall composition may be driven by high plasma triglyceride levels, which have previously been associated with both arterial stiffening and the incidence of CV events.

Keywords: diabetes mellitus; carotid artery; arterial stiffness; triglycerides; radiofrequency signal

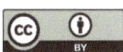

1. Introduction

The incidence of cardiovascular (CV) disease among individuals with type 2 diabetes mellitus (T2DM) is 2–3 times higher than among individuals without diabetes. CV risk factors such as obesity, high blood pressure (BP), and dyslipidemia are common in T2DM patients, placing them in the high-risk category; individuals with diabetes enter the high CV disease risk category (a 10-year risk of 20% or more) 15 years earlier than non-diabetic individuals [1–3].

Arterial stiffness is a strong predictor of future CV events and mortality [4], and T2DM patients experience an accelerated age-related decline in arterial compliance [5–7]. Previous studies have shown that the impact of T2DM is greater in the heart–carotid and heart–femoral segments of the arterial tree (large elastic arteries) than in the heart–brachial and femoral–ankle segments (medium-sized muscular arteries) [8,9]. As a result, T2DM patients exhibit greater aortic and carotid stiffness at any given level of systolic blood pressure (BP) [5–7,10,11], and the aortic stiffness of T2DM patients is comparable to that of non-diabetic individuals who are 15 years older [9].

The elasticity and integrity of the arterial wall are maintained by the extracellular matrix, particularly elastin and collagen, and by vascular smooth muscle cells (VSMCs). Elastin fragmentation, increased collagen synthesis and cross-linking, and VSMC dedifferentiation are all involved in arterial wall stiffening [12–14]. T2DM may accelerate arterial stiffening by several mechanisms, including the formation and accumulation of advanced glycation end-products (AGEs), endothelial dysfunction, inflammation, and dyslipidemia [15–19]. AGEs contribute to vascular stiffening not only by the formation of cross-links on long-lived proteins such as collagen, but also by reducing nitric oxide bioavailability [20], increasing reactive oxygen species (ROS) formation [16], and stimulating endothelin-1 transcription in endothelial cells [21]. An interesting study using ^{18}F-fluorodeoxyglucose positron emission tomography (FDG-PET) revealed a significant impact of T2DM on FDG uptake in the carotid wall, with the degree of uptake increasing with fasting glucose levels [18]. Other studies have also suggested the association between arterial stiffness and plasma lipid levels [19,22,23]. Therefore, targeting the factors contributing to arterial stiffening in patients with T2DM could help to reduce diabetes-related CV morbidity.

Structural alterations in the arterial wall can be detected by ultrasound (US), as the mechanical energy of the propagating US interacts with the material of the arterial media. The information from this ultrasound–tissue interaction is contained in the reflected signal, which is captured by the US transducer and converted into an electrical signal known as a radiofrequency (RF) signal [24]. Arterial wall changes can be assessed either through the densitometric analysis of B-mode images or by analyzing the RF signal. In previous studies, a first-order densitometric analysis of the B-mode carotid images showed a direct correlation between the mean gray level of the carotid plaque shoulder and the content of VSMCs, as assessed by immunocytochemistry (r = 0.58) [25], and the integrated backscatter power of the carotid media was correlated directly with both the elastic fragmentation index and the collagen fiber index, as determined by histological examination [26].

In the present study, we compared the power of the signal reflected from the media layer (media power) of the common carotid artery (CCA), as well as the CCA geometry and stiffness, between T2DM patients and non-diabetic individuals free of CV events. We also assessed the association of CCA media power with body size, BP, plasma glucose and lipid levels, and carotid stiffness.

2. Materials and Methods

2.1. Study Population and Protocol

The study population consisted of 540 individuals without a history of myocardial ischemia (symptoms, ECG), myocardial infarction and percutaneous coronary procedures, transient ischemic attack and ictus, peripheral artery disease, or carotid plaque in the CCA. The participants were voluntarily recruited from the prospective cohort study, "MHeLP, Montignoso Heart and Lung Project", during follow-up visits between December 2015 and January 2022. All participants underwent an examination protocol that included medical history, anthropometry, brachial BP measurements, fasting blood test, ECG, and a high-resolution carotid ultrasound. Diabetes mellitus was defined as fasting glucose $\geq$ 7.0 mmol/L or 2 h plasma glucose $\geq$ 11.1 mmol/L confirmed by a second test, or treatment for diabetes [27]. Type 1 diabetes mellitus was ruled out based on medical history, insulin, and C-peptide plasma levels. Hypertension was defined as systolic BP > 140 mmHg and/or diastolic BP > 90 mmHg [28].

The study protocol adhered to the ethical guidelines of the 1975 Declaration of Helsinki, and was approved by the "Comitato Etico di Area Vasta Nord-Ovest" (CEAVNO), approval code number 2514, approval date 1 September 2008, at the beginning of the MHeLP study. All individuals gave their informed consent to participate.

2.2. Body Size and BP Measurement

Body weight (kg) and height (m) were measured, and body mass index (BMI, kg/m^2) was calculated. Waist circumference (cm) was measured as the narrowest circumference between the lower rib margin and the anterior superior iliac crest. BP was measured at two different visits by a validated digital electronic tensiometer (Omron, model 705cp, Kyoto, Japan). Measurements were taken with participants seated for at least 10 min, using regular or large adult cuffs, depending on arm circumference. Two measurements were taken at each visit, and the average was calculated. The mean of the two visits was used to estimate brachial BP (mmHg). Brachial pulse pressure was calculated as the difference between systolic and diastolic BP.

2.3. CCA Intima–Media Thickness, Luminal Diameter, Wall Tensile Stress, Local Pulse Wave Velocity, Media Thickness and Media Power

Carotid ultrasound was performed on the right CCA by a single operator blinded to the diagnosis of the participants, using an ultrasound scanner equipped with a 10 MHz linear probe (MyLabOne, Esaote, Genova, Italy) and RF-based tracking of the arterial wall (QIMT®, QAS®), which automatically determines far-wall intima–media thickness (IMT), inter-adventitial diameter (IAD) and distension with high spatial and temporal resolution (sampling rate of 550 Hz on 32 lines) [29–31]. CCA structure and function were assessed within a rectangular 1 cm long ROI placed 1 cm before the flow divider. All participants were asked to abstain from cigarette smoking, caffeine and alcohol consumption, and vigorous physical activity for 24 h prior to the examination.

CCA IMT was defined as the distance between the lumen–intima and the media–adventitia interfaces of the CCA far (posterior) wall at diastole, and IAD as the distance between the media–adventitia interfaces of the near and far wall at diastole. CCA luminal diameter (mm) was calculated as IAD-(2*IMT) [32]. Carotid wall tensile stress (WTS; kPa) was calculated according to Laplace's law as pulse pressure*(r/w), where r is the luminal radius (luminal diameter/2) and w is the wall thickness (far-wall IMT) [33]. Local carotid pulse wave velocity (PWV; m/s) was estimated from distension curves using the Bramwell–Hill equation, which relates propagation velocity to arterial distensibility through the following equation: CCA PWV = $\sqrt{\rho \times DC}$, where ρ is the blood density and DC is distensibility coefficient describing the absolute change in vessel diameter (ΔD) during cardiac cycle for a given change in local pressure (Δp) [31,34]. The local carotid pressure used for PWV calculation was estimated by the QAS system, converting the distension curve to pressure curve by a linear conversion factor and assuming that the difference between mean arterial pressure and diastolic pressure is invariant along the arterial tree [35]. The peripheral BP needed for rescaling was measured at the left brachial artery (Omron, Kyoto, Japan) during each acquisition of the distension curves.

The ultrasound system was modified to allow the raw RF signal to be transmitted and stored on a personal computer and later analyzed using MATLAB programming platform (MathWorks, Natick, MA, USA). Peak signal-to-noise ratio (PSNR) of media layer was calculated in the time domain. PSNR, or media power, represents the ratio between the maximum signal power (p) and the signal noise power, defined as variance (var) and calculated in the center of the vessel. Media power was expressed as 10 log(P/var).

RF-derived measures (IMT and distension) represent the average of 6 consecutive cardiac beats. The mean of two acquisitions was used for statistical analysis. Intra- and interindividual variability was assessed in 25 volunteers, with acquisitions performed in two separate sessions 30 min apart, both by the same operator and by two different operators. Brachial pulse pressure was consistent across different acquisitions ($p = 0.88$). Intra- and interindividual variability for IMT and distension measurements were 6.7 ± 4.2 and 8.7 ± 6.4%, and 7.5 ± 4.6 and 9.0 ± 6.9%, respectively.

2.4. Statistical Analysis

Data are expressed as mean ± SD, categorical data as percentages. Variables with skewed distribution were summarized as median (interquartile range), and were logarithmically transformed for parametric statistical analysis. ANOVA was used to compare continuous variables, while the χ^2 test was applied for categorical variables. The association of CCA media power and PWV with variables related to T2DM such as body size and plasma levels of lipids and glucose were assessed by univariate regression analysis. To identify the independent determinants of CCA media power and PWV, multiple regression analysis with backward stepwise removal was performed.

Two multiple regression analyses were conducted; in the first, we tested the independent associations of vascular measures with sex, age, BP, current smoking, hypertensive and lipid-lowering therapy, and the presence of T2DM. In the second analysis, we examined independent associations with sex, age, BP, current smoking, hypertensive and lipid-lowering therapy, and T2DM-related variables that were significantly associated with vascular measures in the univariate analysis ($p < 0.05$). Statistical tests were two-sided, and significance was set at a value of $p < 0.05$. Statistical analysis was performed by JMP software, version 3.1 (SAS Institute Inc., Cary, NC, USA).

3. Results

Characteristics of the study population are reported in Table 1, and the differences in established CV risk factors between individuals with and without T2DM in Table 2. The T2DM patients were more often men, were older, and had higher body size, plasma levels of triglycerides (TGs), and fasting glucose, and lower levels of HDL and LDL cholesterol. They also had a higher prevalence of hypertensive and lipid-lowering treatment. Brachial BP and current smoking did not differ between the two groups.

Table 3 compares the CCA geometry and function between individuals with and without T2DM, after adjustment for sex, age, and BMI. The diabetic patients had significantly higher CCA IMT, media thickness, luminal diameter, media power, and PWV compared to the non-diabetic individuals. The WTS was comparable between the two groups.

In the entire population, the CCA media power increased with waist circumference, pulse pressure, TGs, and fasting glucose (r = 0.15–0.23; $p < 0.005$–0.0001), and decreased with HDL cholesterol (r = −0.22; $p < 0.0001$). The CCA PWV increased with media power (r = 0.29; $p < 0.0001$), as well as with age, waist circumference, pulse pressure, TGs, and fasting glucose (r = 0.14–0.40; $p < 0.005$–0.0001), and decreased with HDL cholesterol (r = −0.14; $p < 0.005$). In addition, the plasma TGs increased and HDL cholesterol decreased with fasting plasma glucose levels (r = 0.25 and −0.29, respectively; $p < 0.0001$ for both).

Table 4 demonstrates the results of the multiple regression analyses for CCA media power and CCA PWV across the entire population. In the first analysis, which included T2DM as the independent variable, media power was independently associated with male sex, pulse pressure, current smoking, and T2DM. In the second analysis, which included T2DM-related variables, media power was independently associated with male sex, pulse pressure, current smoking, and TG levels. CCA PWV was independently associated with age, pulse pressure, media power, and T2DM in the first analysis, and with age, pulse pressure, media power, and fasting glucose levels in the second analysis.

Table 1. Characteristics of Study Population.

	Mean ± SD/Median (IQR)/n (%)	Range
Sex—Male:Female	273 (49):267 (51)	
Age (years)	64 ± 8	41–90
BMI (kg/m^2)	27.2 ± 4.1	15.5–51.7
Waist circumference (cm)	96 ± 12	64–139
Brachial systolic BP (mmHg)	134 ± 20	96–198
Brachial pulse pressure (mmHg)	57 ± 16	25–105
HDL cholesterol (mmo/L)	1.53 ± 0.42	0.44–3.05
LDL cholesterol (mmo/L)	3.15 ± 0.88	0.91–6.43
TGs (mmo/L)	1.06 [0.77]	0.23–4.28
Fasting glucose (mmol/L)	5.70 ± 1.27	2.39–13.39
Current smoker (yes)	94 (17)	
Hypertension therapy (yes)	130 (24)	
T2DM (yes)	115 (21)	
Lipid-lowering therapy (yes)	126 (23)	

Table 2. Established Cardiovascular Risk Factors in Individuals with and without T2DM.

	Mean ± SD/Median (IQR)/n (%)		p *
	T2DM (No)	T2DM (Yes)	
	425	115	
Sex (male)	189 (45)	84 (73)	<0.0005
Age (years)	63 ± 8	67 ± 8	<0.0001
BMI (kg/m^2)	26.8 ± 4.1	28.7 ± 4.0	<0.0005
Waist circumference (cm)	95 ± 12	103 ± 12	<0.0001
Brachial systolic BP (mmHg)	134 ± 20	132 ± 18	0.09
Brachial pulse pressure (mmHg)	57 ± 17	57 ± 15	0.14
HDL cholesterol (mmo/L)	1.60 ± 0.42	1.28 ± 0.34	<0.0001
LDL cholesterol (mmo/L)	3.28 ± 0.83	2.69 ± 0.92	<0.0001
TGs (mmo/L)	0.98 [0.75]	1.23 [0.90]	0.0001
Fasting glucose (mmol/L)	5.27 ± 0.62	7.35 ± 1.70	<0.0001
HbA1c (%)		45.4 [13.2]	
Current smoker (yes)	70 (17)	24 (21)	0.32
Hypertension therapy (yes)	81 (19)	49 (43)	<0.0001
Lipid-lowering therapy (yes)	64 (15)	62 (54)	<0.0001

*: adjusted for sex and age.

Table 3. CCA Geometry and Function in Individuals with and without T2DM.

	Mean ± SD		p *
	T2DM (No)	T2DM (Yes)	
Luminal diameter (mm)	6.12 ± 0.78	6.86 ± 0.96	<0.0005
IMT (microns)	725 ± 135	802 ± 153	<0.005
Media thickness (microns)	652 ± 122	721 ± 138	<0.005
Wall tensile stress (kPa)	32.7 ± 10.4	33.1 ± 10.7	0.25
Media power	36.1 ± 4.8	39.3 ± 4.6	<0.0001
PWV (m/s)	7.65 ± 1.32	8.40 ± 1.89	<0.01

*: adjusted for sex, age and BMI.

Table 4. Independent Determinants of CCA Media Power and PWV.

		Model with T2DM		Model with T2DM-Related Factors	
		Beta ± SE	p	Beta ± SE	p
CCA Media power	Sex (male)	0.28 ± 0.04	<0.0001	0.31 ± 0.04	<0.0001
	PP (mmHg)	0.15 ± 0.04	<0.0005	0.13 ± 0.04	<0.005
	Smoking (yes)	0.14 ± 0.05	<0.01	0.12 ± 0.05	<0.05
	T2DM (yes)	0.24 ± 0.04	<0.0001		
	logTGs			0.14 ± 0.04	0.001
	Cumulative R^2	0.18	<0.0001	0.16	<0.0001
CCA PWV (m/s)	Age (years)	0.13 ± 0.04	<0.005	0.13 ± 0.04	<0.005
	PP (mmHg)	0.33 ± 0.04	<0.0001	0.31 ± 0.04	<0.0001
	CCA media power	0.19 ± 0.03	<0.0001	0.22 ± 0.03	<0.0001
	T2DM (yes)	0.17 ± 0.04	0.0005		
	FPG (mmol/L)			0.12 ± 0.03	<0.005
	Cumulative R^2	0.25	<0.0001	0.25	<0.0001

PP: pulse pressure, FPG: fasting plasma glucose.

4. Discussion

In this study, patients with T2DM exhibited significantly higher CCA media power and PWV compared to non-diabetic individuals. The increase in media power likely reflects alterations in the extracellular matrix of the arterial wall, a hypothesis supported by both experimental and clinical studies. In an "ex vivo" study, the integrated backscatter signal from freshly excised human aortic segments increased from normal to fibrous and calcified regions [36]. In an experimental study on the canine ascending aorta, the backscatter coefficient for elastin-isolated tissue was found to be five times higher than that of collagen-isolated tissue, suggesting that elastin fibers are the primary scattering components within elastic arteries [37]. In a human study, the integrated backscatter value of the carotid media obtained ante mortem was correlated with both the elastic fragmentation index and the collagen fiber index (r = 0.63 and 0.59, respectively) in histological specimens. Additionally, the integrated backscatter was correlated directly with the carotid beta stiffness index [26].

T2DM can induce changes in arterial wall composition through various mechanisms related to its metabolic dysregulation and systemic inflammation [15–23]. In the present study, T2DM was identified as an independent determinant of media power. However, when T2DM-related variables, like body size and plasma lipid and glucose levels, were included in the model, TG levels emerged as independent determinants of media power, which, in turn, was an independent determinant of carotid stiffness.

Hypertriglyceridemia is the most common lipid abnormality in T2DM, and several studies have demonstrated a link between TGs and arterial stiffness [19,22,38,39], as well as between TGs and CV events [22,40]. In healthy men, TG levels were found to be associated with augmentation index independently of other cardiometabolic risk factors [38]. Similarly, in a community-based population in China, plasma TG levels were independently associated with both carotid–femoral and carotid–radial PWV, and changes in TG levels over a 4.8-year period were correlated with changes in carotid–femoral PWV [39]. The impact of TGs on CV events was highlighted in a Danish study of newly diagnosed T2DM patients without previous CV disease, in which TG levels were associated with major adverse cardiac events, starting at a level of 1.0 mmol/L [40]. Moreover, a recent meta-analysis of randomized controlled trials showed that TG-lowering therapy in diabetic patients resulted in a reduced risk of CV events (RR = 0.91, 95% CI 0.87–0.95), independent of the degree of TGs reduction and glycemic control [41].

The mechanisms linking TGs to the structural changes in media and arterial stiffening are not fully understood, but experimental studies offer some potential explanations. TGs are composed of three fatty acids esterified to a glycerol molecule, and elastin has a propensity to associate with fatty acids. The resulting elastin–fatty acid complexes are more susceptible to elastolysis than elastin itself [42–44]. Certain saturated fatty acids, such as palmitic acid, may also promote medial calcification by enhancing the production of reactive oxygen species, which stimulate extracellular-signal-regulated kinase (ERK1/2)-mediated osteogenic gene expression and osteogenic differentiation of VSMCs [45]. In warfarin/vitamin K-treated Wistar rats, the addition of palmitic acid to the diet increased aortic calcification by 2.4-fold, and this increase was associated with a significant rise in aortic PWV [45]. Taken together, these findings suggest that TGs may accelerate elastin fragmentation in the carotid media and induce medial calcification, both of which could enhance the power of reflected signals and increase carotid stiffness. As expected, carotid stiffness also increased with increasing fasting plasma glucose levels [46].

Other independent determinants of media power, aside from T2DM and TGs, include pulse pressure, current smoking, and male sex. Chronic exposure to high pulsatile load exerts a fatiguing effect on the load-bearing elements of the arterial media, mainly on elastin, causing its fracture and fragmentation [13]. Exposure to tobacco smoke has been shown to increase the number of elastin breaks in the thoracic and abdominal aorta of mice [47], as well as to elevate the content of VSMCs and the extracellular matrix in the aortic wall [48]. The impact of sex on the echo-reflectivity of the carotid media is less clear, but it may be explained by the influence of sex hormones on VSMC proliferation and migration, as well as the sex-specific expression of mineralocorticoid receptors (MRs) in VSMCs. Endogenous estrogen and progesterone inhibit VSMC proliferation and migration [49–52], while the MRs in VSMCs may accelerate age-related vascular fibrosis and stiffening, particularly in males [53].

Structural changes in the carotid media can induce arterial remodeling, as the loss of media elastic function leads to luminal enlargement and increases in WTS [54]. Increased tensile stress activates intracellular signaling pathways, which promotes VSMCs proliferation and migration within the media [55], resulting in wall thickening and subsequent stress reduction. Indeed, our T2DM patients exhibited higher CCA PWV and luminal diameter, but comparable WTS due to higher media thickness.

Study Limitations

The T2DM patients and non-diabetic individuals were not comparable for sex, age or body size, all of which contribute to arterial stiffening and remodeling. However, analyses comparing the vascular measures in diabetic and non-diabetic individuals were adjusted for sex, age and BMI. Markers of inflammation, which might contribute to structural changes in the carotid media of T2DM patients, were not assessed.

5. Conclusions

This is the first study to analyze the power of the signal reflected from the carotid wall, with the aim of obtaining information on diabetes-related alterations in the carotid media. Our findings indicate that hypertriglyceridemia, the most common diabetic lipid abnormality, may trigger structural changes in arterial media, leading to arterial stiffening and remodeling. Since arterial stiffness is a strong predictor of CV mortality, and since the T2DM patients had accelerated arterial stiffening, strict TG control could reduce CV risk in diabetic patients.

Author Contributions: M.K. contributed to the conceptualization of the study, data analysis, manuscript drafting, and final approval; C.M., G.P., and D.C. contributed to data acquisition, analysis and interpretation, critical review of the paper, and final approval; C.P. contributed to the conceptualization, data interpretation, manuscript drafting and final approval. All authors are accountable for all aspects of the work in ensuring that questions related to the accuracy or integrity of any part of the work are appropriately investigated and resolved. All authors have read and agreed to the published version of the manuscript.

Funding: This research received no external funding.

Institutional Review Board Statement: The study protocol conformed to the ethical guidelines of the 1975 Declaration of Helsinki, and was approved by the "Comitato Etico di Area Vasta Nord-Ovest" (CEAVNO); approval code number 2514, approval date 1 September 2008.

Informed Consent Statement: All individuals gave their informed consent to participate.

Data Availability Statement: The data presented in this study are available on request from the corresponding author due to legal reasons.

Conflicts of Interest: Michaela Kozakova is responsible for clinical studies at Esaote SpA.

References

1. Raghavan, S.; Vassy, J.L.; Ho, Y.L.; Song, R.J.; Gagnon, D.R.; Cho, K.; Wilson, P.W.F.; Phillips, L.S. Diabetes mellitus-related all-cause and cardiovascular mortality in a national cohort of adults. *J. Am. Heart Assoc.* **2019**, *8*, e011295. [CrossRef] [PubMed]
2. Booth, G.L.; Kapral, M.K.; Fung, K.; Tu, J.V. Relation between age and cardiovascular disease in men and women with diabtes compared with non-diabetic people: A population-based retrospective cohort study. *Lancet* **2006**, *368*, 29–36. [CrossRef] [PubMed]
3. Wong, N.D.; Sattar, N. Cardiovascular risk in diabetes mellitus: Epidemiology, assessment and prevention. *Nat. Rev. Cardiol.* **2023**, *20*, 685–695. [CrossRef]
4. Vlachopoulos, C.; Aznaouridis, K.; Stefanadis, C. Prediction of cardiovascular events and all-cause mortality with arterial stiffness: A systematic review and meta-analysis. *J. Am. Coll. Cardiol.* **2010**, *55*, 1318–1327. [CrossRef]
5. Cruickshank, K.; Riste, L.; Anderson, S.G.; Wright, J.S.; Dunn, G.; Gosling, R.G. Aortic pulse-wave velocity and its relationship to mortality in diabetes and glucose intolerance: An integrated index of vascular function? *Circulation* **2002**, *106*, 2085–2090. [CrossRef]
6. Prenner, S.B.; Chirinos, J.A. Arterial stiffness in diabetes mellitus. *Atherosclerosis* **2015**, *238*, 370–379. [CrossRef] [PubMed]
7. Sharif, S.; Visseren, F.L.J.; Spiering, W.; de Jong, P.A.; Bots, M.L.; Westerink, J.; SMART study group. Arterial stiffness as a risk factor for cardiovascular events and all-cause mortality in people with Type 2 diabetes. *Diabet. Med.* **2019**, *36*, 1125–1132. [CrossRef]
8. Kimoto, E.; Shoji, T.; Shinohara, K.; Hatsuda, S.; Mori, K.; Fukumoto, S.; Koyama, H.; Emoto, M.; Okuno, Y.; Nishizawa, Y. Regional arterial stiffness in patients with type 2 diabetes and chronic kidney disease. *J. Am. Soc. Nephrol.* **2006**, *17*, 2245–2252. [CrossRef]
9. Cameron, J.D.; Bulpitt, C.J.; Pinto, E.S.; Rajkumar, C. The aging of elastic and muscular arteries: A comparison of diabetic and nondiabetic subjects. *Diabetes Care* **2003**, *26*, 2133–2138. [CrossRef]
10. Roca, F.; Zmuda, L.; Noël, G.; Duflot, T.; Iacob, M.; Moreau-Grangé, L.; Prévost, G.; Joannides, R.; Bellien, J. Changes in carotid arterial wall viscosity and carotid arterial stiffness in type 2 diabetes patients. *Atherosclerosis* **2024**, *394*, 117188. [CrossRef]
11. Ahmadizar, F.; Wang, K.; Roos, M.; Bos, M.; Mattace-Raso, F.; Kavousi, M. Association between arterial stiffness/remodeling and new-onset type 2 diabetes mellitus in general population. *Diabetes Res. Clin. Pract.* **2023**, *196*, 110237. [CrossRef] [PubMed]
12. Avolio, A.; Jones, D.; Tafazzoli-Shadpour, M. Quantification of alterations in structure and function of elastin in the arterial media. *Hypertension* **1998**, *32*, 170–175. [CrossRef] [PubMed]
13. Lyle, A.N.; Raaz, U. Killing Me Unsoftly: Causes and mechanisms of arterial stiffness. *Arterioscler. Thromb. Vasc. Biol.* **2017**, *37*, e1–e11. [CrossRef]
14. Lacolley, P.; Regnault, V.; Segers, P.; Laurent, S. Vascular smooth muscle cells and arterial stiffening: Relevance in development, aging, and disease. *Physiol. Rev.* **2017**, *97*, 1555–1617. [CrossRef] [PubMed]
15. Staef, M.; Ott, C.; Kannenkeril, D.; Striepe, K.; Schiffer, M.; Schmieder, R.E.; Bosch, A. Determinants of arterial stiffness in patients with type 2 diabetes mellitus: A cross sectional analysis. *Sci. Rep.* **2023**, *13*, 8944. [CrossRef]
16. Nowotny, K.; Jung, T.; Höhn, A.; Weber, D.; Grune, T. Advanced glycation end products and oxidative stress in type 2 diabetes mellitus. *Biomolecules* **2015**, *5*, 194–222. [CrossRef]
17. Muniyappa, R.; Sowers, J.R. Role of insulin resistance in endothelial dysfunction. *Rev. Endocr. Metab. Disord.* **2013**, *14*, 5–12. [CrossRef]
18. Bucerius, J.; Mani, V.; Moncrieff, C.; Rudd, J.H.; Machac, J.; Fuster, V.; Farkouh, M.E.; Fayad, Z.A. Impact of noninsulin-dependent type 2 diabetes on carotid wall 18F-fluorodeoxyglucose positron emission tomography uptake. *J. Am. Coll. Cardiol.* **2012**, *59*, 2080–2088. [CrossRef]
19. Sekizuka, H.; Hoshide, S.; Kabutoya, T.; Kario, K. Determining the relationship between triglycerides and arterial stiffness in cardiovascular risk patients without low-density lipoprotein cholesterol-lowering therapy. *Int. Heart J.* **2021**, *62*, 1320–1327. [CrossRef]
20. Bucala, R.; Tracey, K.J.; Cerami, A. Advanced glycosylation products quench nitric oxide and mediate defective endothelium-dependent vasodilatation in experimental diabetes. *J. Clin. Investig.* **1991**, *87*, 432–438. [CrossRef]
21. Quehenberger, P.; Bierhaus, A.; Fasching, P.; Muellner, C.; Klevesath, M.; Hong, M.; Stier, G.; Sattler, M.; Schleicher, E.; Speiser, W.; et al. Endothelin 1 transcription is controlled by nuclear factor-kappaB in AGE-stimulated cultured endothelial cells. *Diabetes* **2000**, *49*, 1561–1570. [CrossRef] [PubMed]

22. Pavlovska, I.; Kunzova, S.; Jakubik, J.; Hruskova, J.; Skladana, M.; Rivas-Serna, I.M.; Medina-Inojosa, J.R.; Lopez-Jimenez, F.; Vysoky, R.; Geda, Y.E.; et al. Associations between high triglycerides and arterial stiffness in a population-based sample: Kardiozive Brno 2030 study. *Lipids Health Dis.* **2020**, *19*, 170. [CrossRef] [PubMed]
23. Wen, J.; Huang, Y.; Lu, Y.; Yuan, H. Associations of non-high-density lipoprotein cholesterol, triglycerides and the total cholesterol/HDL-c ratio with arterial stiffness independent of low-density lipoprotein cholesterol in a Chinese population. *Hypertens. Res.* **2019**, *42*, 1223–1230. [CrossRef]
24. Granchi, S.; Vannacci, E.; Biagi, E.; Masotti, L. Multidimensional spectral analysis of the ultrasonic radiofrequency signal for characterization of media. *Ultrasonics* **2016**, *68*, 89–101. [CrossRef]
25. Puato, M.; Faggin, E.; Rattazzi, M.; Paterni, M.; Kozàkovà, M.; Palombo, C.; Pauletto, P.; Study Group on Arterial Wall Structure. In vivo noninvasive identification of cell composition of intimal lesions: A combined approach with ultrasonography and immunocytochemistry. *J. Vasc. Surg.* **2003**, *38*, 1390–1395. [CrossRef]
26. Kawasaki, M.K.; Ito, Y.; Yokoyama, H.; Arai, M.; Takemura, G.; Hara, A.; Ichiki, Y.; Takatsu, H.; Minatoguchi, S.; Fujiwara, H. Assessment of arterial medial characteristics in human carotid arteries using integrated backscatter ultrasound and its histological implications. *Atherosclerosis* **2005**, *180*, 145–154. [CrossRef]
27. World Health Organization. *Definition and Diagnosis of Diabetes Mellitus and Intermediate Hyperglycaemia: Report of a WHO/IDF Consultation*; WHO: Geneva, Switzerland, 2006. Available online: https://www.who.int/publications/i/item/definition-and-diagnosis-of-diabetes-mellitus-and-intermediate-hyperglycaemia (accessed on 1 December 2023).
28. Ramzy, I. Definition of hypertension and pressure goals during treatment (ESC-ESH Guidelines 2018). *E-J. Cardiol. Pract.* **2019**, *22*. Available online: https://www.escardio.org/Journals/E-Journal-of-Cardiology-Practice/Volume-17/definition-of-hypertension-and-pressure-goals-during-treatment-esc-esh-guidelin (accessed on 1 December 2023).
29. Brands, P.J.; Willigers, J.M.; Ledoux, L.A.; Reneman, R.S.; Hoeks, A.P. A noninvasive method to estimate pulse wave velocity in arteries locally by means of ultrasound. *Ultrasound Med. Biol.* **1998**, *24*, 1325–1335. [CrossRef]
30. Brands, P.J.; Hoeks, A.P.; Willigers, J.; Willekes, C.; Reneman, R.S. An integrated system for the non-invasive assessment of vessel wall and hemodynamic properties of large arteries by means of ultrasound. *Eur. J. Ultrasound* **1999**, *9*, 257–266. [CrossRef]
31. Engelen, L.; Bossuyt, J.; Ferreira, I.; van Bortel, L.M.; Reesink, K.D.; Segers, P.; Stehouwer, C.D.; Laurent, S.; Boutouyrie, P.; Reference Values for Arterial Measurements Collaboration. Reference values for local arterial stiffness. Part A: Carotid artery. *J. Hypertens.* **2015**, *33*, 1981–1996. [CrossRef]
32. Henry, R.M.; Kostense, P.J.; Dekker, J.M.; Nijpels, G.; Heine, R.J.; Kamp, O.; Bouter, L.M.; Stehouwer, C.D. Carotid arterial remodeling: A maladaptive phenomenon in type 2 diabetes but not in impaired glucose metabolism: The Hoorn study. *Stroke* **2004**, *35*, 671–676. [CrossRef] [PubMed]
33. Luo, X.; Du, L.; Li, Z. Ultrasound assessment of tensile stress in carotid arteries of healthy human subjects with varying age. *BMC Med. Imaging* **2019**, *19*, 93. [CrossRef] [PubMed]
34. Kozakova, M.; Morizzo, C.; Guarino, D.; Federico, G.; Miccoli, M.; Giannattasio, C.; Palombo, C. The impact of age and risk factors on carotid and carotid-femoral pulse wave velocity. *J. Hypertens.* **2015**, *33*, 1446–1451. [CrossRef] [PubMed]
35. van Bortel, L.M.; Balkestein, E.J.; van der Heijden-Spek, J.J.; Vanmolkot, F.H.; Staessen, J.A.; Kragten, J.A.; Vredeveld, J.W.; Safar, M.E.; Struijker Boudier, H.A.; Hoeks, A.P. Non-invasive assessment of local arterial pulse pressure: Comparison of applanation tonometry and echo-tracking. *J. Hypertens.* **2001**, *19*, 1037–1044. [CrossRef] [PubMed]
36. Barzilai, B.; Saffitz, J.E.; Miller, J.G.; Sobel, B.E. Quantitative ultrasonic characterization of the nature of atherosclerotic plaques in human aorta. *Circ. Res.* **1987**, *60*, 459–463. [CrossRef]
37. Hall, C.S.; Nguyen, C.T.; Scott, M.J.; Lanza, G.M.; Wickline, S.A. Delineation of the extracellular determinants of ultrasonic scattering from elastic arteries. *Ultrasound Med. Biol.* **2000**, *26*, 613–620. [CrossRef]
38. Aznaouridis, K.; Vlachopoulos, C.; Dima, I.; Ioakeimidis, N.; Stefanadis, C. Triglyceride level is associated with wave reflections and arterial stiffness in apparently healthy middle-aged men. *Heart* **2007**, *93*, 613–614. [CrossRef]
39. Wang, X.; Ye, P.; Cao, R.; Yang, X.; Xiao, W.; Zhang, Y.; Bai, Y.; Wu, H. Triglycerides are a predictive factor for arterial stiffness: A community-based 4.8-year prospective study. *Lipids Health Dis.* **2016**, *15*, 97. [CrossRef]
40. Cristensen, F.P.B.; Christensen, D.H.; Mortensen, M.B.; Maeng, M.; Kahlert, J.; Sørensen, H.T.; Thomsen, R.W. Triglycerides and risk of cardiovascular events in statin-treated patients with newly diagnosed type 2 diabetes: A Danish cohort study. *Cardiovasc. Diabetol.* **2023**, *22*, 187. [CrossRef]
41. Yang, X.H.; Tu, Q.M.; Li, L.; Guo, Y.P.; Wang, N.S.; Jin, H.M. Triglyceride-lowering therapy for the prevention of cardiovascular events, stroke, and mortality in patients with diabetes: A meta-analysis of randomized controlled trials. *Atherosclerosis* **2024**, *394*, 117187. [CrossRef]
42. van Vreeswijk, J.; Lyklema, J.; Norde, W. Interaction between fatty acid salts and elastin: Kinetics, absorption equilibrium, and consequences for elasticity. *Biopolymers* **1999**, *50*, 472–485. [CrossRef]
43. Kagan, H.M.; Jordan, R.E.; Lerch, R.M.; Mukherjee, D.P.; Stone, P.; Franzblau, C. Factors affecting the proteolytic degradation of elastin. *Adv. Exp. Med. Biol.* **1977**, *79*, 189–207. [PubMed]
44. Shock, A.; Baum, H.; Kapasi, M.F.; Bull, F.M.; Quinn, P.J. The susceptibility of elastin-fatty acid complexes to elastolytic enzymes. *Matrix* **1990**, *10*, 179–185. [CrossRef] [PubMed]
45. Brodeur, M.R.; Bouvet, C.; Barrette, M.; Moreau, P. Palmitic acid increases medial calcification by inducing oxidative stress. *J. Vasc. Res.* **2013**, *50*, 430–441. [CrossRef]

46. Henry, R.M.; Kostense, P.J.; Spijkerman, A.M.; Dekker, J.M.; Nijpels, G.; Heine, R.J.; Kamp, O.; Westerhof, N.; Bouter, L.M.; Stehouwer, C.D.; et al. Arterial stiffness increases with deteriorating glucose tolerance status: The Hoorn Study. *Circulation* **2003**, *107*, 2089–2095. [CrossRef]
47. Azarbal, A.F.; Repella, T.; Carlson, E.; Manalo, E.C.; Palanuk, B.; Vatankhah, N.; Zientek, K.; Keene, D.R.; Zhang, W.; Abraham, C.Z.; et al. A novel model of tobacco smoke-mediated aortic injury. *Vasc. Endovasc. Surg.* **2022**, *56*, 244–252. [CrossRef]
48. Farra, Y.M.; Matz, J.; Ramkhelawon, B.; Oakes, J.M.; Bellini, C. Structural and functional remodeling of the female Apoe$^{-/-}$ mouse aorta due to chronic cigarette smoke exposure. *Am. J. Physiol. Heart Circ. Physiol.* **2021**, *320*, H2270–H2282. [CrossRef]
49. Orshal, J.M.; Khalil, R.A. Sex hormones and the vascular smooth muscle. *Adv. Mol. Cell Biol.* **2004**, *34*, 85–103.
50. Khalil, R.A. Sex hormones as potential modulators of vascular function in hypertension. *Hypertension* **2005**, *46*, 249–254. [CrossRef]
51. Lee, W.S.; Harder, J.A.; Yoshizumi, M.; Lee, M.E.; Haber, E. Progesterone inhibits arterial smooth muscle cell proliferation. *Nat. Med.* **1997**, *3*, 1005–1008. [CrossRef]
52. DuPont, J.J.; Kim, S.K.; Kenney, R.M.; Jaffe, I.Z. Sex differences in the time course and mechanisms of vascular and cardiac aging in mice: Role of the smooth muscle cell mineralocorticoid receptor. *Am. J. Physiol. Heart Circ. Physiol.* **2021**, *320*, H169–H180. [CrossRef] [PubMed]
53. Kim, S.K.; McCurley, A.T.; DuPont, J.J.; Aronovitz, M.; Moss, M.E.; Stillman, I.E.; Karumanchi, S.A.; Christou, D.D.; Jaffe, I.Z. Smooth muscle cell-mineralocorticoid receptor as a mediator of cardiovascular stiffness with aging. *Hypertension* **2018**, *71*, 609–621. [CrossRef] [PubMed]
54. Eberth, J.F.; Gresham, V.C.; Reddy, A.K.; Popovic, N.; Wilson, E.; Humphrey, J.D. Importance of pulsatility in hypertensive carotid artery growth and remodeling. *J. Hypertens.* **2009**, *27*, 2010–2021. [CrossRef] [PubMed]
55. Cai, Z.; Gong, Z.; Li, Z.; Li, L.; Kong, W. Vascular extracellular matrix remodeling and hypertension. *Antioxid. Redox Signal.* **2021**, *34*, 765–783. [CrossRef]

Disclaimer/Publisher's Note: The statements, opinions and data contained in all publications are solely those of the individual author(s) and contributor(s) and not of MDPI and/or the editor(s). MDPI and/or the editor(s) disclaim responsibility for any injury to people or property resulting from any ideas, methods, instructions or products referred to in the content.

MDPI AG
Grosspeteranlage 5
4052 Basel
Switzerland
Tel.: +41 61 683 77 34

Journal of Clinical Medicine Editorial Office
E-mail: jcm@mdpi.com
www.mdpi.com/journal/jcm

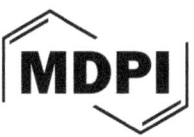

Disclaimer/Publisher's Note: The statements, opinions and data contained in all publications are solely those of the individual author(s) and contributor(s) and not of MDPI and/or the editor(s). MDPI and/or the editor(s) disclaim responsibility for any injury to people or property resulting from any ideas, methods, instructions or products referred to in the content.

www.ingramcontent.com/pod-product-compliance
Lightning Source LLC
LaVergne TN
LVHW070001100526
838202LV00019B/2601